theclinics.com

SURGICAL CLINICS OF NORTH AMERICA

Advances and Controversies in Minimally Invasive Surgery

GUEST EDITORS
Jon Gould, MD
W. Scott Melvin, MD

CONSULTING EDITOR
Ronald F. Martin, MD

October 2008 • Volume 88 • Number 5

SAUNDERS

An Imprint of Elsevier, Inc.
PHILADELPHIA   LONDON   TORONTO   MONTREAL   SYDNEY   TOKYO

W.B. SAUNDERS COMPANY

A Division of Elsevier Inc.

1600 John F. Kennedy Blvd., Suite 1800, Philadelphia, PA 19103-2899

http://www.theclinics.com

SURGICAL CLINICS OF NORTH AMERICA
October 2008
Editor: Catherine Bewick

Volume 88, Number 5
ISSN 0039–6109
ISBN-10: 1-4160-6357-9
ISBN-13: 978-1-4160-6357-5

Surgical Clinics of North America (ISSN 0039–6109) is published bimonthly by Elsevier Inc., 360 Park Avenue South, New York, NY 10010-1710. Months of publication are February, April, June, August, October, and December. Business and Editorial Offices: 1600 John F. Kennedy Blvd., Suite 1800, Philadelphia, PA 19103-2899. Customer Service Office: 6277 Sea Harbor Drive, Orlando, FL 32887-4800. Periodicals postage paid at New York, NY and additional mailing offices. Subscription prices are $238.00 per year for US individuals, $382.00 per year for US institutions, $119.00 per year for US students and residents, $292.00 per year for Canadian individuals, $466.00 per year for Canadian institutions, $309.00 for international individuals, $466.00 per year for international institutions and $154.00 per year for Canadian and foreign students/residents. To receive student/resident rate, orders must be accompanied by name of affiliated institution, date of term, and the *signature* of program/residency coordinator on institution letterhead. Orders will be billed at individual rate until proof of status is received. Foreign air speed delivery is included in all *Clinics* subscription prices. All prices are subject to change without notice. POSTMASTER: Send address changes to *Surgical Clinics*, Elsevier Journals Customer Service, 6277 Sea Harbor Drive, Orlando, FL 32887-4800. **Customer Service: 1-800-654-2452 (US). From outside of the United States, call 1-407-563-6020. Fax: 1-407-363-9661.** E-mail: JournalsCustomerService-usa@elsevier.com.

Reprints. For copies of 100 or more of articles in this publication, please contact the commercial Reprints Department, Elsevier Inc., 360 Park Avenue South, New York, New York 10010-1710; Tel. (212) 633-3812, Fax: (212) 462-1935, E-mail: reprints@elsevier.com.

The Surgical Clinics of North America is also published in Spanish by McGraw-Hill Interamericana Editores S.A., P.O. Box 5-237 06500 Mexico D.F. Mexico; and in Portuguese by Interlivros Edicoes Ltda., Rua Comandante Coelho 1085, CEP 21250, Rio de Janeiro, Brazil; and in Greek by Paschalidis Medical Publications, Athens Greece.

The Surgical Clinics of North America is covered in *MEDLINE/PubMed (Index Medicus)*, *EMBASE/Excerpta Medica*, *Current Contents/Clinical Medicine*, *Current Contents/Life Sciences*, *Science Citation Index*, and *ISI/BIOMED*.

Printed in the United States of America.

CONSULTING EDITOR

RONALD F. MARTIN, MD, Staff Surgeon, Marshfield Clinic, Marshfield; and Clinical Associate Professor, University of Wisconsin School of Medicine and Public Health, Madison, Wisconsin; Lieutenant Colonel, Medical Corps, United States Army Reserve

GUEST EDITORS

JON GOULD, MD, FACS, Associate Professor, Department of Surgery, University of Wisconsin School of Medicine and Public Health, Clinical Science Center, Madison, Wisconsin

W. SCOTT MELVIN, MD, Professor of Surgery; Director, Center for Minimally Invasive Surgery; Chief, Division of General Surgery, The Ohio State University School of Medicine and Public Health, Columbus, Ohio

CONTRIBUTORS

SIMON BERGMAN, MD, Clinical Assistant Professor, Department of Surgery; Center for Minimally Invasive Surgery, The Ohio State University School of Medicine and Public Health, Columbus, Ohio

LARRY C. CAREY, MD, Professor of Surgery, Division of General Surgery, University of South Florida College of Medicine, James A. Haley VA Hospital, Tampa, Florida

BIPAN CHAND, MD, Associate Professor, Department of General Surgery, Cleveland Clinic Lerner College of Medicine, Cleveland, Ohio

S. SCOTT DAVIS, Jr, MD, Assistant Professor of Surgery, Emory Endosurgery Unit, Emory University, Atlanta, Georgia

CHIRAG DHOLAKIA, MD, Department of Surgery, University of Wisconsin School of Medicine and Public Health, Madison, Wisconsin

EMILY T. DURKIN, MD, Resident, Department of Surgery, University of Wisconsin School of Medicine and Public Health, Madison, Wisconsin

E. CHRISTOPHER ELLISON, MD, Robert M. Zollinger Professor and Chairman, Department of Surgery, Ohio State University Medical Center, Columbus, Ohio

JON GOULD, MD, FACS, Associate Professor, Department of Surgery, University of Wisconsin School of Medicine and Public Health, Clinical Science Center, Madison, Wisconsin

LYNN C. HAPPEL, MD, Clinical Assistant Professor, Center for Minimally Invasive Surgery, The Ohio State University, Columbus, Ohio

CHARLES P. HEISE, MD, FACS, FASCRS, Department of Surgery, University of Wisconsin School of Medicine and Public Health, Madison, Wisconsin

JUDY JIN, MD, Surgical Resident, Department of Surgery, University Hospitals Case Medical Center, Cleveland, Ohio

MATTHEW C. KOOPMANN, MD, Department of Surgery, University of Wisconsin School of Medicine and Public Health, Madison, Wisconsin

MATTHEW KROH, MD, Assistant Professor, Department of General Surgery, Cleveland Clinic Lerner College of Medicine, Cleveland, Ohio

JAMES D. MALONEY, MD, Assistant Professor of Surgery, Section of Thoracic Surgery, Division of Cardiothoracic Surgery, University of Wisconsin School of Medicine and Public Health, Madison, Wisconsin

BRENT D. MATTHEWS, MD, Associate Professor of Surgery and Chief, Section of Minimally Invasive Surgery, Washington University School of Medicine, St. Louis, Missouri

LORA MELMAN, MD, Institute for Minimally Invasive Surgery, Department of Surgery, Washington University School of Medicine, St. Louis, Missouri

W. SCOTT MELVIN, MD, Professor of Surgery; Director, Center for Minimally Invasive Surgery; Chief, Division of General Surgery, The Ohio State University School of Medicine and Public Health, Columbus, Ohio

BRADLEY J. NEEDLEMAN, MD, FACS, Assistant Professor of Surgery, Division of General and Gastrointestinal Surgery, Center for Minimally Invasive Surgery, The Ohio State University; Director of Bariatric Surgery, The Ohio State University, Columbus, Ohio

DMITRY OLEYNIKOV, MD, Associate Professor of Surgery; Joseph and Richard Still Faculty Fellow in Medicine; Director, Minimally Invasive and Computer Assisted Surgery, Omaha, Nebraska

MICHAEL J. ROSEN, MD, FACS, Assistant Professor, Department of Surgery; and Director, Case Comprehensive Hernia Center, University Hospitals Case Medical Center, Cleveland, Ohio

AIMEN F. SHAABAN, MD, Associate Professor, Department of Surgery, University of Iowa Carver College of Medicine, Iowa City, Iowa

C. DANIEL SMITH, MD, Professor and Chair, Department of Surgery, Mayo Clinic–Florida, Jacksonville, Florida

TRACEY L. WEIGEL, MD, Professor of Surgery; Chief, Section of Thoracic Surgery, Division of Cardiothoracic Surgery, University of Wisconsin School of Medicine and Public Health, Madison, Wisconsin

CONTENTS

> After 100 years of practice, the face of general surgery changed forever when laparoscopic cholecystectomy was introduced. The impact was felt in how new procedures were taught and learned, proficiency determined, and credentials established. In addition, the revolution of laparoscopic surgery brought to bear ethical considerations and the harsh reality of medical legal and economic ramifications of new technology introduction. Finally, minimally invasive surgery challenged dogma of traditional perioperative care, allowing streamlining of postoperative recovery.

> Antireflux surgery (ARS) is appropriate and effective management for patients who have gastroesophageal reflux disease (GERD) refractory to medical management, who are on lifelong acid suppression, or who are experiencing side effects of the medical management. Over the past 2 decades, the operations have evolved from predominantly open thoracic approaches to a predominantly laparoscopic abdominal approach with similar, if not better, outcomes. The success of ARS in managing GERD lies largely in an understanding of GERD and its diagnosis, proper patient selection, sound surgical technique, and postoperative management.

kind of mesh, open or laparoscopic, extraperitoneal or trans-abdominal, and so forth. Inguinal hernia repairs have morbidity and recurrence rates that are not inconsequential. The search for the gold standard of repair continues.

Ventral hernia repair remains one of the most common operations performed by general surgeons. Despite the frequency with which this procedure is performed, there is little agreement and extensive controversy as to the cause of most of the hernias, or the ideal approach to repair these complicated problems. This article attempts to identify and provide some clarification of these controversial issues in abdominal wall reconstruction after ventral herniation based on the available literature.

Children represent a unique group of patients who are likely to greatly benefit from minimally invasive surgery (MIS). The promise of less postoperative pain, smaller scars, shorter hospital stays, and a faster return to school continues to drive growth in this area. The development of pediatric-specific techniques and documentation of improved outcomes form a critical gateway to widespread application of pediatric MIS. A brief perspective on current approaches to MIS for pediatric congenital and acquired disease is provided in this report. Technical departures from standardized adult MIS and the rationale for their modification are highlighted.

This article discusses the developments that led up to robotic surgical systems as well as what is on the horizon for new robotic technology. Topics include how robotics is enabling new types of procedures, including natural orifice endoscopic translumenal surgery in which one cannot reach by hand under any circumstances, and how these developments will drive the next generation of robots.

This article provides an overview of the currently available animal data on natural orifice translumenal endoscopic surgery (NOTES) on the topics of translumenal access and closure, iatrogenic intra-peritoneal complications, especially infection and overinsufflation, spatial orientation, and the development of enabling technologies. Human trials to date are also reviewed and discussed.

FORTHCOMING ISSUES

RECENT ISSUES

The Clinics are now available online!

www.theclinics.com

SURGICAL
CLINICS OF
NORTH AMERICA

Surg Clin N Am 88 (2008) xi–xiii

Foreword

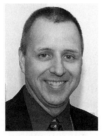

Ronald F. Martin, MD
Consulting Editor

History does not crawl, it jumps.

—Nassim Nicholas Taleb, Author of *The Black Swan: The Impact of the Highly Improbable.*

It may not be possible to adequately assess the impact of minimally invasive surgical (MIS) procedures on the practice and discipline of surgery. One could start nearly anyplace to begin a discussion about how the expansion of videoscopic procedures has changed our practice and go on to develop an entire book of thoughts. But the idea that led to the beginning concept for this issue was, how do we know when something is working out the way we had intended or, at least, hoped for? During discussions, we began to formulate a series of topics to look at advances and controversies in MIS development. Interestingly, many of the people with whom I spoke felt that there were no controversies and that we would probably perform every procedure with videoscopic assistance someday—perhaps all by NOTES (natural orifice translumenal endoscopic surgery) at some point. An outflow of those discussions set the stage for this series of articles that Drs. Gould and Melvin have been kind enough to edit.

Probably the first controversy that should leap to mind regarding MIS procedures is the mechanism by which new technology is introduced to the public. As is well illustrated by Drs. Ellison and Carey in their article in this issue, the introduction of laparoscopic cholecystectomy was a "revolutionary" introduction, not borne out of development after careful development and investigation in academic centers, but arising from community hospitals and

0039-6109/08/$ - see front matter © 2008 Elsevier Inc. All rights reserved.
doi:10.1016/j.suc.2008.07.013   *surgical.theclinics.com*

delivered directly to an eager public. After an initial rebuff from the established academic centers and concurrent rapid market shift of patients to community institutions offering this new procedure, the academic halls scrambled quickly (and some might add desperately) to develop their own MIS capacity. Since that time it seems that many are extremely reluctant to risk delay in embracing new procedures—regardless of their level of development—for fear of getting behind the curve so badly again.

The next, and logically necessary, controversy was who was going to define standards and competencies for MIS procedures. Some might argue that the original pioneers (who by the way had no real oversight during their developmental phase) would be the logical choice to train the next adoptive generation; others argued that the usual large societies and national organizations should place these procedures under their "umbrella" of responsibility. It is hard to say whether this initially constituted an environment of "pulling up the ladder once one is in the life raft" for the pioneers or furthered monopolistic control of "certifying" organizations but, thankfully, the resulting process as endorsed by the American College of Surgeons and other large national and international professional societies have created guidelines that seem reasonable, fair, and beneficial. This may also reflect that the pioneers, or at least the very early generation of followers, were quickly accepted into leadership positions within many of the large established societies, and this new breed of surgeons formed new societies which grew rapidly and became influential as well.

The desire for hospitals and physicians to maintain or expand their positions in a new competitive marketplace drove the need for rapid training of surgeons in these techniques and use of instruments. The creation of these largely technique-based fellowships to create "technical experts" (as opposed to "disease-based experts") in all organ systems has generated yet another controversy. There has been a marked expansion in the number of programs and number of positions in MIS fellowships. In my opinion, this has been short-sighted. One thing that we should have learned from the development of MIS techniques is that any operation can potentially be accomplished by MIS instrumentation and techniques. As we reach a new level of equilibrium and distribution of MIS technology, it may be time to reconsider that MIS training should return in part or whole to sub-specialty fellowships and general surgery residency training as an expectation of competency and proficiency, as opposed to an "additional" skill set. It does not appear that MIS knowledge is optional in any surgical specialty any longer.

The last controversy that I would like to address is that the perceived benefit of videoscopic surgery over open procedures may not be due completely to the newer techniques actually being superior. We may have learned as much about the dogmatic and somewhat errant practice in open surgery as we did about MIS. We certainly learned that one can discharge patients sooner than we thought after many operations, we can feed people sooner after many procedures, and we can use different fastening devices than we were used to using. These realizations do not diminish the value of MIS procedures but they do illustrate how far off the mark we were in some of most clung-to assumptions about surgery in the open era.

The last two decades or so have largely allowed us to push the envelope on what we can do with MIS. I would submit we have done a far poorer job of defining what we should do with MIS. There are still many of us who remember the frenzy of trying to recover position after initially scoffing at people (not even thought of as surgeons) who "operated through keyholes with chopsticks," as one mentor of mine used to put it. And those who remember those days vividly recall how absolutely wrong those unfounded disbeliefs were. Yet, we remain in a position where it should be incumbent upon us all to define what problem we are solving and whether or not adopting new technology is something that truly benefits the patient medically and helps the system to remain fiscally sustainable.

The presence of MIS procedures is and should remain an important part of our practice, as will the development and improvement of these techniques. As surgical history continues to be written, there will inevitably be another jump in our future. In the meantime, we shall have to crawl along with these changes until that new paradigm shift occurs. These excellent articles will hopefully give the reader an opportunity to become better versed in what is possible and what is advisable. I am deeply indebted to Drs. Gould and Melvin, along with their co-contributors, for their excellent effort.

Ronald F. Martin, MD
Department of Surgery
Marshfield Clinic
1000 North Oak Avenue
Marshfield, WI 54449, USA

E-mail address: martin.ronald@marshfieldclinic.org

SURGICAL
CLINICS OF
NORTH AMERICA

Surg Clin N Am 88 (2008) xv–xvi

Preface

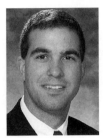
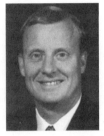

Jon Gould, MD   W. Scott Melvin, MD
Guest Editors

In the 20 years since the first laparoscopic cholecystectomy, we have witnessed an incredible paradigm shift in the surgical treatment of disease. Within 3 short years, laparoscopic cholecystectomy has become commonplace and the preferred approach. Through the "evolution of the laparoscopic revolution" (discussed in the article by Ellison), we have learned many lessons as a result of this experience. The laparoscopic revolution has occurred during a time of tremendous and rapid technologic progress. At the time of the first cholecystectomy, no one had heard of the Internet, cell phones were the size of a brick, and instruments for advanced laparoscopy simply did not exist. Today, robotic technology can enable a surgeon to remove the gallbladder from a patient across the ocean. Gallbladders can be extracted from a patient's mouth with virtually no scars (see the article by Melvin). We may not be far from a day when miniature surgical robots can be deployed into the peritoneal cavity to facilitate or even perform surgery through a natural orifice (as presented in the article by Oleynikov). Antireflux surgery has evolved from open, to laparoscopic, and now to endoscopic and endoluminal therapy (as discussed in the article by Smith).

In this modern era of health care, and looking into the future, we will be forced to consider how far to ride this "tidal wave" of technology and progress. Is it reasonable to violate a vital organ to take out a gallbladder in order to avoid three to four tiny scars? At what cost? At what morbidity? Who should be doing these procedures: surgeons or gastroenterologists? Who should pay for them? Can we as a society afford to pay for this kind

doi:10.1016/j.suc.2008.07.014   *surgical.theclinics.com*

of technology? Is a robotic Nissen fundoplication really better than a laparo-scopic Nissen fundoplication? Is a laparoscopic hernia repair really better than an open hernia repair? The last 20 years of progress in minimally invasive surgery have created as many unanswered questions and dilemmas as have been solved. One thing is for certain: compared to today, the face of General Surgery is likely to look as different in 2028 as it did back in 1988, when that first gallbladder was squeezed out of a tiny laparoscopic port site.

Jon Gould, MD
University of Wisconsin School of Medicine and Public Health
Department of Surgery
H4/726 Clinical Science Center
600 Highland Avenue
Madison, WI 53792, USA

E-mail address: gould@surgery.wisc.edu

W. Scott Melvin, MD
Department of Surgery
Center for Minimally Invasive Surgery
Division of General Surgery
The Ohio State University School of Medicine and Public Health
N729 Doan Hall
410 West 10th Avenue
Columbus, OH 43210, USA

E-mail address: scott.melvin@osumc.edu

ELSEVIER
SAUNDERS

SURGICAL
CLINICS OF
NORTH AMERICA

Surg Clin N Am 88 (2008) 927–941

Lessons Learned from the Evolution of the Laparoscopic Revolution

E. Christopher Ellison, MD[a,*], Larry C. Carey, MD[b]

[a]Department of Surgery, The Ohio State University Medical Center, 327 Means Hall,
1654 Upham Drive, Columbus, OH 43210, USA
[b]Division of General Surgery, University of South Florida College of Medicine,
Tampa General Hospital, P.O. Box 1289, Room F145, Tampa, FL 33601, USA

Introduction of new technology

Evolution versus revolution

Advances in new technology and medications in medicine occur in two ways: evolutionary or revolutionary. The majority of time they are evolutionary, based on discovery and incremental innovation in the scientific community and the academic medical centers. In these instances, there is time to respond with prospective analysis to determine the safety and efficacy of new treatments and to provide appropriate education beginning initially in university medical centers and then with gradual introduction into the medical community through continuing medical education. An example of surgical evolutionary change is cardiopulmonary bypass or the introduction of surgical staplers. Not so with the introduction of laparoscopic cholecystectomy. This was a revolutionary change; there would be no time for the orderly introduction. When first introduced, there was a rush for practicing surgeons to acquire this new technique and incorporate it into their practice. This resulted from the clear advantages that the technique provided patients in terms of reduced abdominal wall scarring, hospitalization, and time off work [1]. It also was driven by economics of surgical practice. Early on it became readily apparent to the public through media coverage, including television, radio, printed material, and even billboards, that there was a new technique for gall bladder removal. Patients needing gall bladder surgery and their referring physicians asked for "laser cholecystectomy." This name became attached to the procedure because at the time

* Corresponding author.
E-mail address: christopher.ellison@osumc.edu (E.C. Ellison).

0039-6109/08/$ - see front matter © 2008 Elsevier Inc. All rights reserved.
doi:10.1016/j.suc.2008.05.007
surgical.theclinics.com

use of lasers was the only way to deliver cutting and coagulating energy to the gallbladder bed. General surgeons who did not do this procedure quickly saw referrals disappear. As cholecystectomy was the most common procedure done by general surgeons at the time, with approximately 500,000 cases per year, the fiscal success of the general surgery practice was in some part dependent of the volume of these procedures. Surgery is not immune to capitalism; hence, there was a frenzy to learn the technique and establish a program at surgeons' hospitals and an equal frenzy to provide courses for training surgeons and their operative teams. There was no organized effort to credential and codify these training programs; the process simply did not exist. Some of these courses were good, including didactic, video, and instruction with inanimate models; the predecessor to simulation was a black box with a laparoscopic camera system and hands-on procedures in animal models that emphasized team training. Others were less comprehensive. All gave a certificate of attendance but usually not proficiency and the course did not certify competence. Surgeons usually ascertained their own proficiency. Studies have shown that students may overestimate their performance and skill level during laparoscopic training courses [2]. In addition, hospitals had limited guidelines for credentialing. They were facing the same economic pressures as the surgeons and wanted a program to be established. Not infrequently, surgeons taking one of these courses would return home and almost immediately schedule patients. Initially, two surgeons usually worked together on the first few cases, but there were no established guidelines or recommendations for preceptoring by surgeons trained in the procedure. Although patient outcomes in most instances were good, they were not good enough. There were all too many complications, resulting in a public outcry.

Training, credentialing, and awarding of privileges of practicing surgeons in new technology

The impact of the perfect storm created by the introduction of laparoscopic cholecystectomy led to a response by academic and organized surgery in partnership with industry to take the lead in training practicing surgeons in new techniques. The Society of American Gastrointestinal Endoscopic Surgeons (SAGES) moved quickly with guidelines for credentialing in laparoscopic cholecystectomy [3]. The guidelines recognized that the procedure was effective and safe but that it required training in animal models and that the first cases should be preceptored by an experienced surgeon [4]. The American College of Surgeons (ACS) responded with reorganization of its Division of Education and the addition of the Committee on Emerging Surgical Technology and Education (Fig. 1). In June of 1994, the ACS published a statement on emerging surgical technologies and guidelines for the evaluation of credentials of individual surgeons for the purpose of awarding surgical privileges (Box 1) [5]. In 1995, the ACS presented

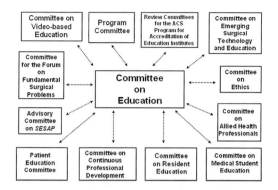

Fig. 1. Standing committees of the ACS Division of Education. The addition of the Committee on Emerging Surgical Technology and Education followed the advent of laparoscopy.

Box 1. American College of Surgeons guidelines for evaluation of credentials of individuals for the purpose of awarding surgical privileges in new technologies

1. The surgeon must be a member in good standing of the department or service from which privileges are to be recommended.
2. A defined educational program in the technology, including didactic and practical elements, must be completed and documented either as a postresidency course of instruction or as a component of an approved residency program.
3. The surgeon must be qualified, experienced, and knowledgeable in the management of the diseases for which the technology is applied—for example, laparoscopic instrumentation would be applied by surgeons who have abdominal or pelvic surgical experience and credentials.
4. The qualifications of the surgeon to apply the new technology must be assessed by a surgeon who is qualified and experienced in the technology and should result in a written recommendation to the department or service head. In the case of a resident trained in the technology during residency, recommendation by the program director is acceptable.
5. Maintenance of skills should be documented through periodic outcomes assessment and evaluation in association with the regular renewal of surgical privileges.

From American College of Surgeons Statements on emerging surgical technologies and the evaluation of credentials. Bull Am Coll Surg 1994;79(6):40–1; with permission.

a statement on issues to be considered before a new surgical technology is applied to the care of patients [6]. This statement considered four fundamental issues:

1. Has the new technology been adequately tested for safety and efficacy?
2. Is the new technology at least as safe and effective as existing, proved techniques?
3. Is the individual proposing to perform the new procedure fully qualified to do so?
4. Is the new technology cost effective?

At its February 1998 meeting, the Board of Regents of the ACS approved a process by which its fellows and associate fellows could be verified for use of emerging technologies. This process was designed to provide surgeons with documentation of educational achievement sufficient to persuade those who are responsible for credentialing/privileging in the local practice setting that the surgeons can be permitted to apply the technology to patients. This was published in 1998 [7]. After the experience with laparoscopic cholecystectomy, the ACS became a leader in establishing guidelines for other new procedures. Additional examples of the effective educational policies and programs are the joint statement of the ACS and the American College of Radiology on physician qualifications for the performance of stereotactic biopsy (1998) and the development of a curriculum and training program in ultrasonography.

In addition, the ACS currently accredits Education Institutes. The definition and goals of these Educational Institutes is outlined in the following quotation from The American College of Surgeons Web site.

> The goal of the ACS Accredited Education Institutes is to focus on competencies and to specifically address the teaching, learning, and assessment of technical skills using state-of-the-art educational methods and cutting-edge technology. All phases of learning (before a course, during a course, and after a course) are addressed by the faculty at the Education Institutes. Leading-edge educational approaches will be used to ensure achievement of competence and development of expertise. The Education Institutes may use a variety of methods to achieve specific educational outcomes, including the use of bench models, simulations, simulators, and virtual reality. The faculty at these institutes will ensure that the participants achieve predetermined levels of skill at the completion of the course. Opportunities for post-course proctoring will be explored, to facilitate transfer of the newly acquired skill to surgical practice. Also, collaborative education research would be pursued by the Education Institutes under the aegis of the College, to advance the science of acquisition and maintenance of surgical competence [8].

These Educational Institutes will, in part, develop a network of advanced training sites for new surgical techniques in the future.

An additional impact of laparoscopic surgery was the development of partnerships between industry and medical institutions. Many academic centers have developed relationships with industry to provide high-quality educational programs that have given practicing surgeons access to learning new techniques. Successes have been achieved in bariatric surgery, sentinel lymph node biopsy, and endovascular procedures. American surgery and industry responded effectively to the publics need for a process by which to introduce new technology.

As the minimally invasive revolution began to evolve, more and more complex procedures adapted to a laparoscopic approach, including inguinal hernia repair, Nissen fundoplication, Roux-en-Y gastric bypass, colon resections, splenectomy, and adrenalectomy. The bad experience with the introduction of laparoscopic cholecystectomy was not repeated because of the efforts of organized surgery, industry, and the surgical profession. The speed of development and widespread acceptance of these more complex procedures was more controlled and less media driven. A mechanism to ensure the appropriate training and preceptoring of surgeons was available in many circumstances. Hospitals and credentialing authorities were more aware of the need for these experiences before awarding surgeons clinical privileges to perform a certain new minimally invasive procedure without supervision. The revolution became an evolution.

Training of new technology to fellows and residents in surgery

Another challenge that arose from laparoscopic cholecystectomy was how to introduce this new procedure into the surgery resident training programs. When the faculty were learning the procedures, residents initially participated as assistants but gradually laparoscopic cholecystectomy was incorporated into residency training. Today, the old paradigm of "see-one, do-one, teach one" has been replaced with curricula to teach basic laparoscopic techniques and gradual introduction of the newer procedures into fellowships and surgical residency. Fundamentals of laparoscopic surgery (FLS) is a program developed by SAGES and designed to teach and evaluate the knowledge, judgment, and skills fundamental to laparoscopic surgery, independent of the surgical specialty. Through rigorous evaluation, the program has been demonstrated a reliable and valid means of developing proficiency in laparoscopic surgery [9]. The manual skills component is based on that developed at McGill University [10]. Many surgery training programs have incorporated FLS or other structured skills training curricula into the residency [11].

Before laparoscopic cholecystectomy, there was little if any mention of surgical simulation in the surgical literature. In many areas of surgery and endoscopy, industry has developed procedure simulation. These have proved valuable adjuncts in training. Recently, however, some authorities have indicated that until the predictive value of simulated testing has been validated further, competence still needs to be determined by expert assessment of observed performance in real cases by measurable outcomes in real procedures [12]. There is no substitute for experience. Hence, the evolution of minimally invasive surgery also has been accompanied the development of procedure-based fellowships.

The focus of these fellowships is to provide in-depth training in advanced minimally invasive procedures. Currently there are approximately 127 minimally invasive surgery fellowships accredited by the Fellowship Council. The Fellowship Council is an oversight body with representatives from several specialty societies created to accredit fellowships in minimally invasive surgery. In 2007, there were 173 positions available and 202 applicants completed the match process (Adrian Park, MD, FACS, personal communication, 2007).

In Fig. 2, a hypothetical illustration of the performance of a new surgical procedure by attending surgeons, fellows, and residents is depicted. Early in the introduction of a new technique, the procedure is done by an attending surgeon, perhaps with another attending surgeon assisting. Then the procedure is introduced to fellows or advanced trainees and finally surgical residents learn the procedure. Supervised laparoscopic cholecystectomy performed by surgical trainees has a complication rate not statistically different from that of the procedure performed by attending surgeons. In addition, the operative time was not different. In one study, the operative time was 57 minutes for trainees and 49 minutes for attending surgeons [13]. Resident case log experience supports the premise that advanced laparoscopic procedures are being introduced in residency programs. The number of complex laparoscopic procedures performed by residents is increasing as attending staff gain greater confidence in these techniques and residents gain greater skills in minimally invasive surgery through well-defined curricula and simulation.

Proficiency

How is proficiency in surgical procedures determined? Historically this has been based on repeated observation of trainees performing a surgical procedure by an experienced faculty member. It is an overall global assessment of trainees based on their understanding of the indications and reasons for surgery, the surgical anatomy, the steps of the procedure, the ability to gain exposure, tissue handling, creative problem solving, and outcome. FLS has been demonstrated to be accurate in assessing proficiency in basic

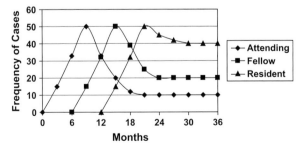

Fig. 2. The learning process of a new procedure. At first the attending surgeons perform the case, followed by fellows and then residents. It may take 18 to 24 months for new procedures to be fully incorporated into residency training programs.

laparoscopic skills. Establishing proficiency in an entire operative procedure with multiple manual steps and various levels of decision making is a different story.

One of the lessons learned from laparoscopy involves the concept of the learning curve. Before 1990 there were few references to the learning curve in surgery. As noted by Subramonian and Muir [14] T.P. Wright introduced the concept of a learning curve in aircraft manufacturing in 1936. He described a basic theory for defining the repetitive process of aircraft assembly. The term was introduced to medicine after the advent of minimal access surgery. Yet there is no standardization of what the term means. The learning curve likely is different for each surgeon and each procedure.

For the Wright learning curve, the underlying hypothesis is that the direct person-hours necessary to complete a unit of production decrease by a constant percentage each time the production quantity is doubled. In manufacturing, the learning curve applies to the time and cost of production. Can a surgeon's learning curve be described on similar lines? It probably is not that simple. The variability introduced by the human factor, patient comorbidity, and disease make simple construction of a learning curve unlikely. It has been proposed that there are two definitions of the learning curve for a surgical procedure: (1) the time taken or the number of procedures an average surgeon needs to be able to perform a procedure independently with a reasonable outcome and (2) the graphic representation of the relationship between experience with a new procedure or technique and outcomes, including operative time, complication rate, hospital stay, and mortality. The former is less objective and depends on defining an average surgeon and a reasonable outcome. Education theorists agree the learning process is cumulative, that is, the effects of experience carry over to aid later performance. There are three main features of a learning curve: (1) the initial or starting point, which defines where the performance of an individual surgeon begins; (2) the rate of learning, which measures how quickly a surgeon reaches a certain level of performance; and (3) the plateau point at which a surgeon's performance stabilizes. The implications for training in laparoscopic procedures are twofold: (1) practice helps improve performance but the most dramatic improvement happens in the first experiences with a procedure and (2) with sufficient practice surgeons can achieve comparable levels of performance.

The way learning curves are calculated is complex and validity is difficult to establish [15]. In minimally invasive surgery, the number of procedures required to reach the summit of the learning curve and achieve proficiency varies based on the type of procedure. The volume of cases for laparoscopic cholecystectomy proficiency is estimated at 50. This is based on the observation that 90% of bile duct injuries occur during the first 30 procedures and the calculated risk for an injury is 1.7% on the first case and 0.17% on the fiftieth case [16]. In contrast, that for laparoscopic Nissen fundoplication is estimated at 20 cases, laparoscopic colon resection 50 cases, and Roux-en-Y gastric bypass 100 cases [17,18]. This does not include factoring in transference of skill of one procedure to another, practice in simulators, and cumulative skill development from other procedures. For example, some procedures are built on basic steps involved with other procedures, such as trocar placement, suturing, use of staplers, and so forth. Also these estimates do not consider individual capabilities. Unfortunately, there is an overall lack of consensus on how many procedures need to be performed to be eligible for the initial awarding of privileges for a procedure or to maintain those privileges. With increasing general laparoscopic experience, it is likely that the asymptote of the learning curve will be reached with fewer cases. Thus, there is no simple formula for credentialing new procedures. It is up to individual hospital credentials committees to decide the threshold of necessary experience to ensure safe and quality patient care and to award privileges.

Ethical considerations in the introduction of new technology

Laparoscopy has stimulated interest in the ethics of new procedure application. In this area there likely are more questions than answers and lessons. Iserson and Chiasson state, "Medical technology itself, including minimally invasive surgery has no morals: our morality revolves around when and how we use the technology" [19]. The primary ethical consideration involving application of new technologies in medicine and surgery over which physicians have control is that of provider proficiency with the procedure or device, information they provide to patients about the risks and benefits of the procedure and alternative treatments. One could argue that such disclosure should include the number of times the new procedure has been performed by a provider or the number of times a new device has been used and what the outcomes have been. As indicated in the previous discussion, the learning curve for new procedures is variable depending on the complexity of an operation, patient factors, the disease process, equipment, and the surgeon skill and judgment.

There are many questions around the process for introduction of new technology. When do providers know they are ready to perform a new procedure without supervision? As discussed previously, surgeons tend to overrate their performance in laparoscopic training programs. Therefore, standard performance metrics, such as FLS, are essential and need to be developed for more complex tasks. Who will determine that surgeons can perform a new procedure safely? In a surgery resident training program, this is determined by assessment by the faculty and the number of cases performed. Ideally, for a practitioner learning a new procedure, a third party should preceptor the individual and verify proficiency. But how many cases are sufficient to know that providers have developed sufficient skill to know that they can perform a procedure independently. How does a single preceptor know that a surgeon is ready to do a procedure independently? Is the preceptor willing to sign off on proficiency? Who is liable should there be a bad outcome: the physician or the certifier of competence? How should these assessments be incorporated into hospital credentialing and the award of privileges? In reality, practitioner credentialing primarily controls the use of a new technology. In the end, however, the ethics of physicians and hospitals ultimately determine how new procedures are introduced. The evolution of laparoscopy has taught the profession to reflect on these issues but has provided few clear-cut answers. Continued attention to the ethical fabric is essential.

Reimbursement for new procedures and the process for applying for a new Current Procedural Terminology code

When laparoscopic cholecystectomy was introduced, physicians did not know how best to interact with medical insurance companies to be reimbursed or the multiple steps required as a new procedure advanced from research concept to the assignment of a code in the American Medical Association (AMA) Current Procedural Terminology (CPT). Today, new procedure development outpaces the development of CPT codes. When a new procedure is introduced, there is an increased need for preauthorization, reporting an unlisted procedure code, and ensuring that complete documentation accompanies the claim. Physicians should be proactive about educating the insurance community where necessary about the results of new treatments and procedures. This proved helpful in avoiding denials for payment when laparoscopic cholecystectomy was introduced.

The process for applying for a new CPT code is outlined on the AMA Web site [20]. There are several questions that should be considered before submitting requests for new CPT codes or changes to existing codes:

1. Is the suggestion a fragmentation or variation of an existing procedure or service?
2. Can the suggested procedure or service be reported by using two or more existing codes?
3. Does the suggested procedure or service represent a distinct service?
4. Is the suggested procedure or service merely a means to report extraordinary circumstances related to the performance of a procedure or service already in CPT?
5. Is this a new procedure or technology?

If the answer to these questions supports a new procedure code, then the requesting physician should contact the appropriate specialty society or the ACS to initiate the process. The best reasons for new codes are (1) new clinical service or technical procedure not found in the current version of CPT (CPT [R]) and not sufficiently represented or reported with existing CPT codes; (2) change of an existing service or procedure when the existing CPT code no longer adequately describes the services or typical patients, and (3) the CPT code generally used for a service or procedure does not represent the technical difficulty or physician work when dealing with a specific population (eg, neonates).

The process to request a new CPT code is outlined in Fig. 3. Once the necessary information is received, the AMA staff reviews the request; then, it is reviewed by the by CPT specialty advisors and then the CPT panel. If a new or revised CPT code is issued, it is referred to the AMA/ Specialty Society Relative Value Scale Update Committee for determination of the new codes value for reimbursement.

Medical lessons learned from laparoscopy

Length of hospitalization

The rapid recovery of patients having laparoscopic cholecystectomy intrigued surgeons and initiated a review of practices with open cholecystectomy. Fast tracking open procedures was reported. In a prospective study in 1991, 500 consecutive patients who had open cholecystectomy were found to have had a mean length of stay of 1.9 days. One fourth of the total group was discharged within 24 hours and more than half within 48 hours [21]. Moss [21] reported 158 of 160 consecutive patients who had open cholecystectomy discharged the day after surgery after a specific protocol and concluded that the shorter length of stay after cholecystectomy primarily may reflect the altered expectations that were derived form the introduction of laparoscopic cholecystectomy. Other studies also reported that conversion of a laparoscopic cholecystectomy resulted in minimal increases in hospitalization [22]. A review of length of stay of elective open cholecystectomy at The Ohio State University showed a similar trend to shortened length of stay (Fig. 4).

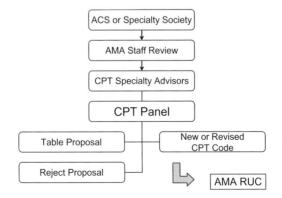

Fig. 3. Process to request a new CPT code.

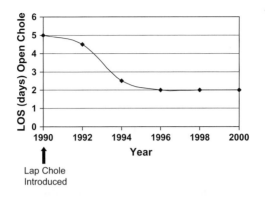

Fig. 4. Length of stay of patients undergoing open cholecystectomy decreased after the experience with laparoscopic cholecystectomy.

Physiologic response to surgery

The observations of quick recovery of laparoscopic cholecystectomy patients stimulated investigation into the physiologic response to surgery in these patients. In addition the application of advanced laparoscopic methods for the resection of cancers has led to research that has made it clear that surgery has important detrimental immune consequences.

Initial studies addressed the effect of open or laparoscopic procures on pulmonary function. Peters and colleagues [23] reported an initial experience. Changes in pulmonary function were studied via standard spirometry in 30 patients after laparoscopic cholecystectomy and compared with those in nine patients after traditional open cholecystectomy. The mean functional vital capacity was found to decrease 23% and 35.2% after laparoscopic and open procedures, respectively. Forced expiratory volume in 1 second (FEV_1) decreased by 24.3% with the minimally invasive approach compared with a 36.2% reduction in FEV_1 after an open operation. Forced expiratory flow was decreased more after open procedures. It was concluded that laparoscopic cholecystectomy provides less decrement in pulmonary function than traditional open cholecystectomy. Many studies have reported similar observations. A recent meta-analysis concluded that pulmonary function is better preserved after laparoscopic procedures [24].

Additional studies have reported that laparoscopic surgery induces less of an acute-phase stress response than open surgical procedures as assessed by measurement of norepinephrine, C-reactive protein, corticotropin, interleukin 6, and tumor necrosis factor α [25]. These findings have been reported in laparoscopic cholecystectomy [26], gynecologic procedures [27], Roux-en-Y gastric bypass [28], and animal models of laparoscopic liver resection [29]. Some studies, however, have found no difference in the stress response. Mendoza-Sagaon and colleagues [30] assessed the stress response in an animal model. The assessment of the stress response was determined by measurement of hepatic mRNA levels of beta-fibrinogen, alpha-1-chymotrypsin inhibitor, metallothionein, heat shock protein, and polyubi-quitin. No differences were found between open and laparoscopic procedures.

The inflammatory response to laparoscopic surgery also is dampened. The peripheral leukocyte function may be better preserved after laparo-scopic cholecystectomy in comparison to open cholecystectomy. Elevations of polymorphonuclear cells (PMN)-elastase and C-reactive protein are bio-markers for the inflammatory response. Elevations are less after laparo-scopic compared with open cholecystectomy [31]. The dampened systemic response may be related to carbon dioxide insufflation during laparoscopy rather than the less traumatic nature of the procedure. Theoretically, this may be related to a suppression of peritoneal macrophage functions induced by carbon dioxide. In vivo data suggest that carbon dioxide also can affect neutrophils (polymorphonuclear cells), the most abundant cell type in the inflamed peritoneal cavity. Shimotakahara and colleagues [32] demonstrated that carbon dioxide incubation directly and temporarily suppressed the proinflammatory functions of polymorphonuclear cells. This effect could contribute to the dampened inflammatory response to laparoscopic surgery. It also raises the question of whether or not the temporary suppression of neutrophil functions could affect the clearance of bacterial contaminations.

The logical extension of the studies (discussed previously) was to investi-gate the impact of traditional open methods and minimally invasive tech-niques on a variety of immune function parameters. Major surgery results in period of cell-mediated immunosuppression that can affect patient recov-ery negatively. Carter and Whelan [33] reviewed the topic and found that studies uniformly show that open methods result in significantly more immu-nosuppression than laparoscopic techniques. It seems that the choice of surgical approach does not have an impact on the absolute number of lymphocytes or lymphocyte subpopulations but is associated with suppressed lymphocyte function. Laparotomy seems to result in greater decreases in monocyte-mediated cytotoxicity while at the same time activating monocytes to elaborate more tumor necrosis factor α and superoxide anion than laparo-scopic methods. Studies on natural killer cell counts and function are conflict-ing and no definitive conclusions can be established. As indicated previously, the majority of the data suggest that open surgery is associated with signifi-cantly higher levels of interleukin 6 and C-reactive protein.

Minimally invasive methods are less stressful, as judged by these param-eters. It seems that one way to avoid or minimize immunosuppression after surgery is to use minimally invasive methods. In theory, laparoscopic cancer resection methods may be associated with less cancer progression. A case in point is the study of Shiromizu and colleagues [34], which showed that laparotomy accelerated pulmonary tumor metastases whereas laparoscopy did not increase the frequency or growth of lung metastases. There is no human evidence to support this hypothesis. Minimally invasive methods may be associated with oncologic advantages that go well beyond less pain, a quicker recovery, and a shorter length of stay. More basic science and human studies are needed on this intriguing topic.

Postoperative gastrointestinal function

Before laparoscopy, nasogastric decompression was used routinely after most major abdominal operations to prevent the consequences of postoperative ileus. Although there are a few studies questioning the necessity of this practice before 1990, many studies followed the introduction of laparoscopy. Ojerskog and coworkers [35] reported 52 patients in whom nasogastric decompression was not used after construction of a continent ileostomy had no increase in complications. In 1984, Reasbeck and colleagues [36] reported a randomized prospective trial of no postoperative nasogastric decompression and reported no differences in complications between the groups. Wolff and colleagues [37] reported a randomized prospective trial of nasogastric decompression in 535 patients. The protocol excluded patients who had emergency surgery and peritonitis, extensive adhesions, enterotomies, previous pelvic radiation, intra-abdominal infection, pancreatitis, chronic obstruction, prolonged operative times or difficult endotracheal intubation. They concluded that even though there was an increase rate of minor symptoms of nausea, vomiting, and abdominal distention, routine nasogastric decompression was not warranted after elective colon and rectal surgery. The practice was not widely accepted until the expectations of postoperative recovery changed with minimally invasive surgery. Increasing numbers of reports challenged the routine use of nasogastric tubes in nearly all elective abdominal procedures. A meta-analysis in 1995 reported on 26 trials (3964 patients) did not support routine nasogastric tube use. Another meta-analysis in 2005 of 28 studies (4194 patients) and 2007 of 33 studies (5240 patients) observed that routine use of nasogastric tubes did not accomplish any of its intended purposes and should be abandoned in favor of selective use [38,39]. Fig. 5 shows the frequency of nasogastric tube use in colorectal procedures.

Traditionally, postoperative oral intake was withheld until the return of bowel function. There was concern that early oral intake could result in

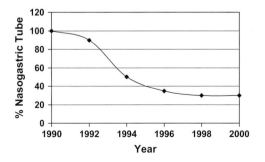

Fig. 5. Frequency of nasogastric tube use after colon and rectal surgery.

vomiting, possibly leading to aspiration, anastomotic leaks, or wound dehis-cence. The shorter stays after minimally invasive gastrointestinal surgery forced early resumption of oral intake and challenged the traditional para-digm. Reissman and colleagues [40] reported a prospective randomized trial of initiation of oral intake on postoperative day 1 after elective colon and rectal surgery in 161 patients. There was no difference in complications or length of stay although the early group had quicker return of bowel function and tolerated a regular diet significantly earlier than the group treated in the traditional manner. A meta-analysis in 2007 reported no significant differ-ence in postoperative ileus, vomiting, abdominal distension, time to passage of flatus, wound complications, and pneumonia with early oral intake [41].

Summary

The evolution of the laparoscopic and minimally invasive surgical revo-lution has taught many lessons that have had an impact on the way physi-cians are trained in new procedures and in caring for patients. It is likely that the continued evolution of minimally invasive surgery will provide additional lessons that will challenge traditional concepts and change the way patients are cared for in the future.

References

[1] Sidhu RS, Vikis E, Cheifetz R, et al. Self-assessment during a 2-day laparoscopic colectomy course: can surgeons judge how well they are learning new skills? Am J Surg 2006;191(5):677–81.
[2] McKernan B. Laparoscopic cholecystectomy. Am Surg 1991;57(5):309–12.
[3] Laparoscopic cholecystectomy. JAMA 1991;265(12):1585–7.
[4] NY State issues guidelines for lap cholecystectomy. New York State Health Department 1. OR Manager 1992;8(7):8–9.
[5] The Bulletin of the American College of Surgeons. 1994;79:40–41.
[6] The Bulletin of the American College of Surgeons. 1995;80:46–47.
[7] The Bulletin of the American College of Surgeons. 1998;83.
[8] American College of Surgeons Website. Available at: http://www.facs.org/. Accessed Janu-ary 15, 2008.
[9] Fried GM. FLS assessment of competency using simulated laparoscopic tasks. J Gastroint-est Surg 2008;12(2):210–2.
[10] Dauster B, Steinberg A, Vassiliou MC, et al. Validity of the MISTELS simulator for lapa-roscopy training in urology. J Endourol. 2005;19:541–5.
[11] Gould JC. Building a laparoscopic skills lab: resources and support. JSLS 2006;10(3):293–6.
[12] Fried GM. Lessons form the surgical experience with simulators: incorporation into training and utilization in determining competency. Gastrointest Endosc Clin N Am 2006;16:425–34.
[13] Koulas SG, Tsimoyiannis J, Koutsourelakis I, et al. Laparoscopic cholecystectomy per-formed by surgical trainees. JSLS 2006;10:484–7.
[14] Subramonian K, Muir G. The learning curve in surgery: what is it, how do we measure it and can we influence it? BJU Int 2004;93(9):1173–4.
[15] Cook JA, Ramsay CR, Fayers P. Statistical evaluation of learning curve effect in surgical trials. Clin Trials 2004;1:421–7.
[16] Moore MJ, Bennett CL. The learning curve for laparoscopic cholecystectomy. The Southern Surgeon Club. Am J Surg 1995;170:55–9.

[17] Watson DI, Baigrie RJ, Jamieson G. A learning curve for laparoscopic fundoplication: definable, avoidable, or a waste of time. Ann Surg 1996;224:198–203.

[18] Iserson KV, Chisaaon PM. The ethics of applying new technologies. Semin Laparosc Surg 2003;9:222–9.

[19] Saltzstein EC, Mercer LC, Peacok JB, et al. Twenty-four hour hospitalization after cholecystectomy. Surg Gynecol Obstet 1991;173:367–70.

[20] American Medical Association. Available at: http://www.ama-assn.org/. Accessed January 15, 2008.

[21] Moss G. Raising the outcome standards for conventional cholecystectomy. Am J Surg 1996; 172:383–5.

[22] Jones K, decamp BS, Mangram AJ, et al. Laparoscopic converted to open cholecystectomy minimally prolongs hospitalization. Am J Surg 2005;190:879–81.

[23] Peters JH, Ortega A, Lehnard SL, et al. The physiology of laparoscopic surgery: pulmonary function after laparoscopic cholecystectomy. Surg Laparosc Endosc 1993;3:370–4.

[24] Damiani G, Pinnarelli L, Sammarco A. Postoperative pulmonary function in open versus laparoscopic cholecystectomy: a meta-analysis of the Tiffenau index. Dig Surg 2008;25:1–7.

[25] Buunen M, Gholghesaei M, veldkamp R, et al. Stress response to laparoscopic surgery: a review. Surg Endosc 2004;18:1022–8.

[26] Haq Z, Rahman M, Siddique MA, et al. Interleukin-6 (IL-6) and tumor necrosis factor–alpha in open and laparoscopic cholecystectomy. Mymensingh Med J 2004;13:153–6.

[27] Marana E, Scambia G, Maussier ML, et al. Neuroendocrine stress response in patients undergoing benign ovarian cyst surgery by laparoscopy, minilaparotomy, and laparotomy. J Am Assoc Gynecol Laparosc 2003;10:159–65.

[28] Nguyen NT, Goldman CD, Ho HS, et al. Systemic stress response after laparoscopic and open gastric bypass. J Am Coll Surg 2002;194:557–66.

[29] Burpee SE, Kurian M, Murakame Y, et al. The metabolic and immune response to laparoscopic versus open liver resection. Surg Endosc 2002;16:899–904.

[30] Mendoza-Sagaon M, Hanly EJ, Talamini MA, et al. Comparison of the stress response after laparoscopic and open cholecystectomy. Surg Endosc 2000;14:1136–41.

[31] Schietroma M, Carlei F, Cappelli S, et al. Effects of cholecystectomy (laparoscopic versus open) on PMN-elastase. Hepatogastroenterology 2007;54:342–5.

[32] Shimotakahara A, Kuebler JF, Vieten G, et al. Carbon dioxide directly suppresses spontaneous migration, chemotaxis, and free radical production of human neutophils. Surg Endosc 2007, in press.

[33] Carter JJ, Whelan RL. The immunologic consequences of laparoscopy in oncology. Surg Oncol Clin N Am 2001;10:655–77.

[34] Shiromizu A, Suematsu T, Yamaguchi K, et al. Effect of laparotomy and laparoscopy on the establishment of lung metastases in a murine model. Surgery 2000;128:799–805.

[35] Ojerskog B, Kock NG, Myrvold HE, et al. Omission of gastric decompression after major intestinal surgery. Ann Chir Gynaecol 1983;72:47–9.

[36] Reasbeck PG, Rice ML, Herbison GP. Nasogastric intubation after intestinal surgery. Surg Gynecol Obstet 1984;158:354–8.

[37] Wolff BG, Pembeton JH, van Heerden JA, et al. Elective colon and rectal surgery without nasogastric decompression. a prospective,randomized trial. Ann Surg 1989;209:670–3.

[38] Nelson R, Edwards S, Tse B. Prophylactic nasogastric decompression after abdominal surgery. Cochrane Database Syst Rev 2005;1:CD004929.

[39] Nelson R, Edwards S, Tse B. Prophylactic nasogastric decompression after abdominal surgery. Cochrane Database Syst Rev 2007;3:CD004929.

[40] Reissman P, Teoh TA, Cohen SM, et al. Is early oral feeding safe after elective colorectal surgery? a prospective randomized trial. Ann Surg 1995;222:73–7.

[41] Charoenkwan K, Phllipson G, Vutyavanich T. Early versus delayed (traditional)oral fluids and food for reducing complications after major abdominal gynaecologic surgery. Cochrane Database Syst Rev 2007;4:CD004508.

ELSEVIER
SAUNDERS

SURGICAL
CLINICS OF
NORTH AMERICA

Surg Clin N Am 88 (2008) 943–958

Antireflux Surgery

C. Daniel Smith, MD

*Department of Surgery, Mayo Clinic–Florida, 4500 San Pablo Road, Jacksonville,
FL 32224, USA*

Antireflux surgery (ARS) is appropriate and effective management for patients who have gastroesophageal reflux disease (GERD) refractory to medical management, who are on lifelong acid suppression, or who are experiencing side effects of the medical management. Over the past 2 decades, the operations have evolved from predominantly open thoracic approaches to a predominantly laparoscopic abdominal approach with similar, if not better, outcomes. The success of ARS in managing GERD lies largely in an understanding of GERD and its diagnosis, proper patient selection, sound surgical technique, and postoperative management. As our understanding of ARS has evolved and newer approaches and techniques have evolved, it is also important to understand how these newer procedures fit in the spectrum of options for GERD management.

Gastroesophageal reflux disease

GERD is defined as the failure of the antireflux barrier, allowing abnormal reflux of gastric contents into the esophagus [1,2]. It is a mechanical disorder that is caused by a defective lower esophageal sphincter (LES), a gastric emptying disorder, or failed esophageal peristalsis. These abnormalities result in a spectrum of disease ranging from the symptom of "heartburn" to esophageal tissue damage with subsequent complications of stricture, bleeding, or metaplastic mucosal changes (Barrett's changes). As diagnostic tools have become more widely available and applied, a host of extraesophageal manifestations of GERD are also increasingly being identified (eg, asthma, laryngitis, dental breakdown) [3,4].

GERD is an extremely common condition, accounting for nearly 75% of all esophageal pathologic findings. Nearly 44% of Americans experience monthly heartburn, and 18% of these individuals use nonprescription

E-mail address: smith.c.daniel@mayo.edu

0039-6109/08/$ - see front matter © 2008 Elsevier Inc. All rights reserved.
doi:10.1016/j.suc.2008.06.003   *surgical.theclinics.com*

medication directed against GERD. With a prevalence of nearly 19 million cases per year with an associated total cost of care of $9.8 billion in the United States, GERD is clearly a significant public health concern [5].

There is considerable debate regarding optimal treatment of GERD. With a significant number of Americans experiencing daily heartburn and the impact that this condition has on an individual's quality of life, it is no surprise that there is a tremendous amount of interest and effort going into understanding this condition and establishing effective treatment algorithms.

Medical therapy is the first line of management for GERD (Fig. 1). Esophagitis heals in approximately 90% of cases with intensive medical therapy; however, medical management does not address the condition's mechanical cause; thus, symptoms recur in more than 80% of cases within 1 year of drug withdrawal [6,7]. Additionally, although medical therapy may effectively treat the acid-induced symptoms of GERD, esophageal mucosal injury may continue because of ongoing alkaline reflux. Finally, for many, medical therapy may be required for the rest of a one's life. The expense and psychologic burden of a lifetime of medication dependence, undesirable life style changes, uncertainty as to the long-term effects of some newer medications, and the potential for persistent mucosal changes despite symptomatic control all make surgical treatment of GERD an attractive option.

Historically, ARS was recommended only for patients who have refractory or complicated gastroesophageal reflux [8,9]. Throughout the early 1990s, several major developments changed our thinking regarding the long-term management of patients who have GERD. First, the introduction of proton pump inhibitors (PPIs) has provided truly effective medical therapy for GERD. Therefore, few patients have "refractory" GERD. Next, laparoscopic surgery became available, thereby significantly changing the morbidity rate and recovery time after an antireflux procedure. Third, the widespread availability and use of ambulatory pH monitoring and esophageal motility testing have dramatically improved our ability to recognize true GERD and select patients for long-term therapy. Finally, we have realized that patients who have GERD have a greatly impaired quality of life that normalizes with successful treatment [10].

With this, the management goals of GERD have changed. Rather than focusing therapy only on controlling symptoms, modern treatment of GERD aims to eliminate symptoms, improve a patient's quality of life, and institute a lifelong plan for management. Surgical correction of the anatomically deficient antireflux barrier is an appealing option when trying to achieve these goals in the management of GERD.

Patient selection for antireflux surgery

Selecting an appropriate patient for any antireflux procedure requires confirming the diagnosis of GERD and searching for any associated

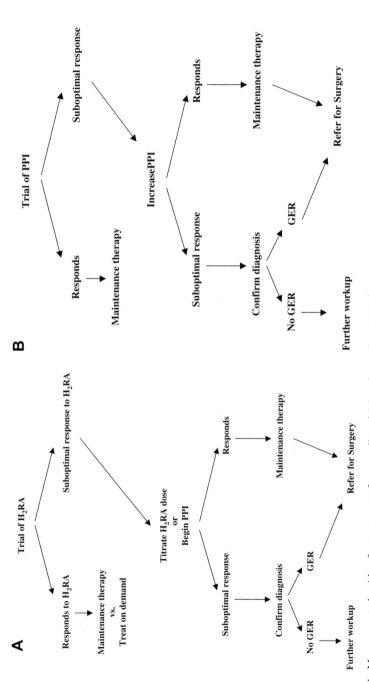
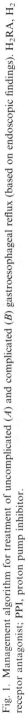

Fig. 1. Management algorithm for treatment of uncomplicated (*A*) and complicated (*B*) gastroesophageal reflux (based on endoscopic findings). H_2RA, H_2 receptor antagonist; PPI, proton pump inhibitor.

conditions that might alter one's surgical approach or options. For example, a patient who has a hiatal hernia may not be a candidate for an endoluminal approach (see section on endoluminal ARS), or a patient who has impaired esophageal clearance should be considered for a partial fundoplication rather than a full fundoplication. Understanding this, the diagnosis and preoperative evaluation are critical to the success of ARS treatment.

The clinical diagnosis of GERD is fairly straightforward if the patient reports the typical symptoms of "heartburn" or regurgitation that are readily relieved after ingesting antacids. Many patients who have this classic presentation have been treated by their primary care physician with an empiric trial of H_2 blockers or PPIs, and resolution of symptoms with such treatment may be diagnostically helpful. In fact, one should be suspicious of the diagnosis of GERD in any patient who reports no improvement in symptoms with any antisecretory regimen or in patients who have atypical or extraesophageal symptoms, such as hoarseness, chronic cough, or asthma.

That being said, it has recently been appreciated that chest pain, asthma, laryngitis, recurrent pulmonary infections, chronic cough, and hoarseness may be associated with reflux, and this association is leading to increasing numbers of patients with these atypical GERD symptoms to be evaluated for reflux. As many as 80% of patients who have asthma have endoscopic evidence of GERD [11], and 50% of patients in whom a cardiac cause of chest pain has been excluded have acid reflux as a cause of their pain. Otolaryngologists are beginning to make primary referrals for the treatment of GERD based on chronic laryngitis and evidence of acid-induced vocal cord damage, and dentists are identifying dental damage from chronic acid reflux.

An objective diagnosis of GERD is mandatory before offering an antireflux operation, and although a barium swallow is often the first test obtained in patients suspected of having GERD, esophagogastroduodenoscopy (EGD) is necessary in all patients who have GERD. Not only can EGD confirm the diagnosis of GERD, but it can rule out other conditions, such as malignancy, stricture, Barrett's esophagus, or eosinophilic esophagitis. During EGD, an esophageal mucosal biopsy should be obtained to confirm esophagitis and esophageal length and the presence of a hiatal hernia or stricture should be assessed. If esophagitis is seen and histologically confirmed during EGD, no other tests beyond EGD are necessary to diagnose GERD. Because most patients are already being empirically treated for GERD with PPIs, however, the results of EGD are normal in many patients. When the diagnosis cannot be confirmed during EGD, esophageal pH testing is necessary to establish the diagnosis of GERD objectively.

The most critical aspects of patient selection are not only objective confirmation of the diagnosis but identifying those who have conditions associated with GERD that may require special consideration. Specifically, those with associated esophageal motor disorders identified by esophageal motility testing, a shortened esophagus, or associated delayed gastric empty-ing may require a tailored approach to GERD. Barrett's esophagus is addressed separately elsewhere in this article. Esophageal body dysfunction (body pressure <30 mm Hg or less than 60% peristalsis with wet swallows) may require a partial fundoplication, a shortened esophagus may require extensive mediastinal dissection to establish adequate esophageal length or a lengthening procedure, and delayed gastric emptying may require tempo-rary postoperative gastric decompression or a drainage procedure (eg, pyloro-plasty). Failure to recognize these associated problems, and surgeon-derived anecdotal "modifications" to proved techniques have led to increasing num-bers of patients "failing" laparoscopic ARS [12,13].

With a thorough understanding of GERD, its associated conditions, and the various objective assessments available today, one should be able to stratify patients to select the best patient for surgery. For example, the ideal patient for ARS is one who has classic symptoms of GERD with heartburn and regurgitation as dominant symptoms, solid objective confirmation of the diagnosis, a good response to PPI therapy, and no other confounding conditions (eg, Barrett's esophagus, impaired esophageal clearance). In this setting, 90% to 95% of patients who have well-done ARS have a good outcome. In contrast, the patient who has primarily atypical symp-toms (eg, chronic cough, hoarseness), has minimal to no improvement with PPIs, has softer data to support the diagnosis of GERD (eg, no acid reflux but impedance pH showing nonacid reflux), or has delayed gastric emptying or impaired esophageal clearance is likely to have a compromised outcome with surgery. With this atypical presentation, only 75% to 85% of patients have good symptom response to surgery, and although many achieve objec-tive control of their acid reflux with surgery (ie, improvement in esophageal acid exposure), many continue to have their preoperative symptoms and are unhappy to have undergone an operation without relief.

Principles and technique of antireflux surgery

The goal of ARS is to establish effective LES pressure. To realize this goal, most surgeons believe it necessary to position the LES within the ab-domen where the sphincter is under positive (intra-abdominal) pressure and to close any associated hiatal defect [14]. To accomplish this, various safe and effective surgical techniques have been developed. In the past 10 years, advances in laparoscopic technology and technique have nearly eliminated open ARS. The laparoscopic techniques reproduce their open counterparts while eliminating the morbidity of an upper midline laparotomy incision [15]. Open ARS remains indicated when the laparoscopic technique is not available or is contraindicated. Contraindications to laparoscopic ARS in-clude uncorrectable coagulopathy, severe chronic obstructive pulmonary disease (COPD), and first-trimester pregnancy. A previous upper abdominal operation and, in particular, prior open ARS are relative contraindications to a laparoscopic approach, and laparoscopic surgery should only be undertaken by experienced laparoscopic surgeons.

The laparoscopic Nissen fundoplication has emerged as the most widely accepted and applied antireflux operation (Fig. 2) [16–21]. In many centers, it is the antireflux procedure of choice in patients who have normal esophageal body peristalsis. Key elements of the procedure include the following:

1. Complete dissection of the esophageal hiatus and both crura
2. Mobilization of the gastric fundus by dividing the short gastric vessels
3. Closure of the associated hiatal defect
4. Creation of a tensionless 360° gastric wrap at the distal esophagus around a 50- to 60-French intraesophageal dilator
5. Limiting the length of the wrap to 1.5 to 2.0 cm
6. Stabilizing the wrap to the esophagus by partial-thickness bites of the esophagus during creation of the wrap

Although widely accepted, these key elements have not been tested in prospective randomized trials.

Early complications have mostly been minor and infrequent. Transient dysphagia occurs in nearly 50% of patients and resolves within 3 weeks of surgery. An infrequent early problem but one of greater concern has been postoperative nausea and retching. During episodes of retching, breakdown of the fundoplication can occur. Therefore, postoperative nausea should be treated aggressively. Late complications of wrap migration and paraesophageal herniation may also be related to postoperative retching

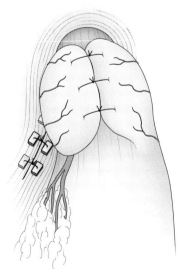

Fig. 2. Depiction of Nissen 360° fundoplication.

but more likely result from failure to close the esophageal hiatus or a shortened esophagus. Long-term dysphagia is emerging in 10% to 15% of patients but is well accepted by patients in the context of GERD symptom control. When a shortened esophagus is encountered, an esophageal lengthening procedure (Collis gastroplasty) may be used. Esophageal lengthening is rarely indicated, however, and its use should be balanced with the findings that 80% of patients develop uncontrollable esophagitis or pathologic esophageal acid exposure [22].

The Toupet fundoplication (Fig. 3) is identical to the Nissen fundoplication except that the fundoplication is a 270° wrap rather than a 360° wrap. The gastric fundus is brought posterior to the esophagus and sutured to either side of the esophagus, leaving the anterior surface bare. This 270° fundoplication has the theoretic advantage of limiting postoperative bloating and dysphagia, especially in those with impaired esophageal body peristalsis. Many centers use the Toupet procedure exclusively in patients who have abnormal esophageal peristalsis identified during preoperative esophageal manometry. Some have advocated the routine use of the Toupet fundoplication in all patients who have GERD, which could eliminate the need for preoperative esophageal manometry in many patients. Nevertheless, it seems that a partial fundoplication is not as durable as a total fundoplication, and its use in the most severe cases (eg, grade IV esophagitis, Barrett's esophagus, stricture) is questionable [23].

Regardless of the technique used, the eightfold increase in the use of ARS over the past decade has also exposed a larger cohort of patients in whom

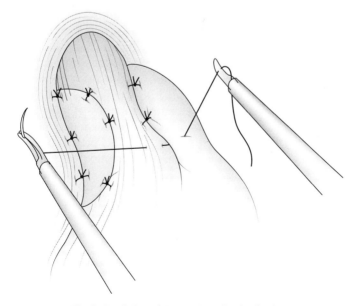

Fig. 3. Depiction of Toupet 270° fundoplication.

the procedure has failed. Failure rates range from 2% to 30% depending on the definition of failure. In select cases (eg, patients with symptomatic recurrent reflux), revisional fundoplication is offered, with most centers reporting a 3% to 5% reoperation rate and a 65% to 90% success rate. Wrap herniation is the leading cause of failure requiring reoperation, whereas wrap disruption, wrap slippage, too tight a fundoplication, and an undiagnosed motility disorder before the initial fundoplication are also frequently observed [13].

Care after antireflux surgery

Patients are allowed to drink liquids immediately after surgery. Carbonated beverages are specifically avoided because of the resulting gastric distention. Because of edema at the fundoplication, patients are maintained on a liquid diet for 5 to 7 days and a soft diet for the next 2 weeks. Hospital dismissal is usually on the first postoperative day, and follow-up is in 3 to 4 weeks. In difficult cases (extensive paraesophageal dissection, redo surgery, or paraesophageal hernia repair), a contrast swallow on postoperative day 1 is recommended to rule out a small leak or other anatomic problem. Patients are released from the hospital with prescriptions for a liquid pain medicine, liquid stool softener, and antiemetic that can be administered rectally should nausea occur. A dietician sees the patients before discharge to instruct them on the soft diet, emphasizing the avoidance of carbonated beverages, breads, and other dry foods, which tend to lodge at the fundoplication. There are no limitations on physical activity unless there has been a paraesophageal hernia that has been repaired, in which case, avoidance of heavy lifting is necessary for approximately 4 to 6 weeks. All preoperative antisecretory or prokinetic medications are stopped.

Postoperative nausea and vomiting or retching remain the most significant and controllable postoperative events associated with significant complications. Most patients receive preemptive antinausea medication, and staff caring for patients after surgery are instructed to respond immediately with medication to any patient complaining of nausea. If any early postoperative retching occurs, a contrast swallow is immediately obtained in case wrap disruption or herniation has occurred. If this occurs and is detected within the first 24 to 48 hours, immediate reoperation can be undertaken to correct the problem. If these anatomic problems are not found until outpatient follow-up, a 6- to 12-week delay is necessary before undertaking reoperation because of the adhesions that have formed by this time.

Outcomes of antireflux surgery

In the 1990s, controlled trials that compared medical and surgical therapy of GERD favored surgical therapy [9]. Within these prospective randomized comparisons, surgical treatment was significantly more effective than medical therapy in improving symptoms and endoscopic signs of esophagitis for as long as 2 years. Other longitudinal studies report good to excellent long-term results in 80% to 93% of surgically treated patients [24–28].

Thousands of patients undergoing laparoscopic Nissen fundoplication have been reported in the world's literature, with 93% of patients free of symptoms at 1 year after surgery. Only 3% have required some medical therapy to control their symptoms. Overall, 97% of these patients are satisfied with their results. Transient dysphagia occurs in nearly 50% of patients and resolves within 3 weeks of surgery. Late complications of wrap migration and paraesophageal herniation may also be related to postoperative retching but are more likely attributable to failure to close the esophageal hiatus or a shortened esophagus. Long-term dysphagia is emerging in 10% to 15% of patients but is frequently well accepted by patients in the context of the excellent GERD symptom control they experience. In 3% to 4% of patients, unremitting dysphagia or recurrent reflux symptoms require reoperation for correction. When redo fundoplication is undertaken, 93% of patients experience good to excellent results. Troubling long-term side effects, such as gas bloat, have been virtually eliminated by the "floppy" nature of the fundoplication.

Although the goal of eliminating symptoms remains the primary concern, long-term follow-up of the controlled trials of the 1990s has raised questions regarding the durability of symptom control after ARS. In a follow-up to their original publication in 1992, Spechler and colleagues [29] noted that 62% of those patients in the surgical treatment group participating in follow-up analysis took antireflux medications regularly. Additionally, they found no significant difference between the medical and surgical groups in the rate of esophagitis, esophageal strictures, esophageal cancer, or overall satisfaction. Others have noted a similar number of patients requiring antisecretory medications longer than 10 years after surgery [27,30,31]. Given a small but not insignificant mortality rate of 0.3% and the known associations with medium- to long-term postprandial bloating and diarrhea in up to 30% to 45% of patients, this has led to a reappraisal of the role of ARS [32]. Ultimately, these data have helped patients to become more informed about their choices in instituting a lifelong management plan.

To summarize, ARS is indicated in any patient who has GERD refractory to medical management or who has symptom recurrence when medicine is withdrawn. In many patients who have classic symptoms, EGD and esophageal manometry are all the preoperative testing necessary. Additional tests are confirmatory in difficult cases. The laparoscopic Nissen fundoplication is safe and effective in the long-term management of nearly all patients who have chronic GERD. The Toupet fundoplication may be best used in patients who have impaired esophageal body peristalsis.

Endoscopic endoluminal therapy

Despite the advances made with the advent of laparoscopy, an ideal treatment for GERD that permanently alleviates symptoms, protects against esophageal erosion, and prevents malignant progression while minimizing the risk associated with therapy remains elusive. Recently, the search for this ideal therapy has led to the development of less invasive alternatives to medical and surgical therapy using endoscopy-based or endoluminal approaches. Now, those patients searching for a nonpharmacologic solution who wish to avoid surgery can opt for procedures that require no skin incision and are often performed on an outpatient basis. The inherent allure of this approach has led several groups within industry to develop therapies designed to alter the anatomy or physiology of the gastroesophageal junction by means of the delivery of radiofrequency energy to the gastroesophageal junction, injection or implantation of devices into the cardia and LES, or suture plication of the proximal stomach [33].

The clinical uses of radiofrequency energy have been well known for decades, ranging from the treatment of benign prostatic hyperplasia to hepatic tumor ablation. The delivery of radiofrequency energy to the esophagus and gastric cardia at a temperature of 65°C has been shown to cause collagen contraction and eventual tissue shrinkage, leading to scarring at the gastroesophageal junction and neurolysis in the same region. Although a clear understanding of the mechanism of action remains to be determined, it is thought that these anatomic changes induced by radiofrequency energy delivery decrease the frequency of transient LES relaxation episodes by means of interference of afferent nerve signals to the brain or by decreasing the stimulation of gastric cardia mechanorcceptors through fibrosis or direct ablation [34]. The Stretta procedure characterizes this technique.

In 1984, O'Conner injected Teflon paste into the esophagogastric (EG) junction of five dogs with a surgically incompetent LES in an attempt to reverse GERD from within the distal esophagus. He noted that all reversed the preinjection levels of esophagitis with an improvement in reflux volume. Since that time, the concept of reversing GERD using an injectable substance at the LES has been actively investigated. Like radiofrequency ablation, no clear mechanism of action has been established. Studies using an ethylene vinyl alcohol copolymer with tantalum dissolved in dimethyl sulfide (Enteryx; Boston Scientific Corporation, Natick, Massachusetts) injected into a porcine model led to an initial inflammatory reaction with eventual circumferential granulation and fibrous capsule formation (around the implant), however. It is hypothesized that this decreased the compliance of the distal esophagus and gastric cardia, preventing shortening of the LES and possibly decreasing the number of transient lower esophageal relaxation episodes [35]. Placement of hydrogel implants into the submucosal space at the level of the LES (Gatekeeper; Medtronic, Minneapolis, Minnesota) increases the volume of the LES and is thought to create a barrier to gastric refluxate [36].

The creation of intraluminal gastric pleats at the gastroesophageal junction is intended to mimic the effects of a gastric fundoplication by revising the anatomic alterations affecting the gastric cardia caused by chronic GERD. This is done by means of the deployment of staples or stitches through unique devices designed to work in tandem with standard esophagogastroscopes. Partial- and full-thickness gastropexy techniques have been described under the trade names of Endocinch (Bard, Murray Hill, New Jersey), Plicator (NDO, Mansfield, Massachusetts), and Esophyx (Endogastric Solutions, Redmond, Washington) [37–39]. The physiologic impact of intraluminal gastroplication has been observed in animals and people, with an immediate increase in LES pressure, decrease in acid sensitivity, and decrease in the number of transient esophageal relaxation episodes detected.

Evidence regarding the effectiveness and safety of these procedures is still accumulating, primarily in the setting of proof-of-concept, small case-study, cohort, or sham-comparison studies. Early results from cohort studies are promising, with therapies demonstrating improvements in quality of life (between 50% and 75% improvement), postprocedure symptom scores, PPI use (up to 40%–75%), 24-hour pH (16%–33% time pH <4 improvement), and LES pressure. Randomized data reveal a trend in improvement of quality-of-life scores and medication use, with two studies noting improvements on objective evaluation (pH, EGD/esophagitis score/manometry). These findings suggest that endoluminal therapy may primarily play a future role in reducing symptoms and medication use, with further evaluation required to understand fully the effects on the histopathologic changes associated with GERD. Follow-up has been limited, thereby limiting conclusions as to the durability of the therapeutic effect. To date, one case-control comparison of endoscopic suturing with laparoscopic Nissen fundoplication has been published [40]. Other sham controlled trials have been completed on several of the techniques [41–43].

As with any new therapy, questions of efficacy remain. US Food and Drug Administration (FDA) phase III and IV data are only recently being evaluated. Perhaps more telling and importantly, market forces are also having an impact on the availability of these therapies. Of the six companies offering some form of endoluminal therapy for GERD, four have gone out of business or pulled their product from the market. Two remain, the first to enter this market (Endocinch, Bard) and the last to enter this market (Esophyx, Endogastric Solutions). Until more data are accumulated, recommendations regarding the widespread use of endoluminal therapies for GERD outside of clinical trials cannot be made. Consistent across all the proposed endoluminal therapies has been the limitation that they are not suited to patients who have hiatal herniation, Barrett's esophagus, or multiple comorbidities.

There is still promise that endoluminal therapies may serve as a means of symptom control as a bridge to definitive therapy, as an alternative in mild to moderately symptomatic patients who do not desire surgery, as a more permanent therapeutic option for those who cannot tolerate surgical intervention, or as a less involved method of helping patients who have recurrent reflux after ARS.

Barrett's esophagus

Special mention is necessary for Barrett's esophagus. In 1950, Norman Barrett described the condition in which the tubular esophagus becomes lined with metaplastic columnar epithelium that is at risk for adenocarcinoma. Most recently, it has been recognized that the specialized intestinal metaplasia (not gastric type columnar changes) constitutes true Barrett's esophagus, with a risk for progression to dysplasia and adenocarcinoma [44].

This abnormality occurs in 7% to 10% of people with GERD and may represent the end stage of the natural history of GERD. Clearly, Barrett's esophagus is associated with a more profound mechanical deficiency of the LES, severe impairment of esophageal body function, and marked esophageal acid exposure [45]. In contrast, some patients are asymptomatic and have only short segments of columnar-lined epithelium in the distal esophagus (<3 cm), which does not have this same strong association with GERD. Additionally, there seems to be a lower incidence of metaplastic epithelium in these "short segments" of Barrett's esophagus, and therefore a lower malignancy potential. There remains considerable debate regarding the significance of short-segment Barrett's esophagus, and identifying those patients with so-called "short-segment" Barrett's esophagus remains problematic, because endoscopically localizing the precise anatomic esophagogastric junction is difficult and metaplastic epithelium (and therefore malignant potential) can exist even in these short segments. The endoscopic feature most strongly associated with intestinal metaplasia is the finding of long segments of esophageal columnar lining, with more than 90% of patients with greater than 3 cm of esophageal columnar lining having intestinal metaplasia.

Endoscopically obvious Barrett's esophagus with intestinal metaplasia is a major risk factor for adenocarcinoma of the esophagus, with the annual incidence of adenocarcinoma in this condition estimated at approximately 0.8%, 40 times higher than in the general population. Once high-grade dysplasia is identified in more than one biopsy from columnar-lined esophagus, nearly 50% of patients already harbor foci of invasive cancer. This frequency is the basis for recommending careful endoscopic surveillance in patients who have Barrett's esophagus with intestinal metaplasia and esophagectomy when high-grade dysplasia is identified [46,47].

Treatment goals for patients who have Barrett's esophagus are similar to those for patients who have GERD, that is, relief of symptoms and arrest of ongoing reflux-mediated epithelial damage. Additionally, those with Barrett's esophagus, regardless of type of treatment (surgical or medical), require long-term endoscopic surveillance with biopsy of columnar segments to identify progressive metaplastic changes or progression to dysplasia [48].

Several studies have compared medical and surgical therapy in patients who have Barrett's esophagus. These data support the notion that Barrett's esophagus is associated with more severe and refractory GERD and ARS is effective at alleviating these symptoms in 75% to 92% of patients. Many patients are asymptomatic (perhaps explaining why they have such advanced sequelae of GERD), however, and there is mounting evidence to suggest that an alkaline refluxate may be as damaging as acid reflux [49]. For these reasons, correction of the mechanically defective antireflux barrier may be especially important in these patients.

Although symptom control in these patients suggests control of ongoing damage, the ultimate goal in therapy is to change the natural history in Barrett's esophagus of progression to adenocarcinoma. With this goal, several questions arise:

1. Does ARS result in regression of Barrett's epithelium?
2. Does ARS prevent progression of metaplastic changes?
3. Is there a role for ARS accompanied by other therapies for metaplastic or dysplastic epithelium?

Does ARS result in regression of Barrett's epithelium? Operative therapy corrects the mechanically defective antireflux barrier, and therefore might be expected to have a higher likelihood than medical therapy alone of inducing regression of Barrett's epithelium. In reviewing the results regarding regression with medical treatment, there is no substantial evidence that medical therapy results in regression. In a summary of several series, complete regression occurred in only 6 patients, with all but 1 coming from one series. Thirty-one patients showed some decrease in the length of Barrett's epithelium, but only 6 had a decrease in length of more than 1 cm. Furthermore, 6 patients went on to develop adenocarcinoma of the esophagus. In contrast, several studies are now showing regression with surgical therapy. In some series, up to 60% of patients have experienced visual regression and 40% have experienced histologic regression [50,51].

Does ARS prevent progression of metaplastic changes? There is growing evidence suggesting that ARS may prevent progression of Barrett's changes, and thereby protect against dysplasia and malignancy. In a series reported by McDonald and colleagues [52] from the Mayo Clinic, three cancers occurred over an 18.5-year follow-up period, all within the first 3 years after operation. The clustering of these three cases within the first 3 years of follow-up suggests that these patients may have already progressed to dysplasia at the time of operation. These are strong data in support of the favorable impact of operative therapy on the natural history of Barrett's esophagus.

Is there a role for ARS accompanied by other therapies for metaplastic or dysplastic epithelium? Combination therapy, that is, pharmacologic or operative control of acid reflux plus endoscopic ablation of Barrett's mucosa, is having encouraging preliminary results. These early experiences suggest that the ablated areas re-epithelialize with more normal squamous mucosa. Ablative therapies have included laser ablation, photodynamic therapy, and cryotherapy. A promising newer therapy is radiofrequency ablation delivered by means of a tightly wound wire array around a balloon that can be inflated in the esophagus, thereby providing esophageal mucosal effacement with the deliver wires. When a short burst of high energy is delivered in this way, there seems to be uniform ablation of the esophageal mucosa without deep injury to the submucosa. With this, the ablation of the esophageal mucosa involved with Barrett's esophagus can be more uniform and predictable and can result in complete ablation with minimal risk for stricture or complications. Early studies using this technique are promising [53,54]. This exciting early work needs further study before becoming a clinical standard.

References

[1] Patti MG, Bresadola V. Gastroesophageal reflux disease: basic considerations. Problem in General Surgery 1996;13:1–8.

[2] Wetscher GJ, Redmond EJ, Vititi LMH. Pathophysiology of gastroesophageal reflux disease. In: Hinder RA, editor. Gastroesophageal reflux disease. Austin (TX): R.G. Landes Company; 1993. p. 7–29.

[3] Dore MP, Pedroni A, Pes GM, et al. Effect of antisecretory therapy on atypical symptoms in gastroesophageal reflux disease. Dig Dis Sci 2007;52:463–8.

[4] Long MD, Shaheen NJ. Extra-esophageal GERD: clinical dilemma of epidemiology versus clinical practice. Curr Gastroenterol Rep 2007;9:195–202.

[5] Richter JE. The many manifestations of gastroesophageal reflux disease: presentation, evaluation, and treatment. Gastroenterol Clin North Am 2007;36:577–99.

[6] Klingman RR, Stein HJ, DeMeester TR. The current management of gastroesophageal reflux. Adv Surg 1991;24:259–91.

[7] Pace F, Tonini M, Pallotta S, et al. Systematic review: maintenance treatment of gastro-oesophageal reflux disease with proton pump inhibitors taken 'on-demand' [see comment]. Aliment Pharmacol Ther 2007;26:195–204.

[8] Richter JE, Castell DO. Gastroesophageal reflux: pathogenesis, diagnosis and therapy. Ann Intern Med 1989;97:93–103.

[9] Spechler SJ. Comparison of medical and surgical therapy for complicated gastroesophageal reflux disease in veterans. N Engl J Med 1992;326:786–92.

[10] Laycock WS, Mauren S, Waring JP. Improvement in quality of life measures following laparoscopic antireflux surgery. Gastroenterology 1995;108:A244.

[11] Sontag SJ. Gastroesophageal reflux and asthma. Am J Med 1997;103:84S–90S.

[12] Hunter JG, Smith CD, Branum GD, et al. Laparoscopic fundoplication failures: patterns of failure and response to fundoplication revision. Ann Surg 1999;230:595–604 [discussion: 604–6].

[13] Smith CD, McClusky DA, Rajad MA, et al. When fundoplication fails: redo? Ann Surg 2005;241:861–9 [discussion: 69–71].

[14] Smith CD, Fink AS, Applegren K. Guidelines for surgical treatment of gastroesophageal reflux disease (GERD). Society of American Gastrointestinal Endoscopic Surgeons (SAGES). Surg Endosc 1998;12:186–8.

[15] Eshraghi N, Farahmand M, Soot SJ, et al. Comparison of outcomes of open versus laparoscopic Nissen fundoplication performed in a single practice. Am J Surg 1998;175: 371–4.

[16] Anvari M, Allen C. Laparoscopic Nissen fundoplication: two-year comprehensive follow-up of a technique of minimal paraesophageal dissection. Ann Surg 1998;227:25–32.

[17] Anvari M, Allen C, Borm A. Laparoscopic Nissen fundoplication is a satisfactory alternative to long-term omeprazole therapy. Br J Surg 1995;82:938–42.

[18] Bloomston M, Zervos E, Gonzalez R, et al. Quality of life and antireflux medication use following laparoscopic Nissen fundoplication. Am Surg 1998;64:509–13 [discussion: 13–4].

[19] Champault G, Volter F, Rizk N, et al. Gastroesophageal reflux: conventional surgical treatment versus laparoscopy. A prospective study of 61 cases. Surg Laparosc Endosc 1996;6: 434–40.

[20] Hinder RA, Filipi CJ, Wetscher G, et al. Laparoscopic Nissen fundoplication is an effective treatment for gastroesophageal reflux disease. Ann Surg 1994;220:472–81 [discussion: 81–3].

[21] Hunter JG, Trus TL, Branum DG, et al. A physiologic approach to laparoscopic fundoplication for gastroesophageal reflux disease. Ann Surg 1996;223:673–87.

[22] Lin E, Swafford V, Chadalavada R, et al. Disparity between symptomatic and physiologic outcomes following esophageal lengthening procedures for antireflux surgery. J Gastrointest Surg 2004;8:31–9 [discussion: 38–9].

[23] Farrell TM, Smith CD, Archer SB, et al. Heartburn is more likely to recur after Toupet fundoplication than Nissen fundoplication. Am J Surg 2000;66:229–36 [discussion 236–7].

[24] Macintyre IM, Goulbourne IA. Long-term results after Nissen fundoplication: a 5–15-year review. J R Coll Surg Edinb 1990;35:159–62.

[25] Mark LA, Okrainec A, Ferri LE, et al. Comparison of patient-centered outcomes after laparoscopic Nissen fundoplication for gastroesophageal reflux disease or paraesophageal hernia. Surg Endosc 2008;22:343–7.

[26] Morgenthal CB, Lin E, Shane MD, et al. Who will fail laparoscopic Nissen fundoplication? Preoperative prediction of long-term outcomes. Surg Endosc 2007;21:1978–84.

[27] Morgenthal CB, Shane MD, Stival A, et al. The durability of laparoscopic Nissen fundoplication: 11-year outcomes. J Gastrointest Surg 2007;11:693–700.

[28] Pope CE II. The quality of life following antireflux surgery. World J Surg 1992;16:355–8.

[29] Spechler SJ, Lee E, Ahnen D, et al. Long-term outcome of medical and surgical therapies for gastroesophageal reflux disease: follow-up of a randomized controlled trial [see comment]. JAMA 2001;285:2331–8.

[30] Liu JY, Woloshin S, Laycock WS, et al. Late outcomes after laparoscopic surgery for gastroesophageal reflux. Arch Surg 2002;137:397–401.

[31] Zaninotto G, Portale G, Costantini M, et al. Long-term results (6–10 years) of laparoscopic fundoplication. J Gastrointest Surg 2007;11:1138–45.

[32] Richter JE. Let the patient beware: the evolving truth about laparoscopic antireflux surgery [comment]. Am J Med 2003;114:71–3.

[33] Falk GW, Fennerty MB, Rothstein RI. AGA Institute technical review on the use of endoscopic therapy for gastroesophageal reflux disease. Gastroenterology 2006;131: 1315–36.

[34] Utley DS, Kim M, Vierra MA, et al. Augmentation of lower esophageal sphincter pressure and gastric yield pressure after radiofrequency energy delivery to the gastroesophageal junction: a porcine model. Gastrointest Endosc 2000;52:81–6.

[35] Mason RJ, Hughes M, Lehman GA, et al. Endoscopic augmentation of the cardia with a biocompatible injectable polymer (Enteryx) in a porcine model [see comment]. Surg Endosc 2002;16:386–91.

[36] Fockens P, Bruno MJ, Gabbrielli A, et al. Endoscopic augmentation of the lower esophageal sphincter for the treatment of gastroesophageal reflux disease: multicenter study of the Gatekeeper Reflux Repair System. Endoscopy 2004;36:682–9.

[37] Cadiere GB, Rajan A, Rqibate M, et al. Endoluminal fundoplication (ELF)—evolution of EsophyX, a new surgical device for transoral surgery. Minim Invasive Ther Allied Technol 2006;15:348–55.

[38] Mahmood Z, McMahon BP, Arfin Q, et al. Endocinch therapy for gastro-oesophageal reflux disease: a one year prospective follow up [see comment]. Gut 2003;52:34–9.

[39] Tam WC, Holloway RH, Dent J, et al. Impact of endoscopic suturing of the gastroesophageal junction on lower esophageal sphincter function and gastroesophageal reflux in patients with reflux disease [see comment]. Am J Gastroenterol 2004;99:195–202.

[40] Chadalavada R, Lin E, Swafford V, et al. Comparative results of endoluminal gastroplasty and laparoscopic antireflux surgery for the treatment of GERD. Surg Endosc 2004;18:261–5.

[41] Corley DA, Katz P, Wo JM, et al. Improvement of gastroesophageal reflux symptoms after radiofrequency energy: a randomized, sham-controlled trial [see comment]. Gastroenterology 2003;125:668–76.

[42] Deviere J, Costamagna G, Neuhaus H, et al. Nonresorbable copolymer implantation for gastroesophageal reflux disease: a randomized sham-controlled multicenter trial [see comment]. Gastroenterology 2005;128:532–40.

[43] Montgomery M, Hakanson B, Ljungqvist O, et al. Twelve months' follow-up after treatment with the EndoCinch endoscopic technique for gastro-oesophageal reflux disease: a randomized, placebo-controlled study. Scand J Gastroenterol 2006;41:1382–9.

[44] Van Blankenstein M, Looman CW, Kruijshaar ME, et al. Modelling a population with Barrett's oesophagus from oesophageal adenocarcinoma incidence data. Scand J Gastroenterol 2007;42:308–17.

[45] Peters JH. The surgical management of Barrett's esophagus. Gastroenterol Clin North Am 1997;26:647–68.

[46] Edwards MJ, Gable DR, Lentsch AB, et al. The rationale for esophagectomy as the optimal therapy for Barrett's esophagus with high-grade dysplasia. Ann Surg 1996;223:585–9 [discussion: 89–91].

[47] Heitmiller RF, Redmond M, Hamilton SR. Barrett's esophagus with high-grade dysplasia. An indication for prophylactic esophagectomy. Ann Surg 1996;224:66–71.

[48] Society for Surgery of the Alimentary T. SSAT patient care guidelines. Management of Barrett's esophagus. J Gastrointest Surg 2007;11:1213–5.

[49] Dixon MF, Neville PM, Mapstone NP, et al. Bile reflux gastritis and Barrett's oesophagus: further evidence of a role for duodenogastro-oesophageal reflux? Gut 2001;49:359–63.

[50] Rossi M, Barreca M, de Bortoli N, et al. Efficacy of Nissen fundoplication versus medical therapy in the regression of low-grade dysplasia in patients with Barrett esophagus: a prospective study [see comment]. Ann Surg 2006;243:58–63.

[51] Sharma P. Barrett esophagus: will effective treatment prevent the risk of progression to esophageal adenocarcinoma? Am J Med 2004;117(Suppl 5A):79S–85S.

[52] McDonald ML, Trastek VF, Allen MS, et al. Barretts's esophagus: does an antireflux procedure reduce the need for endoscopic surveillance? J Thorac Cardiovasc Surg 1996; 111:1135–8 [discussion: 39–40].

[53] Dunkin BJ, Martinez J, Bejarano PA, et al. Thin-layer ablation of human esophageal epithelium using a bipolar radiofrequency balloon device. Surg Endosc 2006;20:125–30.

[54] Smith CD, Bejarano PA, Melvin WS, et al. Endoscopic ablation of intestinal metaplasia containing high-grade dysplasia in esophagectomy patients using a balloon-based ablation system. Surg Endosc 2007;21:560–9.

SURGICAL
CLINICS OF
NORTH AMERICA

ELSEVIER
SAUNDERS

Surg Clin N Am 88 (2008) 959–978

Current Controversies in Paraesophageal Hernia Repair

S. Scott Davis, Jr, MD

*Emory Endosurgery Unit, Emory University, Emory Clinic Building A,
1365 Clifton Road, Suite H-124, Atlanta, GA 30322, USA*

The management of paraesophageal hernia (PEH) has become one of the most widely debated and controversial areas in surgery. PEH's are relatively uncommon, often presenting in patients entering their seventh or eighth decades of life. These patients often bear complicating medical comorbidities making them potentially poor operative candidates. Taking this into account makes surgical management of these patients all the more complex. Many considerations must be taken into account in formulating a management strategy for patients with PEH, and these considerations have led surgeons into ongoing debates in recent decades (Box 1).

Common to all these discussions are the agreed-on tenets of PEH repair: reduction of the stomach to an intra-abdominal location, achieving adequate intra-abdominal esophageal length, excision of the hernia sac, and sound closure of the esophageal hiatus. This article reviews in detail a few of the major controversies in the evolution of the surgical approach to PEHs. Given the profile of the patients in whom these hernias occur, the indication for operation is perhaps the most important. Also discussed is the choice of surgical approach. Often the case in controversies of this sort, this debate typically blurs lines of subspecialty. Recently, the optimal technique for hiatal closure has been the most discussed topic, spurred by the revolution in hernia reinforcement by prosthetic and biologic materials. This progression was predictable as the use of mesh has spread from inguinal hernias to include repair of all manner of abdominal wall and even thoracic defects. This article does not pursue the discussion of the importance of "short esophagus" or preoperative evaluation, as these are discussed in detail in a previous issue in this series [1,2].

E-mail address: s.scott.davis@emoryhealthcare.org

**Box 1. Current controversies in surgical management
of paraesophageal hernias**

Indications for surgery
Approach to surgery
  • Transthoracic versus transabdominal
  • Open versus Laparoscopic
Need for esophageal lengthening procedure
Closure of hiatus
  • Simple suture
  • Pledget reinforced
  • Mesh-reinforced onlay or interpositiion tension-free
    • Prosthetic mesh
    • Biologic mesh
Need for antireflux procedure
Need for gastropexy
  • Fundoplication
  • Gastrostomy
  • Anterior gastropexy

Classification of paraesophageal hernias

Perhaps one of the most agreed-on aspects within the PEH literature is their classification, as they generally are classified into four types ranging in extent and probably existing over a spectrum [3].

Type I: sliding hiatal hernias

Sliding hiatal hernias are the most common, accounting for 90% to 95% of cases. They are characterized by the migration of the gastroesophageal junction above the diaphragm with associated laxity of the phrenoesophageal ligament. These typically have a small, herniated peritoneal sac that can be reduced with gentle caudal retraction on the stomach. Patients typically suffer from typical symptoms of gastroesophageal reflux disease (GERD) resulting from a distortion of the anatomic characteristics of a normal hiatus, namely the absence of adequate intra-abdominal esophagus, and an altered angle of His. These hernias most likely are the consequence of increased intra-abdominal pressure and thus are seen more frequently in obese or pregnant patients, among others.

Type II: true paraesophageal hernias

Type II is "true" PEHs, characterized by herniation of the fundus of the stomach with an intact location of the gastroesophageal junction below the diaphragm. They are considered relatively uncommon and probably account for less than 5% of patients diagnosed with PEH. They probably occur as a weakening of the pleuroperitoneal membrane, which allows the anterior wall the stomach to herniate into the potential space between the esophagus and the phrenoesophageal ligament. They typically are seen originating in the 12- or 4-o'clock position viewed transabdominally and in a minority of cases can become quite large. These hernias classically are associated with symptoms of dysphagia owing to compression of the lower esophagus by the herniated fundus. The gastroesophageal junction itself is considered intact so GERD symptoms frequently are not absent.

Type III: combined sliding and paraesophageal hernias

These generally are believed to account for the majority of PEHs. They are characterized by a combination of characteristics of types I and II, with the gastroesophageal junction located above the diaphragmatic crus and the upper portion of the stomach herniated into the posterior mediastinum. Like type II hernias, these can become large and likely represent the majority of large or "massive" PEHs. The upper portion of the stomach typically rolls into the posterior mediastinum, also originating at the 12- and 4-o'clock positions. Patients suffer the typical symptoms or GERD often, owing to the derangement of typical hiatal anatomy and the intrathoracic location of the gastroesophageal junction. In addition, atypical symptoms, such as regurgitation, chest pain, dysphagia, and respiratory symptoms, frequently are present due to the mechanical effects of the herniated stomach in the mediastinal space.

Type IV: complex paraesophageal hernias

Type IV is the rarest of the PEHs and defined by the intrathoracic migration of other intra-abdominal organs. This results from a combination of increased intra-abdominal pressure and a large hiatal defect. These are extreme examples of type II or type III hernias and manifest from the same process. They may or may not be associated with an abnormal location of the gastroesophageal junction; thus, patients may present with any of the typical or atypical symptoms seen in the other three hernia types, including symptoms attributable to organs herniated other than the stomach, often colon.

Indications for surgical treatment

The recommendations for surgery for patients were significantly affected by reports by Hill [4] and Skinner and Belsey [5] almost 4 decades ago. These articles raised concerns of significant complication rates suffered by patients left untreated. Skinner described 21 asymptomatic patients, six (29%) of whom developed potentially catastrophic complications of bleeding, perforation, and strangulation when left untreated. In addition, operative mortality for emergent operations was estimated as high as 17%. The combination of these two observations led to surgical teaching that any patient who was medically fit for surgery should have the hernia repaired [6–10]. This dictum is based on small series largely from a different era, although little currently is known about the true natural history of PEHs. With careful history, some investigators suggest that nearly all patients who have PEHs are symptomatic [11]. Maziak and colleagues [11] described 94 patients undergoing thorough preoperative evaluation and found 94% had some degree of symptoms and further that 36% of the patients had erosive esophagitis. Modern pharmacotherapy may be sufficient for symptom control in a segment of patients, and these have been termed "minimally symptomatic."

In the past several years, investigators have questioned past surgical dictum and revisited defining the natural history of PEHs. Few studies exist that describe outcomes in unoperated patients. Allen and colleagues [12] described nonoperative management in 23 patients, who were followed for a mean of 78 months, with none developing acute complications requiring emergent operation. In this cohort, four patients did proceed to develop symptoms requiring repair, and there was one death from aspiration. They also included a cohort of 124 patients managed operatively, five of whom had surgery for emergent indications. Despite performing five emergent operations in that subset, they concluded from the nonoperative cohort that gastric strangulation was rare. Treacy and colleagues [13] evaluated progression of symptoms in 29 patients followed nonoperatively and found that 13 (45%) went on to require elective operations for progressive symptoms, although none was emergent.

Given the relative paucity of available data describing natural history, Stylopoulos and colleagues [14] designed a population-based decision analysis model used to determine if elderly asymptomatic, or minimally symptomatic, patients benefit from elective PEH repair. The model examined existing literature regarding mortality and hernia progression rates and modeled 5 million patients who were 65 years old and asymptomatic. They concluded that the mortality rate of emergency repair of PEHS likely was overestimated by early studies, likely only 5.4% versus the 17% quoted previously. Based on current literature, they also estimated that the mortality rate of elective PEH repair likely was 1.4% whereas the annual likelihood of developing gastric complications from the hernias was only 1.1%. This analysis indicated that fewer than one in five asymptomatic patients 65 years and older benefit from elective PEH repair and fewer than 1 in 10 patients at age of 85 and older.

These studies have led some to redefine their indications for repair [15]. The original observations inherent to the previous surgical dictum have changed. Although elective surgery clearly has improved mortality rates over emergency surgery, outcomes have improved for emergent operations. This is likely because of better understanding and care of elderly, comorbid patients. Improved pharmacotherapy also offers the opportunity for improved symptom control for minimally symptomatic patients. Lastly, symptom progression is slow and less likely to evolve to emergent operation than previously believed. Many investigators now support conservative management for selected patients, agreeing that it is reasonable to follow asymptomatic, or minimally symptomatic, patients who are elderly and possess comorbidities.

Surgical approach

After the initial description of the PEH repair by Akerlund in 1926, patients who had PEH were managed for many decades via thoracotomy or laparotomy, with morbidity approximating 20% and mortality 2% [12,16–18]. Before the current era of minimally invasive surgery, debate was waged as to whether or not these repairs were approached best through the abdomen or thorax. The advent of minimally invasive techniques has revolutionized the approach to many surgical diseases and redefined gold standards of care. These techniques nearly universally improve morbidity and mortality significantly without degradation of efficacy, addressing a concern surgeons had with open approaches.

Transthoracic versus transabdominal

In general, excellent results have been reported with both open approaches (Table 1). As expected, the debate often follows the lines of subspecialty. Published series in the thoracic surgery literature are published predominantly by thoracic groups, whereas general surgeons publish the majority of transabdominal series.

Reviewing these series, proponents of the thoracic approach tout superior ability to mobilize the esophagus and ease of access to perform a Collis-Nissen gastroplasty as the main advantages to the thoracic approach [11,17,18]. They typically note a high incidence of short esophagus and report using an esophageal lengthening procedure in 69% to 97% of cases [11,12,25]. This is in contradistinction to investigators describing the transabdominal approach, who seem to find shortened esophagus rarely, citing that extensive mobilization of the esophagus allows for adequate intra-abdominal esophageal length and the need for Collis-Nissen to be minimal [20–22]. These data suggest that there is perhaps some aspect of the transthoracic exposure that lends itself to the appearance of a short esophagus, if not different sets of beliefs between thoracic and general surgeons. Recurrence rates typically are lowest in the transthoracic series, ranging from 0.8% to 2.6% [12,25]. Only one group critically studied patients postoperatively who had radiography or endoscopy, with most groups reporting

Table 1
Selected published series of open paraesophageal hernia repairs

Author	No. of patients	Mean follow-up (mo)	Mean length of stay (d)	Morbidity (%)	Symptomatic recurrence (%)	Radiographic recurrence (%)	Notes
Abdominal							
Ellis, et al [17]	55	52	9.5	24	9.1	NS	—
Williamson, et al [19]	124	61.5	NS	12	10.1	NS	Rarely need antireflux
Rakic, et al [20]	40	30	NS	5	2.5	NS	—
Geha, et al [21]	82	NS	NS	6	2	NS	—
Low and Unger [22]	72	30	4.5	23.6	NS	18	No Collis needed
Thoracic							
Allen, et al [12]	119	42	9	27	0.8	NS	Collis 69%
Maziak, et al [11]	94	72	NS	19	2.1	NS	Collis 80%
Altorki, et al [23]	47	45	NS	42	NS	NS	Collis 0%
Rogers, et al [24]	60	19	9	8	1.6	NS	—
Patel, et al [25]	240	42	7	8	2.6	7.9	Collis 97%

symptomatic recurrence as the principal outcome analyzed. In the lone study with objective follow-up, Patel and colleagues [25] reported 240 patients repaired transthoracically, with 97% requiring Collis gastroplasty. These patients were evaluated at 1-, 3-, and 5-year intervals with barium radiographs and of the 153 who had available reports, there were 19 recurrences (7.9%), considerably higher than the symptomatic recurrence rates reported other studies. Overall morbidity rates are highest in the transthoracic series, ranging from 8% to 42%, and mortality ranging from 0% to 2% [11,23,24,26]. Most concerning were reported leaks from the esophageal staple line at the site of the Collis gastroplasty, which occurred in as many as 4% of cases in these series [27]. Lengths of stay (LOS) usually are in excess of 7 days [11,24].

Those favoring the transabdominal approach cite less morbidity because of avoidance of the thoracotomy incision [21,28]. Post-thoracotomy pain syndrome is described in as many as 8% of patients undergoing thoracotomy [29]. Because far fewer patients undergo Collis gastroplasty, the risk for staple line leak can be avoided. Pulmonary complications also are believed fewer with the abdominal approach, as there in no need for single lung ventilation and easier pulmonary toilet postoperatively. Large series describing the transabdominal approach are available for review [17,20–22]. Symptomatic recurrence rates generally are excellent, although perhaps slightly higher than those reported in the thoracic literature, ranging from 2.5% to 13% [19,20]. It is again notable that in only one published series were these patients evaluated critically for recurrences with postoperative barium studies. Low and Unger recently described 72 patients approached transabdominally, with none requiring Collis gastroplasty [22]. After a mean follow-up of 29.8 months, 88% of patients underwent objective assessment with endoscopy or radiography. They found recurrences in 10 patients (18%) and emphasized that eight of them were small sliding hernias, which were asymptomatic. Reported morbidity rates for transabdominal approaches range from 5% to 24% [17,20]. Reported LOS ranges from 4.5 to 9.5 days [17,22].

These series contain many factors that confound interpretation. Simple analysis of recurrence rates, morbidity, and mortality is difficult because of the varied nuances of technique. The primary outcome in most early series was symptom recurrence, not critical analysis with objective studies. In more recent literature, spurred by intense investigation into the efficacy of minimally invasive techniques, recurrences typically are sought by radiographic follow-up. There is only one series published for each open approach bearing this type of data, and in both series, objective follow-up revealed significantly higher recurrence rates than previously published. It generally is accepted that morbidity rates for transabdominal approaches are less than those for trans-thoracic and that hospital LOS are shorter. It seems this also is true of mortality rates; however, this in not borne out in the literature.

Open versus laparoscopic

The first laparoscopic PEH repair was described by Cuschieri and colleagues [30] in 1992. Since that time this approach has been widely adopted, driven by patients and physicians desiring a less morbid repair. Recent years have seen the transabdominal laparoscopic approach gain rapid acceptance as standard, principally because of several studies that demonstrate significant improvement in morbidity rates versus the open approaches [31,32]. This notion is consistent with findings comparing outcomes of open and laparoscopic approaches for the management of other surgical diseases. Given this, there would be no debate if outcomes were measured solely in the early postoperative period. The initial concerns raised by advocates of open approaches cited the alarmingly high recurrence rates reported in laparoscopic series (Table 2) [33,37]. Unfortunately, there are surprisingly few series comparing the results of open and laparoscopic approaches directly, and there are no randomized controlled series [31–33]. These studies are difficult to interpret because they often report on heterogenous patient populations with varying lengths of follow-up and severity of disease and presentation [32]. Operative techniques (ie, use of gastropexy, fundoplication, and esophageal lengthening procedures) vary between series.

The most commonly cited series by proponents of open approaches was put forth by Hashemi and colleagues [33]. This is one of the few that directly compares open and laparoscopic approaches. They compared 54 patients undergoing PEH repair, 27 by laparoscopy and 27 by open approaches (13 thoracotomy and 14 laparotomy), with mean follow-up of 35 months in the open group and 17 months in the laparoscopic group. This series was one of the first to include symptomatic questionnaires and objective radiologic follow-up. They found 12 out of 41 patients had recurred and of these nine were in the laparoscopic group, yielding a radiographic recurrence rate of 42% versus 15% in the open group. They noted that patients repaired laparoscopically reported good symptomatic outcomes equivalent to those repaired open, although they expressed concern for high radiographic recurrence rates. Later, Khaitan and colleagues [37] reported on 25 patients treated laparoscopically, with follow-up in 15 patients at a mean of 25 months. These patients also underwent barium esophagram in addition to symptom analysis. They reported one patient having a recurrent PEH and five patients having migration of the wrap above the diaphragm for a total recurrence rate of 40%. Only two of the patients who had wrap migration were symptomatic and these were managed with proton pump inhibitors, with one patient requiring reoperation.

Early literature describing the feasibility of minimally invasive repair used symptomatic questionnaires to evaluate for recurrence and reported rates ranging from 5% to 21%, significantly lower than rates reported when anatomic recurrence is sought by barium esophagram, which range

Table 2
Selected published series of laparoscopic paraesophageal hernia repairs

Author	N	Follow-up (m)	Morbidity (%)	Mortality (%)	OR time (min)	Lenth of stay (d)	Anatomic recurrence (%)	Symptomatic recurrence (%)	Reoperation (%)
Gantert, et al [6]	55	11	14.4	1.8	219	2.4	NR	5.4	4
Hashemi, et al [33]	27	17	11	0	184	3	42	NR	NR
Luketich, et al [34]	100	12	28	1	220	2	NR	NR	1
Dahlberg, et al [35]	37	15	28	5.4	179	4	14	NR	5.4
Wiechmann, et al [10]	54	13	NR	1.8	202	NR	5.5	5.5	5.5
Jobe, et al [36]	56	37	19	0	186	2.6	32	19	4.2
Khaitan, et al [37]	25	25	16	0	268	5.5	40	12	4
Mattar, et al [38]	136	136	10.2	2.2	218	40	33	4.4	2
Diaz, et al [39]	116	116	4.3	1.7	162	NR	22	11	2.6
Targarona, et al [40]	37	37	11	2.1	196	4	20	21	NR
Andujar, et al [41]	166	15	8.4	0	160	3.8	28	NS	6
Aly, et al [42]	100	48	14	0	87	3.6	30	20	7

from 5.5% to 42% [6,10,33,40]. A recent review by Mehta and colleagues [43] analyzed studies reporting on laparoscopic PEH repairs with radiographic follow-up. They found an average recurrence rate of 27%, again largely assessed objectively. They noted that only 30% of these reported cases were true PEHs, with the remainder sliding hernias or wrap migration. These data compare with only two studies, reviewed previously in this article, with radiographic follow-up in patients repaired using open techniques [22,25]. These reported 7.9% and 18% recurrence rates.

Both approaches seem to have excellent symptomatic results [6,10,41]. The literature shows that quality-of-life measures are improved with patients undergoing laparoscopic repair [40,44]. Velanovich and Karmy-Jones analyzed quality-of-life data in 44 patients undergoing repair, three emergently for ischemia or gastric necrosis. In this series 31 patients were repaired laparoscopically with five conversions to open. They found higher quality-of-life scores in patients repaired laparoscopically, but these data were difficult to interpret given the emergent nature of many of the open operations and that five operations were converted. Targarona and colleagues evaluated 37 patients with Short Form 36 (SF-36) Health Survey and the Gastrointestinal Quality of Life Index and found improved to normal population with both instruments. Similar data exist for open procedures, as described by Low and Unger [21]. They noted in their series that SF-36 scores were better than age-matched population controls in eight of eight categories.

Advocates of minimally invasive approaches cite many other benefits, including improved visualization of the hiatus, easier esophageal mobilization high into the mediastinum, and decreased pulmonary complications. They also suggest that the impact of surgery is lessened in these elderly patients who have frequent medical comorbidities. Draaisma and colleagues [45] reviewed 32 published studies and found a significantly shorter LOS (3 days laparoscopic versus 10 days open). Postoperative complication rates were significantly lower for laparoscopic repairs (0% to 14% versus 5.3% to 25%) and lower median mortality rate (0.3% versus 1.7%), although the ranges for these values overlapped significantly. It seems generally accepted that recovery and complication rates immediately related to surgery are lower when minimally invasive techniques are used.

Techniques for hiatal closure

Critical analysis of recurrence rates led much of recent debate to focus on technique of hiatal closure. Historically, simple sutures, occasionally with the use of Teflon pledgets, were used to reapproximate the hiatal defect. Similar to the argument regarding surgical approach, investigators sought to decrease recurrence rates, knowing that the most common cause of failure for these procedures was intrathoracic wrap migration [46,47]. In the past decades, this discussion has evolved to include the use of synthetic or biologic prostheses for reinforcing or even bridging the crural closure. Standard hernia repairs were anatomic based and used available autologous tissues to close and reinforce defects. The concept of tension-free repair, originally described by Lichtenstein and colleagues [48] for the repair of inguinal hernias, was popularized and applied more broadly to all other hernias. Prosthetic materials bridging defects in a tension-free manner were shown to lower recurrence rates and improve recurrence rates of inguinal hernia repairs [49–51]. Later this was applied widely to incisional hernia repair, becoming standard [52–54]. Because all PEHs were considered an indication for surgery in fit patients, it was only natural that the use of these materials at the hiatus would be investigated.

Prosthetic mesh

The first report of mesh at the hiatus was put forth by Kuster and Gilroy [55] in 1993. They described placing a patch of polyester mesh anterior to the esophagus in six patients whose crura were unable to be closed primarily during laparoscopic PEH repair. In short-term follow-up of 8 to 22 months, there were no mesh-related complications although two had herniation of the posterior portion of the fundus on radiographic studies that were asymptomatic. They concluded that this was not only feasible but safe in selected patients. Subsequently, many series were published reporting the use of a variety of materials and surgical techniques (Table 3). Early series were characterized by small numbers of patients who had large hiatal defects that were unable to be closed primarily. Only two prospective randomized trials have been done evaluating mesh hiatoplasty for PEHs and both demonstrated markedly lower recurrence rates [56,63]. Carlson and colleagues [56] repaired the hiatus with a keyhole-shaped polytetraflouroethylene (PTFE) patch in 15 patients and found no recurrences compared with three recurrences (18.8%) in the control group, although this did not reach statistical significance. Later, Frantzides and colleagues [27] randomized 72 patients who had hiatal defects larger than 8 cm to primary suture repair or keyhole PTFE graft. They studied all patients at 6-month intervals with esophagogastroduodenoscopy (EGD) or barium swallow, with a mean follow-up of 3.3 years. They found eight recurrences (22%) in the primary repair group versus none (0%) in the mesh hiatoplasty group and reported no mesh-related complications. In a third randomized study of fundoplications done for GERD, Granderath and colleagues [64] used a polypropylene onlay to the crural closure and found a significantly reduced wrap migration rate (8% versus 26%). These trials form the basis of the compelling argument made by several investigators that mesh hiatoplasty not only markedly decreases recurrence rates but also is safe with minimal mesh-related complications.

There are several limitations in interpreting the literature with regards to the use of mesh at the hiatus. Foremost is the lack of level 1 data, in particular regarding long-term outcomes. Most data come from small series with

Table 3
Selected published series of prosthetic mesh hiatoplasty

Author	Follow-up	No mesh		Mesh used		Material	Placement	Recurrence
		No. of patients	Recurrence (%)	No. of patients	Recurrence (%)			
Carlson, et al [56]	24	16	18.7	44	0	Polypropylene	Keyhole	NA
Champion and Rock [57]	25	—	—	52	1.9	Polypropylene	Onlay	Symptomatic
Hui [57]	37	12	0	12	8.3	PTFE	Onlay	Symptomatic
Frantzides [27]	39.6	36	22.7	36	0	PTFE	Keyhole	Radiologic
Basso [59]	22.5	65	13.8	70	0	Polypropylene	Interposition	Symptomatic
Leeder [60]	51	37	2.7	14	14.3	Polypropylene	Anterior	Symptomatic
Keidar [61]	58	23	17.3	10	10	Composite	Keyhole	Symptomatic
Horstmann [62]	14	—	—	16	0	Polypropylene	Onlay	Radiologic

short follow-up and reflects not only a variety of different prostheses but also a wide range of surgical techniques, making comparison difficult if not impossible. This was highlighted in a review by Targarona and colleagues [39], who illustrated at least nine different techniques for hiatal closure described. Many prosthetic materials have been investigated, including polypropylene, polyester, PTFE, and composite materials [57,58,61,65].

Some reports indicate a higher rate of dysphagia associated with mesh repair of the hiatus. In one nonrandomized series there was a significantly higher rate of dysphagia 3 months after surgery; however, this decreased at 1 year to a rate similar to that for nonmesh repairs. Granderath and colleagues [66] later investigated this finding in a randomized controlled trial looking at 40 patients undergoing laparoscopic Nissen fundoplication for GERD. The mesh repair performed was a posterior buttress of the crural closure with a 1 × 3 cm only a polypropylene mesh. Objective studies were performed at 3 months and 1 year after surgery. They found that resting lower esophageal sphincter (LES) pressure was higher in the mesh group at 1 year (13.9 versus 8.9 mm Hg); however, there was neither evidence for esophageal dysmotility nor any differences in LES length or relaxation. They again showed that at 1 year reported dysphagia rates were 5% in both groups, although early dysphagia rates again were higher (15%). They concluded that the earlier increased rate of dysphagia reported in mesh repairs resolves in longer-term follow-up with no evidence for induced esophageal dysmotility.

The most concerning issue related to the use of prosthetics near the esophagus is safety. History teaches consequences of previous attempts to place devices near the gastroesophageal junction [67]. The use of Teflon pledgets is associated with erosions into the viscera, foreign body reaction, and gastroesophageal fistula [68–70]. Thus far, reports of esophageal erosion of prosthetic mesh are few but nonetheless increasing [68,71–75]. This event can be catastrophic for these patients for whom in most cases an esophago-gastrectomy is the only solution. In others, significant fibrosis of the hiatus leading to progressive dysphagia requiring esophagectomy is reported [9,47,76]. Animal studies confirm that these suspicions are warranted. Jansen and colleagues [77] studied the effect of two prosthetic mesh materials placed using a keyhole technique in rabbits. They found migration into the esophageal wall at 1 year in 5 of 6 animals using polypropylene and 5 of 9 animals using polypropylene-polyglecaprone composite material. It is of great concern that despite the marked improvement in recurrence rates reported in mesh hiatoplasty series, there is vast underreporting of the associated complications, leading to an illusion of safety.

Biologic mesh

The introduction of biologic mesh materials may provide a superior alternative to prosthetic for hiatal reinforcement. Surgeons agree that the ideal material would form minimal adhesions, incorporate into the hiatal closure without inducing significant fibrosis, and provide sound closure, with no mesh-related complications. To date, porcine small intestinal submucosa (SIS) and acellular human dermis (AHD) have been used to repair or reinforce the hiatal closure (Table 4) [78–83]. Ample scientific evidence exists to support the increasingly popular notion that these materials might be ideal for PEH repair. Investigators have shown that SIS initially degrades but then is replaced over time by a remodeling process, which leads to tissue strength which exceeds that of native tissue over time [85,86]. Similar findings are demonstrated with AHD [87]. In addition, these materials are shown to be resistant to infection and to have strength similar to that of PTFE at the time of placement in surgery [87].

The most critical issue driving the use of biologics at the hiatus is whether or not esophageal erosion, or fibrosis leading to progressive dysphagia, can be avoided. This likely would eliminate the potential for patients to require esophagogastrectomy as a consequence of implant-related complications. Animal studies again support that biologics might prove useful. Desai and colleagues [88] performed laparoscopic PEH repair using porcine SIS on six canines with histologic analysis at 1 year. They found no clinical evidence for dysphagia or weight loss and histologically noted good reinforcement of the hiatus and circumferential ingrowth of connective tissue and skeletal muscle into the graft, concluding the graft may act as a scaffold for tissue ingrowth and does not lead to erosion.

The initial clinical report of PEH repair supplemented with a biologic mesh was by Oelschlager and colleagues [78], who described the use of SIS in nine patients as a feasibility study. That group later followed this case series with a multicenter, prospective randomized trial in which 108 patients were randomized to repair with or without onlay crural reinforcement with the biologic graft, placed in a keyhole fashion [82]. Although follow-up was short (6 months), 90% of patients were available for objective assessment with upper gastrointestinal (UGI) series. They found a significant decrease in recurrence rates (9% mesh versus 24% nonmesh), and moreover, reported no mesh-related complications. In addition, the patients had no difference in symptom severity scores, in particular for dysphagia, which previously was shown to be an issue in the short-term with prosthetic mesh closures. In reviewing other series, reported recurrence rates have ranged from 0% to 11.8%, with studies characterized by small numbers and short-term follow-up. These series, however, include objective follow-up with EGD or UGI in the majority of patients, allowing for complete early assessment of results.

Do recurrences matter?

Many causal factors are proposed, including tension on the crural repair, large hiatal defects, attenuated muscle fibers at the hiatus, and inappropriate diaphragmatic stressors in the early postoperative period [89]. In a review,

Table 4
Selected published series of biologic mesh hiatoplasty

Author	n	Follow-up (m)	Material	Placement	Morbidity (%)	Mortality (%)	Radiographic recurrence (%)	Symptomatic recurrence (%)
Oelschlager, et al [78]	9	8	SIS	Keyhole	11	11	11	0
Strange [79]	12	6	SIS	Keyhole	0	0	0	0
Wisbach, et al [80]	11	12	Alloderm	Onlay-Y	9	0	9	0
Ringley, et al [81]	22	6.7	Alloderm	Onlay-U	4	0	0	0
Oelschlager, et al [82]	51	6	SIS	Onlay- Keyhole	24	0	9	NR
Lee, et al [83]	17	14.4	Alloderm	Onlay-V	6	0	11.8	6
St. Peter, et al [84]	12	36	SIS	Onlay-Keyhole	0	0	0	0

Puri and colleagues [90] found that surgeon inexperience, retention of the hernia sac, early postoperative vomiting, and heavy lifting were the only factors supported by the literature to lead to increased recurrence rates. They also suggest that some of these problems might be augmented by the quicker recovery seen after minimally invasive approaches. It is known that recurrences occur usually soon after surgery and usually are the result of intrathoracic migration of the fundoplication [91–93]. This also is the most likely reason for patients requiring revisional surgery.

The significance of these recurrences must be addressed. The short answer to the question is that, yes, anatomic recurrence must be considered a technical failure. Despite this, data support that many radiographic recurrences are not clinically significant. Many patients who have anatomic recurrences are asymptomatic and require no further therapy [33,38]. Mehta and colleagues [43] reviewed the available literature and found that the majority of recurrences represented intrathoracic wrap migration or wrap disruption but indicated that only 3% of patients who had radiographic recurrence required revisional procedures. With this data in mind, it also seems that most of those patients who are symptomatic can be easily managed with conservative therapy, averting need for further operation. This notion also is supported by the generally excellent results reported in patients by quality-of-life questionnaires and GERD-specific questionnaires, despite many of whom having known anatomic recurrences. The reoperation rates for laparoscopic and open series are less than 5%, indicating that many of the identified anatomic recurrences are unlikely to be clinically significant. Long-term data as to the natural history of these anatomic recurrences are lacking.

Summary

PEHs remain a complex and challenging disorder to treat in a patient population that has many confounding medical factors. Excellent outcomes are reported using a variety of different approaches and a variety of nuances to those approaches. At the author's institution, laparoscopic approach is believed to offer recovery advantages to patients that are difficult to ignore. With this in mind, maximization of the efficacy of this technique has the potential for superior outcomes generally. The literature regarding this topic is replete with small studies and few randomized data. Given the infrequency of this disease, it is likely this characteristic will not change. The use of mesh at the hiatus to supplement the use of minimally invasive techniques is encouraging and likely represents the best choice for patients. That said, the use of prosthetics introduces a potentially catastrophic outcome for patients, which, the author believes, is greatly underreported. This notion likely will bear out in time. Biologic materials offer a safer and equally effective alternative for bolstering the crural repair that eliminates this risk and likely will become the standard of care.

References

[1] Hoang CD, Koh PS, Maddaus MA. Short esophagus and esophageal stricture. Surg Clin North Am 2005;85:433.

[2] Landreneau RJ, Del Pino M, Santos R. Management of paraesophageal hernias. Surg Clin North Am 2005;85:411.

[3] Landreneau RJ, Johnson JA, Marshall JB, et al. Clinical spectrum of paraesophageal herniation. Dig Dis Sci 1992;37:537.

[4] Hill LD. Incarcerated paraesophageal hernia. A surgical emergency. Am J Surg 1973; 126:286.

[5] Skinner DB, Belsey RH. Surgical management of esophageal reflux and hiatus hernia. Long-term results with 1,030 patients. J Thorac Cardiovasc Surg 1967;53:33.

[6] Gantert WA, Patti MG, Arcerito M, et al. Laparoscopic repair of paraesophageal hiatal hernias. J Am Coll Surg 1998;186:428.

[7] Halpin VJ, Soper NJ. Paraesophageal hernia. Curr Treat Options Gastroenterol 2001;4:83.

[8] Hawasli A, Zonca S. Laparoscopic repair of paraesophageal hiatal hernia. Am Surg 1998; 64:703.

[9] van der Peet DL, Klinkenberg-Knol EC, Alonso Poza A, et al. Laparoscopic treatment of large paraesophageal hernias: both excision of the sac and gastropexy are imperative for adequate surgical treatment. Surg Endosc 2000;14:1015.

[10] Wiechmann RJ, Ferguson MK, Naunheim KS, et al. Laparoscopic management of giant paraesophageal herniation. Ann Thorac Surg 2001;71:1080.

[11] Maziak DE, Todd TR, Pearson FG. Massive hiatus hernia: evaluation and surgical management. J Thorac Cardiovasc Surg 1998;115:53.

[12] Allen MS, Trastek VF, Deschamps C, et al. Intrathoracic stomach. Presentation and results of operation. J Thorac Cardiovasc Surg 1993;105:253.

[13] Treacy PJ, Jamieson GG. An approach to the management of para-oesophageal hiatus hernias. Aust N Z J Surg 1987;57:813–7.

[14] Stylopoulos N, Gazelle GS, Rattner DW. Paraesophageal hernias: operation or observation? Ann Surg 2002;236:492.

[15] Floch NR. Paraesophageal hernias: current concepts. J Clin Gastroenterol 1999;29:6.

[16] Akerlund A, Ohnell A, Key E. Hernia diaphragmatica hiatus oesophagei vom anatomischen und rontgenologischen gesichtspunkt. Acta Radiol 1926;6:3.

[17] Ellis FH Jr, Crozier RE, Shea JA. Paraesophageal hiatus hernia. Arch Surg 1986;121:416.

[18] Pearson FG, Cooper JD, Ilves R, et al. Massive hiatal hernia with incarceration: a report of 53 cases. Ann Thorac Surg 1983;35:45.

[19] Williamson WA, Ellis FH Jr, Streitz JM Jr, et al. Paraesophageal hiatal hernia: is an antireflux procedure necessary? Ann Thorac Surg 1993;56:447.

[20] Rakic S, Pesko P, Dunjic MS, et al. Paraoesophageal hernia repair with and without concomitant fundoplication. Br J Surg 1994;81:1162.

[21] Geha AS, Massad MG, Snow NJ, et al. A 32-year experience in 100 patients with giant paraesophageal hernia: the case for abdominal approach and selective antireflux repair. Surgery 2000;128:623.

[22] Low DE, Unger T. Open repair of paraesophageal hernia: reassessment of subjective and objective outcomes. Ann Thorac Surg 2005;80:287.

[23] Altorki NK, Yankelevitz D, Skinner DB. Massive hiatal hernias: the anatomic basis of repair. J Thorac Cardiovasc Surg 1998;115:828.

[24] Rogers ML, Duffy JP, Beggs FD, et al. Surgical treatment of para-oesophageal hiatal hernia. Ann R Coll Surg Engl 2001;83:394.

[25] Patel HJ, Tan BB, Yee J, et al. A 25-year experience with open primary transthoracic repair of paraesophageal hiatal hernia. J Thorac Cardiovasc Surg 2004;127:843.

[26] Myers GA, Harms BA, Starling JR. Management of paraesophageal hernia with a selective approach to antireflux surgery. Am J Surg 1995;170:375.

[27] Frantzides CT, Madan AK, Carlson MA, et al. A prospective, randomized trial of laparoscopic polytetrafluoroethylene (PTFE) patch repair vs simple cruroplasty for large hiatal hernia. Arch Surg 2002;137:649.

[28] Menguy R. Surgical management of large paraesophageal hernia with complete intrathoracic stomach. World J Surg 1988;12:415.

[29] Stirling MC, Orringer MB. Continued assessment of the combined Collis-Nissen operation. Ann Thorac Surg 1989;47:224.

[30] Cuschieri A, Shimi S, Nathanson LK. Laparoscopic reduction, crural repair, and fundoplication of large hiatal hernia. Am J Surg 1992;163:425.

[31] Ferri LE, Feldman LS, Stanbridge D, et al. Should laparoscopic paraesophageal hernia repair be abandoned in favor of the open approach? Surg Endosc 2005;19:4.

[32] Schauer PR, Ikramuddin S, McLaughlin RH, et al. Comparison of laparoscopic versus open repair of paraesophageal hernia. Am J Surg 1998;176:659.

[33] Hashemi M, Peters JH, DeMeester TR, et al. Laparoscopic repair of large type III hiatal hernia: objective followup reveals high recurrence rate. J Am Coll Surg 2000;190:553.

[34] Luketich JD, Raja S, Fernando HC, et al. Laparoscopic repair of giant paraesophageal hernia: 100 consecutive cases. Ann Surg 2000;232:608.

[35] Dahlberg PS, Deschamps C, Miller DL, et al. Laparoscopic repair of large paraesophageal hiatal hernia. Ann Thorac Surg 2001;72:1125.

[36] Jobe BA, Aye RW, Deveney CW, et al. Laparoscopic management of giant type III hiatal hernia and short esophagus. Objective follow-up at three years. J Gastrointest Surg 2002; 6:181.

[37] Khaitan L, Houston H, Sharp K, et al. Laparoscopic paraesophageal hernia repair has an acceptable recurrence rate. Am Surg 2002;68:546.

[38] Mattar SG, Bowers SP, Galloway KD, et al. Long-term outcome of laparoscopic repair of paraesophageal hernia. Surg Endosc 2002;16:745.

[39] Diaz S, Brunt LM, Klingensmith ME, et al. Laparoscopic paraesophageal hernia repair, a challenging operation: medium-term outcome of 116 patients. J Gastrointest Surg 2003; 7:59.

[40] Targarona EM, Novell J, Vela S, et al. Mid term analysis of safety and quality of life after the laparoscopic repair of paraesophageal hiatal hernia. Surg Endosc 2004;18:1045.

[41] Andujar JJ, Papasavas PK, Birdas T, et al. Laparoscopic repair of large paraesophageal hernia is associated with a low incidence of recurrence and reoperation. Surg Endosc 2004;18:444.

[42] Aly A, Munt J, Jamieson GG, et al. Laparoscopic repair of large hiatal hernias. Br J Surg 2005;92:648.

[43] Mehta S, Boddy A, Rhodes M. Review of outcome after laparoscopic paraesophageal hiatal hernia repair. Surg Laparosc Endosc Percutan Tech 2006;16:301.

[44] Velanovich V, Karmy-Jones R. Surgical management of paraesophageal hernias: outcome and quality of life analysis. Dig Surg 2001;18:432.

[45] Draaisma WA, Gooszen HG, Tournoij E, et al. Controversies in paraesophageal hernia repair: a review of literature. Surg Endosc 2005;19:1300.

[46] Carlson MA, Frantzides CT. Complications and results of primary minimally invasive antireflux procedures: a review of 10,735 reported cases. J Am Coll Surg 2001;193:428.

[47] Trus TL, Bax T, Richardson WS, et al. Complications of laparoscopic paraesophageal hernia repair. J Gastrointest Surg 1997;1:221.

[48] Lichtenstein IL, Shulman AG, Amid PK, et al. The tension-free hernioplasty. Am J Surg 1989;157:188.

[49] Brown JH, Khaira HS. Early results with the Lichtenstein tension-free hernia repair. Br J Surg 1995;82:419.

[50] Davies N, Thomas M, McIlroy B, et al. Early results with the Lichtenstein tension-free hernia repair. Br J Surg 1994;81:1478.

[51] Hinson EL. Early results with Lichtenstein tension-free hernia repair. Br J Surg 1995;82:418.

[52] Korenkov M, Sauerland S, Arndt M, et al. Randomized clinical trial of suture repair, polypropylene mesh or autodermal hernioplasty for incisional hernia. Br J Surg 2002;89:50.

[53] Millikan KW. Incisional hernia repair. Surg Clin North Am 2003;83:1223.

[54] Utrera Gonzalez A, de la Portilla de Juan F, Carranza Albarran G. Large incisional hernia repair using intraperitoneal placement of expanded polytetrafluoroethylene. Am J Surg 1999;177:291.

[55] Kuster GG, Gilroy S. Laparoscopic technique for repair of paraesophageal hiatal hernias. J Laparoendosc Surg 1993;3:331.

[56] Carlson MA, Richards CG, Frantzides CT. Laparoscopic prosthetic reinforcement of hiatal herniorrhaphy. Dig Surg 1999;16:407.

[57] Champion JK, Rock D. Laparoscopic mesh cruroplasty for large paraesophageal hernias. Surg Endosc 2003;17:551.

[58] Hui TT, Thoman DS, Spyrou M, et al. Mesh crural repair of large paraesophageal hiatal hernias. Am Surg 2001;67:1170.

[59] Basso N, De Leo A, Genco A, et al. 360 degrees laparoscopic fundoplication with tension-free hiatoplasty in the treatment of symptomatic gastroesophageal reflux disease. Surg Endosc 2000;14:164.

[60] Leeder PC, Smith G, Dehn TC. Laparoscopic management of large paraesophageal hiatal hernia. Surg Endosc 2003;17:1372.

[61] Keidar A, Szold A. Laparoscopic repair of paraesophageal hernia with selective use of mesh. Surg Laparosc Endosc Percutan Tech 2003;13:149.

[62] Horstmann R, Klotz A, Classen C, et al. Feasibility of surgical technique and evaluation of postoperative quality of life after laparoscopic treatment of intrathoracic stomach. Langenbecks Arch Surg 2004;389:23.

[63] Frantzides CT, Richards CG, Carlson MA. Laparoscopic repair of large hiatal hernia with polytetrafluoroethylene. Surg Endosc 1999;13:906.

[64] Granderath FA, Schweiger UM, Kamolz T, et al. Laparoscopic Nissen fundoplication with prosthetic hiatal closure reduces postoperative intrathoracic wrap herniation: preliminary results of a prospective randomized functional and clinical study. Arch Surg 2005; 140:40.

[65] Granderath FA, Schweiger UM, Pointner R. Laparoscopic antireflux surgery: tailoring the hiatal closure to the size of hiatal surface area. Surg Endosc 2007;21:542.

[66] Granderath FA, Kamolz T, Schweiger UM, et al. Impact of laparoscopic nissen fundoplication with prosthetic hiatal closure on esophageal body motility: results of a prospective randomized trial. Arch Surg 2006;141:625.

[67] Purkiss SF, Argano VA, Kuo J, et al. Oesophageal erosion of an Angelchik prosthesis: surgical management using fundoplication. Eur J Cardiothorac Surg 1992;6:517.

[68] Arendt T, Stuber E, Monig H, et al. Dysphagia due to transmural migration of surgical material into the esophagus nine years after Nissen fundoplication. Gastrointest Endosc 2000;51:607.

[69] Baladas HG, Smith GS, Richardson MA, et al. Esophagogastric fistula secondary to Teflon pledget: a rare complication following laparoscopic fundoplication. Dis Esophagus 2000; 13:72.

[70] Dally E, Falk GL. Teflon pledget reinforced fundoplication causes symptomatic gastric and esophageal lumenal penetration. Am J Surg 2004;187:226.

[71] Carlson MA, Condon RE, Ludwig KA, et al. Management of intrathoracic stomach with polypropylene mesh prosthesis reinforced transabdominal hiatus hernia repair. J Am Coll Surg 1998;187:227.

[72] Casabella F, Sinanan M, Horgan S, et al. Systematic use of gastric fundoplication in laparoscopic repair of paraesophageal hernias. Am J Surg 1996;171:485.

[73] Coluccio G, Ponzio S, Ambu V, et al. [Dislocation into the cardial lumen of a PTFE prosthesis used in the treatment of voluminous hiatal sliding hernia, a case report]. Minerva Chir 2000;55:341 [in Italian].

[74] Hergueta-Delgado P, Marin-Moreno M, Morales-Conde S, et al. Transmural migration of a prosthetic mesh after surgery of a paraesophageal hiatal hernia. Gastrointest Endosc 2006; 64:120 [discussion: 121].

[75] Tatum RP, Shalhub S, Oelschlager BK, et al. Complications of PTFE Mesh at the Diaphragmatic Hiatus. J Gastrointest Surg 2007;12:953–7.

[76] Edelman DS. Laparoscopic paraesophageal hernia repair with mesh. Surg Laparosc Endosc 1995;5:32.

[77] Jansen M, Otto J, Jansen PL, et al. Mesh migration into the esophageal wall after mesh hiatoplasty: comparison of two alloplastic materials. Surg Endosc 2007;21:2298.

[78] Oelschlager BK, Barreca M, Chang L, et al. The use of small intestine submucosa in the repair of paraesophageal hernias: initial observations of a new technique. Am J Surg 2003; 186:4.

[79] Strange PS. Small intestinal submucosa for laparoscopic repair of large paraesophageal hiatal hernias: a preliminary report. Surg Technol Int 2003;11:141.

[80] Wisbach G, Peterson T, Thoman D. Early results of the use of acellular dermal allograft in type III paraesophageal hernia repair. JSLS 2006;10:184.

[81] Ringley CD, Bochkarev V, Ahmed SI, et al. Laparoscopic hiatal hernia repair with human acellular dermal matrix patch: our initial experience. Am J Surg 2006;192:767.

[82] Oelschlager BK, Pellegrini CA, Hunter J, et al. Biologic prosthesis reduces recurrence after laparoscopic paraesophageal hernia repair: a multicenter, prospective, randomized trial. Ann Surg 2006;244:481.

[83] Lee E, Frisella MM, Matthews BD, et al. Evaluation of acellular human dermis reinforcement of the crural closure in patients with difficult hiatal hernias. Surg Endosc 2007;21:641.

[84] St Peter SD, Ostlie DJ, Holcomb GW III. The use of biosynthetic mesh to enhance hiatal repair at the time of redo Nissen fundoplication. J Pediatr Surg 2007;42:1298.

[85] Badylak S, Kokini K, Tullius B, et al. Strength over time of a resorbable biosc.affold for body wall repair in a dog model. J Surg Res 2001;99:282.

[86] Gloeckner DC, Sacks MS, Billiar KL, et al. Mechanical evaluation and design of a multilayered collagenous repair biomaterial. J Biomed Mater Res 2000;52:365.

[87] Choe JM, Kothandapani R, James L, et al. Autologous, cadaveric, and synthetic materials used in sling surgery: comparative biomechanical analysis. Urology 2001;58:482.

[88] Desai KM, Diaz S, Dorward IG, et al. Histologic results 1 year after bioprosthetic repair of paraesophageal hernia in a canine model. Surg Endosc 2006;20:1693.

[89] Kakarlapudi GV, Awad ZT, Haynatzki G, et al. The effect of diaphragmatic stressors on recurrent hiatal hernia. Hernia 2002;6:163.

[90] Puri V, Kakarlapudi GV, Awad ZT, et al. Hiatal hernia recurrence: 2004. Hernia 2004;8:311.

[91] Hatch KF, Daily MF, Christensen BJ, et al. Failed fundoplications. Am J Surg 2004; 188:786.

[92] Hunter JG, Smith CD, Branum GD, et al. Laparoscopic fundoplication failures: patterns of failure and response to fundoplication revision. Ann Surg 1999;230:595.

[93] Soper NJ, Dunnegan D. Anatomic fundoplication failure after laparoscopic antireflux surgery. Ann Surg 1999;229:669.

ELSEVIER
SAUNDERS

Surg Clin N Am 88 (2008) 979–990

SURGICAL
CLINICS OF
NORTH AMERICA

Minimally Invasive Esophagectomy for Malignant and Premalignant Diseases of the Esophagus

James D. Maloney, MD*, Tracey L. Weigel, MD

*Division of Cardiothoracic Surgery, Section of Thoracic Surgery,
University of Wisconsin School of Medicine and Public Health, H4/320 CSC,
600 Highland Avenue, Madison, WI 53792, USA*

The incidence of esophageal adenocarcinoma continues to increase, and survival remains poor in comparison to other stage-matched malignancies [1]. Early detection and aggressive intervention are demonstrated to provide optimal results for patients who have early esophageal cancer or Barrett's esophagus with high-grade dysplasia [2]. Mortality statistics for esophageal resection in institutions with low volume have led to comparisons showing significantly improved mortality in institutions with high volume [3,4]. Morbidity, however, remains high at most centers and has provided the impetus for adopting a minimally invasive surgical (MIS) approach. Development of laparoscopic and thoracoscopic techniques for fundoplication, giant paraesophageal hernia repair, and esophageal myotomy and pulmonary lobectomy have given surgeons the tools necessary for MIS esophageal resection. MIS techniques developed for benign esophageal pathology have been refined and now are applied selectively to patients who have malignant esophageal disease. Esophagectomy is also the treatment of choice in Barrett's esophagus, or metaplasia of the squamous epithelium at the gastroesophageal junction once high-grade dysplasia (HGD) has developed. Endoscopic therapies have been advocated for early malignant and premalignant disease in patients who are not candidates for surgery. Controversy remains regarding use of endoscopic treatments in patients who are operative candidates. A significant percentage of patients with Barrett's esophagus and high grade dysplasia may have occult malignancy at the time of diagnosis and a higher percentage may develop cancer during observation [5].

* Corresponding author.
E-mail address: maloney@surgery.wisc.edu (J.D. Maloney).

0039-6109/08/$ - see front matter © 2008 Elsevier Inc. All rights reserved.
doi:10.1016/j.suc.2008.05.016   *surgical.theclinics.com*

Differentiating the grade of dysplasia in Barrett's esophagus has proved problematic, as has identification of intramucosal malignancies [6]. Pathologic specimens do not include lymph node analysis in endoscopic therapy. Endoscopic ultrasound (EUS) has become a mainstay in the workup of esophageal cancer and is now advocated as confirmation that endoscopic ablative therapy is appropriate. The potential for under-staging exists in these patients as EUS in combination with other radiologic studies may miss malignant adenopathy [7]. In a study by Shimpi and colleagues [8] the accuracy of EUS for Tumor (T) stage and Nodal (N) stage were 76% and 89%, respectively. Minimally invasive esophagectomy (MIE) maintains the oncologic principles of resection and pathologic staging while reducing the associated morbidity.

Open esophagectomy

Several techniques have been used for operative treatment of esophageal cancer. Both right and left thoracic exposure, thoracoabdominal incision, and techniques avoiding thoracotomy entirely, such as a transhiatal approach, have been used successfully. The best approach to esophagectomy remains controversial [9,10]. The two most frequently performed operations are the transthoracic esophagectomy (TTE) and the transhiatal esophagectomy (THE). Transhiatal esophagectomy was popularized by Orringer at the University of Michigan. This approach avoids thoracotomy and involves a cervical esophagogastric anastomosis, with the purported advantage of pain reduction, subsequently minimizing respiratory complications [11]. In some series, the cervical anastomosis has decreased morbidity and mortality if anastomotic leak occurs [10]. Recently, authors have questioned the belief that anastomotic leak in the chest has a higher mortality if adequate drainage is achieved [12].

An Ivor-Lewis TTE approach includes a thoracotomy in addition to a laparotomy. The former enables esophageal mobilization under direct vision, and an extended lymphadenectomy with an intrathoracic anastomosis. Disadvantages include increased incisional pain with potentially greater respiratory complications and greater potential morbidity from an intrathoracic anastomotic leak [13]. Recent comparison in large meta-analysis has shown no significant differences in mortality and morbidity between the two approaches [9]. Exposure of the esophagus through the right chest is excellent up to and above the azygous vein, but a neck incision may be necessary in some patients who have more proximal disease. Neither approach has been shown to have a superior oncologic outcome, as overall survival is the same [14]. Similarly, a Mckeown or three-field approach (laparotomy, right chest, left neck) has not been shown to have a definitive oncologic advantage [15].

Minimally invasive esophagectomy

This approach has increased in use in the thoracic surgical community significantly in recent years [16]. MIE can be performed with either a cervical or intrathoracic anastomosis. All or part of the procedure may be performed in a minimally invasive manner. The authors have applied minimally invasive techniques in a selective way based on pathology and patient anatomy. Thoracoscopic esophagectomy, laparoscopic gastric mobilization, and cervical esophagogastrostomy, however, have been their most common approaches in patients who have early malignant and premalignant disease. There has been an evolution in the approach to minimizing morbidity from esophagectomy: first with THE, then minimally invasive surgery. As minimally invasive techniques have progressed, there has been a resurgence of interest in intrathoracic anastomosis accomplished with a thoracoscopic exposure. The strength of the MIS approach is that the extent of resection and ability to assess adenopathy or other potential sites of disease remains intact.

Indications for minimally invasive esophagectomy

At the University of Wisconsin, the authors have used MIE in various stages of disease. It is the procedure of choice in patients who have Barrett's esophagitis with high-grade dysplasia and T1 (carcinoma invading the lamina propria or submucosa) or T2 (carcinoma invading the muscularis propria) tumors without evidence of adenopathy. Neoadjuvant therapy is not an absolute contraindication to a minimally invasive approach. The authors, however, would not recommend a completely minimally invasive approach in a suspected T4 (carcinoma invading local structures) tumor. Still, portions of the surgery may be minimally invasive, such as performing thoracoscopic esophageal mobilization and mediastinal nodal dissection for larger Siewert type 2 gastroesophageal junction malignancies straddling the gastroesophageal junction emanating from the cardia of the stomach [17]. Multiple previous abdominal procedures and other anatomic considerations may deter from a totally endoscopic approach and favor a laparotomy rather than laparoscopy for the abdominal nodal dissection and gastric conduit creation. The authors have a series of patients with esophageal cancer and aberrant right subclavian arteries for which blunt transhiatal intrathoracic esophageal mobilization is contraindicated. This example emphasizes the need for selective approach in which minimally invasive techniques should be tailored to individual patients. Patients must have adequate cardiac and pulmonary reserve to proceed with either MIE, TTE, or THE, and these parameters do not differ from patients planned for an open esophagectomy, because MIE may be associated with significant physiologic stress because of potentially longer operative times or one-lung ventilation. Reversible ischemia on nuclear study or evidence of congestive heart failure despite appropriate medical therapy would preclude patients from surgery. Patients who have reduced functional expiratory volume (FEV1) in combination with other comorbid medical conditions have an increased risk of cardiac arrhythmia and respiratory complications [18]. Careful patient selection is appropriate for all esophagectomies, whether open or minimally invasive.

Minimally invasive esophageal resection techniques

Thoracoscopic–laparoscopic esophagectomy with cervical anastomosis

With a totally endoscopic, Mckeown approach, thoracoscopic mobilization of the esophagus and mediastinal nodal dissection are the initial steps. The patient is intubated with a double-lumen endotracheal tube for selective left lung ventilation. The patient is placed in the left lateral decubitus position with his or her arms in the praying position, supported with pillows on a bean bag mattress with the table flexed at the level of the anterior superior iliac spine. Accurate thoracoport site placement is integral for effective esophageal mobilization. Four working ports are used. 10 mm camera provides optimal lighting and visualization. This port is placed in the seventh intercostal space. Posteriorly, two 5 mm ports are inserted and available for both retraction and dissection with the ultrasonic coagulating shears immediately posterior to the tip of the scapula and approximately 5 cm caudal to this in the posterior axillary line. A second 5 mm port is inserted in the fifth intercostal space posteriorly, just below the tip of the scapula. A 5 mm port is placed anteriorly in the fourth space for lung and esophageal retraction (Fig. 1).

Once port access is obtained, the patient is rotated slightly prone, and the right lung is retracted superiorly as the inferior pulmonary ligament divided. The mediastinal pleura is divided along the anterior border of the esophagus, posterior to the pulmonary vein, elevating the esophagus off of the left atrium. The periesophageal (level #8), inferior pulmonary ligament (level #9), and subcarinal (level #7) nodal packets are easily and completely dissected out thoracoscopically with this approach. The pleura overlying the

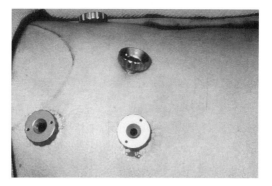

Fig. 1. Four working ports are used for accurate thoracoport site placement in esophageal mobilization.

posterior border of the esophagus then is incised anterior to the azygous vein, and the esophagus is mobilized circumferentially. A Penrose drain then can be placed around the esophagus and stapled into a small loop to facilitate esophageal retraction out of the mediastinum. The azygous vein is divided as it courses anteriorly to join the superior vena cava with a vascular load of the Endo-GIA vascular stapler (Endo-GIA II, Covidien, Norwalk, Connecticut). Wide excision of the esophagus, pleura, and mediastinal nodes is performed up to and including the carina nodal region. Cephalad to this point dissection is kept close to the esophagus to avoid the posterior membranous trachea. Most dissection is accomplished with ultrasonic coagulating shears. The authors (and others), however, recently have been more liberal with applying clips in areas with nodal tissue, as they are uncertain how effectively ultrasonic energy sources seal thin-walled lymphatic vessels. Dissection continues with the ultrasonic shears to the thoracic inlet, and the Penrose drain is left around the esophagus and tucked up into the left neck, which facilitates the cervical esophageal dissection later on. The superior mediastinal (level #4) lymph nodes also are easily dissected out after division of the azygous vein. A single chest 28 French chest tube or 24 French Blake drain is left for drainage through the anterior seventh intercostal thoracoport site. The remaining incisions are closed with absorbable sutures after local anesthesia is achieved with intercostal nerve blocks with 0.25% bupivicaine.

If the anastomosis is planned in the thoracic cavity, the laparoscopic portion is completed first. Typically, the intrathoracic anastomosis is created in a stapled fashion. An 28 mm circular stapler or a 30 mm Endo-GIA stapler (Covidien) stapler may be used. The Endo-GIA stapler is inserted through a 10 mm port. Anterior extension of the lower, posterior axillary line port site incision is necessary for insertion of the circular stapler because of its larger diameter. When using the Endo-GIA, the anastomosis is fashioned in a side-to-side functional end- to-end manner between the posterior wall of the esophagus and anterior wall of the gastric conduit as popularized by Orringer in cervical anastomosis. A double-staple technique or suture closure is used to complete the anterior wall of the esophagogastric anastomosis. Robotic-assisted techniques with a sutured anastomosis have been reported and may be helpful in completing the anastomosis in a side-to-side stapled technique [19]. When using the circular stapler, the authors recommend a 25 mm or greater stapler. The anvil is inserted through the extended port and placed within the open lumen of the divided proximal esophagus. A purse string suture is placed to secure the anvil within the esophagus. The circular stapler is advanced though the side of the gastric conduit, exiting anteriorly close to the apex. After the stapler is fired, it is imperative to have two complete donut rings within the device from the conduit and the esophagus. The lateral entry site for the circular stapler in the gastric conduit then is closed with the Endo-GIA stapler. The authors drain the chest with a Blake drain and a standard right angled chest tube along the anastomosis . Postoperative care is similar to that for an open Ivor-Lewis approach (Fig. 2).

Laparoscopic esophagectomy

At the University of Wisconsin, the authors use a similar approach to that described by Luketich and colleagues [20]. The patient is placed in a supine position. The authors do not use lithotomy or Nissen table position for the surgeon to stand between the legs. The surgeon stands on the patient's right, and the assistant stands on the left. Five port sites are inserted: two paramedian 10 mm ports, and three additional 5 mm ports are placed in bilateral subcostal midaxillary lines and right flank position just below the tip of the 10th rib at approximately the anterior axillary line. The left lobe of the liver is retracted to expose the esophageal hiatus using a flexible retractor and held in place with a self-retaining system. Alternatively, a Nathanson retractor may be positioned through a subxyphoid incision to retract the liver (Fig. 3).

Steep reverse Trendelenberg positioning with a footboard in place provides added exposure of the upper abdomen. The ultrasonic coagulating shears is the principle tool for dissection. The lesser sack is entered by dividing the gastrohepatic ligament, and the right crus of the diaphragm is

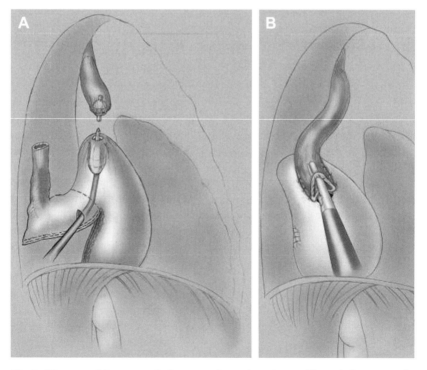

Fig. 2. Diagrams of thoracoscopic–laparoscopic esophagectomy with cervical anastomosis.

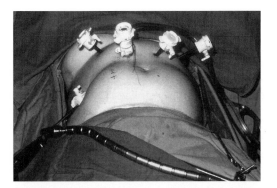

Fig. 3. Five port sites are inserted for laparoscopic esophagectomy. Three paramedian 10 mm ports and three additional 5 mm ports are placed in bilateral subcostal midaxillary lines and right flank position just below the tip of the 10th rib at approximately the anterior axillary line.

identified. At this time, nodal tissue seen on CT scans or positron emission tomography (PET) may be sampled along the common hepatic artery or near the left gastric artery. The authors then identify and preserve the right gastroepiploic artery, divide the gastrocolic ligament, and continue caudal to the vessel along the greater curve of the stomach to the duodenum. A formal Kocher maneuver to mobilize the duodenum is not necessary and rarely performed. The short gastric vessels are divided with the ultrasonic shears, and dissection continues superiorly to the left crus. Endoclips should be available but rarely are used or necessary. The stomach is retracted superiorly, for visualization of the left gastric artery. Nodal dissection at the base of this vessel down to the celiac artery is performed before division of the vessel, reflecting the nodal packet up onto the specimen by incising the peritoneum. The left gastric artery and vein then are divided simultaneously with the Endo-GIA vascular stapler. The authors find that more length for the conduit is obtained by division of the bridging omental vessels at the anterior aspect of the gastrocolic omentum. They do not perform a pyloroplasty or pyloromyotomy routinely [21].

The gastric conduit then is created using an Endo-GIA 3.5 or 4.8 mm load; the latter is used if the stomach is thickened secondary to neoadjuvant chemoradiation. The right gastric artery is preserved. The staple line is completed, staying parallel to the greater curve with a conduit width of approximately 5 cm. The authors do not oversew the gastric staple line routinely. The gastric conduit then is sutured to the esophagogastric specimen. A 7 French needle jejunostomy tube is placed for feeding. The ligament of Treitz is identified by lifting the transverse colon, and a mobile loop of jejunum is identified approximately 25 to 30 cm distal to the ligament. The selected loop of jejunum is a attached to the anterior abdominal wall with suture. A needle catheter kit is inserted percutaneously into the peritoneal cavity. Under laparoscopic guidance, it is directed into the proximal loop of jejunum. The guide wire and catheter are threaded into the jejunum using the

Seldinger technique. The jejunum is tacked to the anterior abdominal wall
with a total of three sutures around the jejunostomy tube entry site, and
an additional stitch a few centimeters distally to prevent torsion of the effer-
ent jejunal limb. The feeding tube is secured to the skin with two 2-0 nylon
sutures. Finally the phrenoesophageal ligament is incised circumferentially
across the anterior surface of the esophagus and down the left crus. The dissection is carried up the hiatus after dividing a few slips of the right crus. If
this is done before this point, pneumoperitoneum may be difficult to maintain. The Achilles heal of esophagectomy is the gastric conduit, and if there
is any question of compromise, conversion to open laparotomy is warranted. A curvilinear incision is made transversely across the base of the
neck, running up the left sternocleidomastoid muscle for a total length of
approximately 5 cm. The dissection is carried anterior to the carotid sheath
down to the cervical spine. This dissection is facilitated by the pneumome-
diastinum, and the Penrose encircling the esophagus is easily retrieved and
used to deliver the esophagus into the field. The specimen is removed
through this cervical incision. The conduit is advanced up the mediastinum
under direct, laparoscopic vision as the esophagogastrectomy specimen is
retrieved from the neck. A cervical esophagogastrostomy then is completed
in the standard fashion. The authors perform a hand-sewn anastomosis with
4-0 Vicryl in a single interrupted transmural layer or a stapled side-to-side,
functional end-to-end anastomosis as described previously.

Results of minimally invasive esophagectomy

A large meta-analysis review was performed demonstrating the widening
application of minimally invasive approaches to esophagectomy. Twenty-
three articles concerning the topic met the stringent requirement for review
and included 1398 patients. Overall mortality (2.3%), morbidity (46%), and
leak rate (7.7%) were similar to open procedures and confirm the safety and
feasibility of the technique. Lymph node yield for an R0 resection (complete
surgical excision) for these patients was similar to published results of open
series [16]. Long-term follow up is needed to confirm that these values trans-
late into satisfactory oncologic outcomes. Initial reports related to survival
(3 years) suggest that it is comparable to open surgery in a highly selected
group [22]. Adequate randomized data is not currently available to statistically confirm quality-of-life improvement from a minimally invasive
approach in direct comparison with open approaches. Some authors believe
that the improved quality of life after minimally invasive resection techniques may be best with a high thoracic anastomosis [23].

Endoscopic therapy for Barrett's esophagitis and esophageal cancer

Endoscopic approaches to Barrett's esophagus with dysplasia have
grown in popularity over the past decade. Photodynamic therapy (PDT)

first was described in 1996; there are currently 81 publications describing its application to this disease [24]. Initially proposed for patients who were not candidates for surgical therapy, there is now a push for more aggressive implementation of PDT and other endoscopic treatments for Barrett's esophagus and superficial (T1) esophageal cancers. The two newer modes of endoscopic therapy are radiofrequency ablative (RFA) therapy and endoscopic mucosal resection (EMR). These techniques often are used in combination if malignancy (intramucosal T1 lesion) is present. Both modalities are performed with a flexible endoscope under conscious sedation.

Photodynamic therapy, unlike RFA or EMR, requires intravenous administration of a photosensitizing agent given before the procedure. Porfimer sodium is activated by a nonthermal, 630 nanometer light directed at the esophageal tissue during endoscopy using a 3 to 5 cm probe with or without a centering balloon. Mucosa is damaged by reactive, unstable singlet oxygen species formed in conjunction with the endoscopic light source [25]. As an ablative therapy, PDT is completely reliant upon EUS for selection of appropriate patients, for example T0 or T1N0 lesions. Rampado and colleagues [7] reported on the predictive value of EUS for determining invasion of the submucosa. Overall accuracy was only 75%, and the negative predictive value was 86%. This report suggests that up to 14% of patients may be understaged and therefore undertreated with ablative therapy. Although EUS is now virtually standard of care to estimate cancer depth, its accuracy, especially for the differentiation of T0 and T1 lesions, has varied in different studies. Standard EUS at 7.5 or 12 MHz accurately predicts the depth of invasion in only 50% to 60% cases, and high-frequency (20 MHz) catheter probes tend to overstage early lesions [26].

Complications of PDT include photosensitivity, fever, chest pain, and odynophagia, pleural effusion, but the most important is esophageal strictures. This has been reported in up to 36% of treated patients [25]. In a retrospective analysis of 131 patients who underwent PDT, 27% had strictures; EMR followed by PDT has a higher rate of stricture and was identified as a risk factor for stricture formation [27]. Subsquamous buried Barrett's mucosa occurs in a significant percentage of patients, and neoplastic elements are seen in up to 25% of patients treated with PDT for early esophageal malignancy [28]. In addition, persistent genetic abnormalities in residual esophageal mucosa have been documented and suggest that the potential for malignancy remains in those patients [29]. Pathologic tumor staging is not obtained in ablative therapy such as PDT or RFA, and this may be an advantage of EMR over these modalities in patients who cannot undergo surgery.

Endoscopic mucosal resection

EMR involves local snare excision of the region of HGD and has been used increasingly in recent years. EMR has been used for diagnosis, staging, and therapeutic treatment of HGD or intramucosal esophageal adenocarcinoma (EAC). EMR has been advocated for tumors confined to the mucosa (EAC), and clear margins of resection (lateral and deep) are obtained. Ell and colleagues [30] recently reported on EMR in 100 patients who had low-risk esophageal adenocarcinoma. There were no major complications. During a relatively short follow-up period of only 36.7 months, however, recurrent or metachronous cancer was found in 11% of patients; all of these patients required a second procedure but were successfully treated with endoscopic resection. The overall calculated 5-year survival rate was 98%. Fifty one patients had successful EMR that did not require additional ablative therapy. A positive margin was seen in 33% of patients and an indeterminate margin in 33%. Forty nine patients were ablated with argon or PDT for incomplete local therapy with EMR [31]. Circumferential EMR and complete removal of Barrett's epithelium in patients who have HGD or early EAC has been attempted to reduce recurrence rates. Peters and colleagues reported on complete eradication in multiple EMR sessions of mucosal abnormalities. Complete removal of Barrett's esophagus was achieved in 89% of patients and early malignancy cleared in 100% with no reported recurrences [31]. Esophageal stenosis, requiring multiple endoscopic dilatations, was seen in 30% to 40% of patients. Data on the long-term success of this approach are not available. Follow-up in the study by Ell and colleagues [30] was exhaustive, including endoscopic surveillance at: 1, 2, 3, 6, 9, 12 months and then every 6 months for 5 years. In addition, EUS, CT scans, and abdominal ultrasound were performed at every other visit, significantly adding to the cost of this therapy. Piecemeal resection often is required for larger lesions. Pathologic tumor staging and confirmation of complete resection in this setting are inaccurate. Not surprisingly, EMR is associated with up to a 20% risk of recurrent neoplasia (either metachronous or synchronous) during follow-up [31].

Oncologic perspectives

Survival data for patients undergoing MIE appear similar to standard open approaches. Additional data are necessary for survival and cancer-free survival after endoscopic therapy for malignant and premalignant disease of the esophagus. At present, esophagectomy remains the gold standard for treating early esophageal cancer and Barrett's esophagus with HGD in patients who are appropriate candidates for surgery. Quality of life as measured by the Short Form 36 (SF-36) obtained after esophagectomy demonstrated that increasing cancer risk is associated with decreased health-related quality of life [32]. Uncertainty over ongoing cancer risk, emphasized by the rigorous follow-up needed following endoscopic therapy, may affect patients' sense of well being and reduce quality of life. A minimally invasive approach allows for complete resection and complete pathologic assessment of the esophagus and lymph nodes for accurate staging and may provide improved quality of life with similar or improved morbidity and mortality compared with a standard open esophagectomy. This approach should be used in a selective way and does not replace open esophagectomy. Minimally invasive surgery may decrease morbidity and allow quicker return to preoperative functioning without compromising oncologic principles.

References

[1] Botterweck AA, Schouten LJ, Volovics A, et al. Trends in incidence of adenocarcinoma of the oesophagus and gastric cardia in ten European countries. Int J Epidemiol 2000;29(4):645–50.
[2] Eloubeidi MA, Mason AC, Desmond RA, et al. Temporal trends (1973–1997) in survival of patients with esophageal adenocarcinoma in the United States: a glimmer of hope? Am J Gastroenterol 2003;98:1627–33.
[3] Birkmeyer JD, Siewers AE, Finlayson EV. Hospital and surgical mortality in the United States. N Engl J Med 2002;346:1128–37.
[4] Connors RC, Reuben BC, Neumayer LA, et al. Comparing outcomes after transthoracic and transhiatal esophagectomy: a 5-year prospective cohort of 17,395 patients. J Am Coll Surg 2007;205(6):735–40 [Epub 2007 Sep 20].
[5] Castells A. Barrett's esophagus and esophageal cancer. Gastroenterol Hepatol 2006;29 (Supl 3):62–6.
[6] Kerkhof M, van Dekken H, Steyerberg EW, et al. Grading of dysplasia in Barrett's esophagus: substantial interobserver variation between general and gastrointestinal pathologists. Histopathology 2007;50(7):920–7.
[7] Rampado S, Bocus P, Battaglia G, et al. Endoscopic ultrasound: accuracy in staging superficial carcinomas of the esophagus. Ann Thorac Surg 2008;85(1):251–6.
[8] Shimpi RA, George J, Jowell P, et al. Staging of esophageal cancer by EUS: staging accuracy revisited. Gastrointest Endosc 2007;66(3):475–82.
[9] Hulscher JB, Tijssen JG, Obertop H, et al. Transthoracic versus transhiatal resection for carcinoma of the esophagus: a meta-analysis. Ann Thorac Surg 2001;72:306–13.
[10] Boyle MJ, Franceschi D, Livingstone AS. Transhiatal versus transthoracic esophagectomy: complication and survival rates. Am Surg 1999;65:1137–42.
[11] Orringer MB, Marshall B, Iannettoni MD. Transhiatal esophagectomy: clinical experience and refinements. Ann Surg 1999;230:392–403.
[12] Martin LW, Swisher SG, Hofstetter W, et al. Intrathoracic leaks following esophagectomy are no longer associated with increased mortality. Ann Surg 2005;242(3):392–9 [discussion: 399–402].
[13] Rentz J, Bull DA, Harpole D, et al. Transthoracic versus transhiatal esophagectomy: a prospective study of 945 patients. J Thorac Cardiovasc Surg 2003;125:1114–20.
[14] Bailey SH, Bull DA, Harpole DH, et al. Outcomes after esophagectomy: a ten-year prospective cohort. Ann Thorac Surg 2003;75:217–22.
[15] Altorki N. En-bloc esophagectomy—the three-field dissection. Surg Clin North Am 2005; 85(3):611–9, xi.
[16] Gemmill EH, McCulloch P. Systematic review of minimally invasive resection for gastro–esophageal cancer. Br J Surg 2007;94(12):1461–7.
[17] Stein HJ, Sendler A, Siewert JR. Site-dependent resection techniques for gastric cancer. Surg Oncol Clin N Am 2002;11(2):405–14.
[18] Ferguson MK, Durkin AE. Preoperative prediction of the risk of pulmonary complications after esophagectomy for cancer. J Thorac Cardiovasc Surg 2002;123(4):661–9.
[19] van Hillegersberg R, Boone J, Draaisma WA, et al. First experience with robot-assisted thoracoscopic esophagolymphadenectomy for esophageal cancer. Surg Endosc 2006;20(9):1435–9.

[20] Luketich JD, Alvelo-Rivera M, Buenaventura PO, et al. Minimally invasive esophagectomy: outcomes in 222 patients. Ann Surg 2003;238(4):486–94 [discussion: 494–5].

[21] Velanovich V. Esophagogastrectomy without pyloroplasty. Dis Esophagus 2003;16(3): 243–5.

[22] Braghetto I, Csendes A, Cardemil G, et al. Open transthoracic or transhiatal esophagectomy versus minimally invasive esophagectomy in terms of morbidity, mortality, and survival. Surg Endosc 2006;20(11):1681–6.

[23] Nakajima M, Kato H, Miyazaki T, et al. Comprehensive investigations of quality of life after esophagectomy with special reference to the route of reconstruction. Hepatogastroenterology 2007;54(73):104–10.

[24] Gossner L, Ell C. [Photodynamic therapy of dysplasia and early cancer of the esophagus]. Leber Magen Darm 1996;26(3):132,135–7 [in German].

[25] Sharma Prateek, Wani Sachin, Rastogi Amit. Endoscopic therapy for high-grade dysplasia in Barrett's esophagus: ablate, resect, or both? Gastrointest Endosc 2007;66(3):469–74.

[26] Waxman I, Raju GS, Critchlow J, et al. High-frequency probe ultramucosal carcinoma: a case series. Am J Gastroenterol 2006;101:1773–9.

[27] Prasad GA, Wang KK, Buttar NS, et al. Predictors of stricture formation after photodynamic therapy for high-grade dysplasia in Barrett's esophagus. Gastrointest Endosc 2007; 65:60–6.

[28] Mino-Kenudson M, Ban S, Ohana M, et al. Buried dyplasia and early adenocarcinoma arising in Barrett esophagus after porfimer–photodynamic therapy. Am J Surg Pathol 2007; 31(3):403–9.

[29] Krisihnadath KK, Wang KK, Taniquchi K, et al. Persistent genetic abnormalities in Barrett's esophagus after photodynamic therapy. Gastroenterology 2000;119:624–30.

[30] Ell C, May A, Pech O, et al. Curative endoscopic resection of early esophageal adenocarcinomas (Barrett's cancer). Gastrointest Endosc 2007;65:3–10.

[31] Peters FP, Kara MA, Rosmolen WD, et al. Endoscopic treatment of high-grade dysplasia and early stage cancer in Barrett's esophagus. Gastrointest Endosc 2005;61:506–14.

[32] Gerson LB, Ullah N, Hastie T, et al. Does cancer risk affect health-related quality of life in patients with Barrett's esophagus? Gastrointest Endosc 2007;65(1):10–25.

ELSEVIER
SAUNDERS

SURGICAL
CLINICS OF
NORTH AMERICA

Surg Clin N Am 88 (2008) 991–1007

Bariatric Surgery: Choosing the Optimal Procedure

Bradley J. Needleman, MD, FACS[a],*,
Lynn C. Happel, MD[b]

[a]Division of General and Gastrointestinal Surgery, Center for Minimally Invasive Surgery,
The Ohio State University, N 745 Doan, 410 W 10th Avenue, Columbus, OH 43210, USA
[b]Center for Minimally Invasive Surgery, The Ohio State University, 410 West 10th Avenue,
Doan Hall Room 558, Columbus, OH 43210, USA

Obesity is pandemic in the United States and in many countries around the world. It is estimated that in 20 years obesity and its related comorbidities will represent the number one health care concern around the world. The prevalence of obesity has steadily increased over the years among genders, all ages, all racial and ethnic groups, all educational levels, and all smoking levels [1]. From 1960 to 2000, the prevalence of obesity (body mass index [BMI] ≥ 30) more than doubled from 13.3% to 30.9% [2]. From 1988 to 2000, the prevalence of extreme obesity (BMI ≥ 40) increased from 2.9% to 4.7% [3,4]. In 1991, only four states had obesity rates of 15% or higher and none had obesity rates above 16%. By 2000, every state except Colorado had obesity rates of 15% or more and 22 states had obesity rates of 20% [5].

The rationale for weight loss surgery

The health risks associated with obesity are complex, multifactorial, and related to the myriad of comorbidities associated with being overweight, having a diminished quality of life, and the risks from impairment in mobility that lead to accidents and injury. An estimated 70% of diabetes risk in the United States can be attributed to excess weight [6], and the prevalence of hypertension in adults who are obese (BMI ≥ 30) is 41.9% for men and

* Corresponding author. Department of Surgery, The Ohio State University, N747 Doan Hall, 410 W 10th Avenue, Columbus, OH 43210.
E-mail address: bradley.needleman@osumc.edu (B.J. Needleman).

0039-6109/08/$ - see front matter © 2008 Elsevier Inc. All rights reserved.
doi:10.1016/j.suc.2008.05.013
surgical.theclinics.com

37.8% for women. The prevalence of high cholesterol for adults who are obese (BMI ≥30) is 22.0% for men and 27.0% for women [7]. In both men and women, a higher BMI is associated with higher death rates from cancers of the esophagus, colon and rectum, liver, gallbladder, pancreas, and kidney. The same trend applies to cancers of the stomach and prostate in men and cancers of the breast, uterus, cervix, and ovaries in women [8,9].

Most studies demonstrate that obese individuals (BMI ≥30) have a 50% to 100% increased risk of death from all causes when compared with normal weight individuals (BMI ≤25), mostly due to cardiovascular causes [10]. The life expectancy of a moderately obese person may be shortened by 2 to 5 years. White men between 20 and 30 years old with a BMI ≥45 may shorten their life expectancy by 13 years; white women in the same category may lose up to 8 years of life. Young African American men with a BMI ≥45 may lose up to 20 years of life and African American women up to 5 years [11,12].

Medical treatment for obesity is met with discouraging results. Results of the 1991 National Institutes of Health (NIH) Consensus Development Conference found that approximately 95% of people who begin weight loss programs with or without behavior modification regain their weight within 2 years of their maximal weight loss. As a result, the NIH conference recommended two treatments for the durable control of excess body weight—the vertical banded gastroplasty (VBG) and the Roux-en-Y gastric bypass (RYGB). Candidates for bariatric surgery include patients with a BMI ≥40 who have failed conventional weight loss attempts and are properly educated and motivated for surgery and patients with a BMI >35 and <40 who have comorbidities related to their obesity that are imminently life-threatening or causing severe lifestyle limitations. The NIH findings, the feasibility of a minimally invasive approach to weight loss surgery [13], and the media exposure of celebrity successes have led to the markedly increased popularity of bariatric surgery as a way to treat severe obesity and its metabolic consequences.

Evaluation of the obese patient for bariatric surgery

In 2004 the American Society for Bariatric Surgery, now the American Society for Metabolic and Bariatric Surgery (ASMBS), published a consensus statement that all patients undergoing bariatric surgery need to be well informed and motivated, compliant with lifestyle changes, and understand the need to participate in long-term follow-up [14]. Most programs now offer a multidisciplinary team approach to patient evaluation and selection, including comprehensive medical, dietary, and psychologic evaluations by a variety of specialists, and provide educational programs and counseling to help prepare the individual for the anticipated effects of surgery. Employing a multidisciplinary program has been further reinforced by organizations that credential bariatric programs as "centers of excellence," such as the American College of Surgeons and the ASMBS as implemented by the Surgical Review Corporation. The evaluation of the obese patient for surgery is geared toward obtaining information that may help the bariatric team determine the patient's candidacy for weight loss surgery and which operation may best serve that individual.

The medical evaluation of the obese patient should include a detailed history and physical examination documenting the patient's comorbidities and often includes diagnosing previously unrecognized problems. During the evaluation, the practitioner should document satisfaction of the basic NIH criteria and ask questions that may influence patient selection and the type of operation. The questions may include the following: "Does this patient have any medical contraindications to weight loss surgery?" "Will this patient be able to tolerate general anesthesia?" "Are there any medical conditions that would make one operation better suited for this individual?" "Will this patient be able to tolerate the most common complications associated with a given operation?" Medical conditions that may influence the procedure choice include age, BMI, gender, cardiopulmonary risk factors, diabetes, severe steatohepatitis, a history of cancer, inflammatory bowel disease, and previous abdominal surgery, as well as the desire for future pregnancies or organ transplantation.

Dietary evaluations should garner information that answers questions regarding the patient's current eating habits, assess prior attempts at weight loss, make recommendations for immediate dietary changes to prepare for an operation, and initiate preparations to optimize success after surgery. The dietary assessment of the patient's ability to make meaningful changes after surgery may be important in helping to determine the chances of success after surgery. Although stress and sweet eating may not have a role in success after surgery, a history of past weight loss success that includes the ability to make meaningful dietary changes may identify patients who are more likely to do well, especially those undergoing purely restrictive operations [15,16].

Although psychologic evaluations are recommended, psychiatric diagnoses have not been able to demonstrate a predictive effect of success after surgery. Although the presence of mental illness is not an absolute contraindication to weight loss surgery, it may be beneficial to diagnose and manage mental health disorders that could influence successful outcomes and influence the surgery team toward a particular type of operation, especially if there is concern regarding the potential of harm caused by noncompliance.

The ASMBS suggestions for a presurgical psychologic assessment recommend the identification of eating behaviors such as binge eating, overeating, grazing, and night eating that may have an emotional component and therefore respond to behavioral counseling. In addition, it may be important to assess the patient's ability to cope with the significant lifestyle changes, their potential for abusive behaviors, and their ability to make informed decisions regarding their health care and potentially permanent alterations of the gastrointestinal tract.

Although the presence of psychopathology has not been found to correlate with surgical outcomes, discussion with the surgery team may help to influence procedure choices. Recommendations may be made to patients to help modify their behaviors to achieve more success and identify patterns that may help steer them toward a particular procedure and prevent problems related to their inability to successfully cope with the significant lifestyle alterations [17].

Operations that are offered to a patient should reflect an understanding of the patient's dietary and psychologic history, medical and surgical history, surgeon experience, patient comfort and expectations, and the ability of the medical facility to handle most known complications related to the specific operation and to obesity. Objective criteria to help choose an operation for a given patient were proposed by Buchwald in 2002. The algorithm is based upon the assumptions that there is no gold standard operation, that a surgeon should be able to perform more than one operation, and that a patient can be matched to a specific procedure. It includes patient variables such as BMI, age, gender, race, body habitus, and the presence of major comorbidities; outcome variables such as safety, the resolution of comorbidities, and patient satisfaction; and operative variables including gastric banding, VBG, RYGB (short- and long-limb), and biliopancreatic diversion with duodenal switch (BPD/DS). By following the algorithm a patient can be broadly matched to an operation based upon these factors, but the ultimate decision is determined by surgeon experience and patient preference [18].

Minimally invasive options for bariatric surgery

Bariatric surgery can be performed safely and is a highly effective means of producing meaningful weight loss, with a profound effect on comorbidities, often leading to their amelioration and resolution. The most commonly performed procedures have the ability to be performed laparoscopically, offering the same operation with lower morbidity, often due to a large abdominal incision. In the United States, more than 200,000 primary operations are performed for weight loss each year, including the most commonly performed procedures of RYGB, the laparoscopic adjustable gastric band (LAGB), BPD/DS, and, more recently, sleeve gastrectomy.

There is no one best operation for all patients, and the paucity of well-controlled, randomized trials comparing all operations makes it difficult to determine which operation is the gold standard for an individual patient. Nevertheless, data are available to help steer the surgeon and patient toward an operation that may best fit their needs based on their history and expectations. Patients should be offered a comprehensive multidisciplinary evaluation to gather information and educate them on what procedures offer them the best chance of weight loss success, aid in the resolution of specific comorbidities, an acceptable quality of life, and a favorable risk-to-benefit ratio.

Patients are considerably knowledgeable regarding their options for bariatric surgery and can readily obtain this information from television, magazines, support groups, and especially the Internet, where they have access to medical Web sites, online support groups, chat rooms, and even scientific literature and videos of operations. Surgeons performing bariatric surgery are encouraged to understand the advantages and disadvantages of most available procedures to be able to answer patients' questions and dispel misconceptions. It is also recommended that a bariatric surgery practice recognize there is not one operation that is best for all patients, offer more than one operation, and select and refer patients for their optimal or desired operation accordingly. Additionally, the decision to offer a patient an operation performed by a minimally invasive approach should depend on the surgeon's training, outcomes, and level of comfort in performing the desired operation. This information should be shared with the patient as part of the informed consent process.

The laparoscopic Roux-en-Y gastric bypass

The RYGB was first described by Mason and Ito in 1966 [19] and has since become the most commonly performed weight loss operation in the United States (Fig. 1). The components of a successful operation include a small proximal gastric pouch typically less than 30 cm^3 based on the lesser curve, a small gastrojejunostomy approximately 12 mm in diameter, and a Roux limb that has ranged from 60 to 250 cm or more in length to alter malabsorption depending on patient factors and surgeon preference.

This restrictive operation imparts a change of appetite and feeling of early satiety causing the individual to eat significantly less food at a given time. Patients must make changes in their eating habits to comply with their new anatomy that include chewing their food well, eating slowly, and stopping when they sense their new feeling of being "full"; otherwise, they may encounter symptoms such as discomfort, nausea, and vomiting. The operation may also impact food tolerances and the potential for dumping syndrome, which is the reaction to foods high in sugar content causing cramping, abdominal pain and diarrhea, diaphoresis, and light-headedness. As a result, some studies have suggested that RYGB may be better than the purely restrictive operations for patients identified as "sweet eaters" [20], but more recent studies have not been able to confirm this result [21].

Malabsorption may be added to RYGB to potentiate the weight loss effects by varying the length of the Roux and biliopancreatic limb. In general, the data suggest that, for a BMI > 50, a 150-cm Roux limb may impart

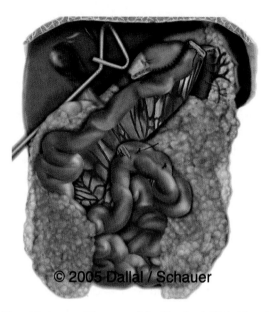

Fig. 1. Roux-en-Y gastric bypass. (*Courtesy of* the Cleveland Clinic Foundation, Cleveland, Ohio; with permission.)

greater weight loss than a 75-cm limb without increasing the metabolic consequences. When the BMI is less than 50, there is no significant weight loss advantage between a Roux limb of 75 and 150 cm. A longer Roux limb may be recommended for patients who have more than 200 lbs of excess body weight [22].

The advantages of RYGB include its longevity with the availability of long-term results, the permanence of the operation, and the multiple factors that impart weight loss. Because diet is restricted immediately, weight loss is immediate and can continue for 18 to 24 months after operation. Mean excess body weight loss (EBWL) is estimated to range from 60% to 75% during this time, with improvements in or resolution of many weight-related comorbidities [23]. The resolution of comorbidities is well documented after gastric bypass, including the amelioration of diabetes and improvements in insulin resistance and glucose tolerance. Bypassing the antrum, duodenum, and jejunum during RYGB may provide additional benefits in the treatment of diabetes by altering gut signaling mechanisms that are beneficial to treating insulin resistance or glucose tolerance when compared with restrictive operations alone [24]. Additional beneficial effects are a reduction in other cardiovascular risk factors and mortality [25]. The systematic review and meta-analysis reported by Buchwald and colleagues [23] in 2003 demonstrated significant improvement in comorbidities. Diabetes resolved in 76.8% of patients, hypertension resolved in 61.7%, obstructive sleep apnea resolved in 85.7%, and hyperlipidemias improved in 70%.

Disadvantages of RYGB may be the short- and long-term complications related to the procedure, such as leakage at the gastrojejunal anatomosis, pouch, remnant stomach, or jejunojejunostomy. Others include gastrojejunal stricture, marginal ulceration, internal hernias, and a variety of metabolic derangements, most commonly of vitamin B_{12}, iron, and calcium. Another consideration in choosing the gastric bypass should be the loss of access to the distal stomach and duodenum, making the diagnosis of pathology and the performance of endoscopic retrograde cholangiopancreatography (ERCP) difficult without undergoing additional surgical intervention. Patients at high risk for future gastric and duodenal pathology, those requiring use of non-steroidal anti-inflammatory drugs (NSAIDs) or other ulcerogenics, or those at highest risk for vitamin and mineral deficiencies may not be ideal candidates for RYGB. Weight gain after maximal weight loss may occur between 2 and 5 years and lead to failure judged by not maintaining more than 50% of EBWL. This number is evident 10 years after RYGB as the failure to maintain $>50\%$ EBWL may be as high as 20.4% for morbidly obese patients and 34.9% in super morbidly obese patients [26].

In an effort to predict the best candidates, one study looked at 180 consecutive patients over a 30-month period and found that preoperative BMI had a significant effect on EBWL, with patients with a BMI <50 achieving a higher percentage of EBWL than those with a BMI >50 (91.7% versus 61.6%, respectively; $P = .001$). Marriage status was also a significant predictor of successful outcome, with single patients achieving a higher percentage of EBWL than married patients (89.8% versus 77.7%, respectively; $P = .04$). Married patients had more than two times the risk of failure when compared with those who were unmarried (OR, 2.6; 95% CI, 1.1–6.5; $P = .04$). Race had a noticeable but not statistically significant effect, with Caucasian patients achieving a higher percentage of EBWL than African Americans (82.9% versus 60%, respectively; $P = .06$). These findings suggest that weight loss achieved at 1 year after LAGB is suboptimal in super obese patients, and that single patients with a BMI <50 have the best chance of achieving greater weight loss [27].

The RYGB continues to be the most commonly performed operation for weight loss in the United States. An abundance of long-term data demonstrates its success in weight loss and the resolution of obesity-related comorbidities. It can usually be performed using minimally invasive techniques with excellent rates of morbidity and mortality. The presence of dumping syndrome in addition to restriction may be attractive to some patients who are known sweet eaters. The RYGB may place some patients at risk for certain vitamin and mineral deficiencies, including the risk of osteoporosis, and may not be the ideal operation for those at high risk for noncompliance related to necessary dietary supplementation. In addition, the risk of marginal ulceration may discourage patients who must take NSAIDs and those who are at highest risk for distal gastric or duodenal pathology.

The laparoscopic adjustable gastric band

The laparoscopically placed adjustable gastric band has been approved by the US Food and Drug Administration since June 2001 and has been increasing in popularity, becoming the second most commonly performed operation for weight loss in the United States (Fig. 2). The LAGB was first described by Belachew and colleagues [28] in 1993 and became the most commonly performed weight loss operation in Europe, Australia, and Latin America. Two types of bands are currently available in the United States: the Lap-Band adjustable gastric banding system distributed by Allergan (Irvine, California) and the Realize Personalized Banding Solution distributed by Ethicon (Cincinnati, Ohio) Endo-Surgery. The relative ease of placement laparoscopically, with short operating room times (<1 hour), low morbidity and mortality ($<0.1\%$), and short hospital stays (<1 day), makes this an attractive option for patients and surgeons and has led to this procedure essentially replacing the VBG as the purely restrictive operation of choice.

During this procedure an inflatable silicon band is placed around the stomach to create a small gastric pouch (usually <20 cm^3). Tubing connects the band to an access port which is implanted in the subcutaneous tissue within the abdominal wall. Access to this port, performed with or without radiologic guidance by a non-coring needle, allows adjustment to the band. The instillation of saline tightens the stoma between the proximal pouch and distal stomach, thereby creating earlier satiety. Negative symptoms including significant food intolerances, symptoms of reflux, pain, and patient request can be treated by aspirating fluid, opening the stoma,

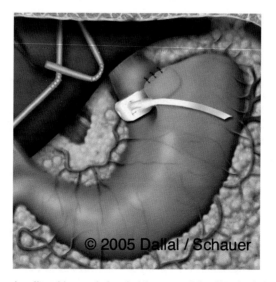

Fig. 2. Laparoscopic adjustable gastric band. (*Courtesy of* the Cleveland Clinic Foundation, Cleveland, Ohio; with permission.)

and relieving these symptoms. Adjustments can be made as often as needed to optimize weight loss by tightening the band sufficiently to achieve a prolonged sensation of satiety while letting the patient tolerate a variety of healthful foods without having adverse symptoms. Weight loss is usually in the range of 0.5 to 1 kg per week. Maximal EBWL generally occurs over a period of 18 months to 3 years [29].

Weight loss results seen with the band can be variable. Without malabsorption or dumping syndrome, it is generally accepted that food selection can have a greater role in the success of restrictive operations like the LAGB, although there is also evidence suggesting the presence of behaviors such as sweet eating before surgery will not predict failure [30]. A systematic review and meta-analysis of a large body of data describing the Swedish adjustable gastric band and Lap-Band was published in 2008 by Cunneen and colleagues [31]. The data showed that the 3-year mean EBWL for the Lap-Band system was 50.20% and the BMI reduction 11.81 kg/m^2 from baseline. The rate of resolution of comorbidities after the procedure was 60.29% for diabetes and 43.58% for hypertension.

In an attempt to profile the best candidates for LAGB, a nationwide survey was performed in France. The greatest success in gastric banding occurred in patients 40 years old with an initial BMI <50 kg/m^2 who were willing to change their eating habits and to recover or increase their physical activity after surgery and who had their operation performed by a team usually performing more than two bariatric procedures per week. This study emphasized that obesity surgery, and LAGB specifically, requires significant experience of the surgical team and a multidisciplinary approach to improve behavioral changes [32].

In another attempt to predict successful outcomes, 85 morbidly obese patients undergoing LAGB were analyzed according to several possible predictive characteristics for success. At 27 months follow-up, significant success predictors included baseline absolute body weight, BMI with a threshold value of 50 kg/m^2 ($P = .02$), and female sex ($P = .02$), as well as postoperative vomiting ($P = .02$), eating behavior, and physical activity ($P < .01$). Baseline EBWL and a change in eating behavior after surgery were identified as independent predictors in multivariate analysis. Patients with a lower excess body weight who improve their eating behavior after surgery have the highest chance of success after LAGB [15].

Complications at the time of band placement are infrequent and may include injury to the stomach and esophagus, bleeding, splenic injury, and poor placement of the band. Complications from LAGB may be unique, and reoperations may be required 10% to 13% of the time owing to port displacement, infection, gastric slippage, erosion, and explantation [33]. In a study of 573 patients in Italy followed up for 5 years after LAGB, complications included migration of the band (4.1%), erosion (2.1%), mortality (0.87%), and conversion to other bariatric procedures (1.9%). Band removal was performed in 5.7% of patients due to gastric pouch dilation and band erosion [34]. In another study in Portugal of 591 patients with follow-up, EBWL at 10 years was 82.7% ± 4.2, with band failure in 9.3%, slippage in 5.3%, and erosion 4.6% [35].

Patients who may benefit from LAGB have comorbidities that put them at the highest risk for perioperative and surgical complications but still would see significant benefit from meaningful weight loss. Patients who have extremes of age, prior abdominal operations with extensive adhesive disease, or a history of inflammatory bowel disease such as Crohn's disease (in which an anastomosis may not be desirable), patients in whom any malabsorption would be disadvantageous, and patients in whom there is a potential for future medical problems or interventions that would benefit from an adjustable operation may be considered better candidates for LAGB over RYGB or BPD/DS.

LAGB may not be the most desirable operation for patients in whom the presence of a foreign body would be contraindicated. It is also not desirable in a patient who is not able to participate in follow-up enough to have the necessary adjustments for optimal success or in some patients with a large hiatal or paraesophageal hernia. In addition, patients with super morbid obesity or who are unable or unwilling to make lifestyle changes related to their diet and activity may benefit more from a more aggressive weight loss intervention.

Laparoscopic biliopancreatic diversion with duodenal switch

BPD, a malabsorptive procedure, was first described by Scopinaro in 1976 [36] as an operation that included a partial gastrectomy leaving a 250 to 500 cm^3 gastric pouch emptying into a 250-cm Roux limb with a 50-cm common channel for absorption. To decrease the incidence of marginal ulceration and metabolic derangements, Marceau and Hess described a modification of the BPD called the duodenal switch (BPD/DS), creating a gastric sleeve and preserving the pylorus (Fig. 3) [37,38]. The BPD/DS is currently being performed by minimally invasive techniques and creates a gastric sleeve 100 to 200 cm^3 in volume while preserving the pylorus anastomosed to an alimentary limb 200 to 300 cm in length and a common channel between 50 and 100 cm in length. Lengthening the limb from 50 to 100 cm in BPD/DS seems to decrease the incidence of metabolic complications such as iron deficiency anemia and protein malnutrition.

Long-term results after BPD/DS reported by Marceau and colleagues demonstrated that 82% of patients had greater than 50% EBWL, with a mean EBWL of 73% ± 19. The 30-day mortality rate was 1.1% and the 90-day mortality rate 1.3%. BPD/DS may have more success in patients who have a higher starting BMI. In patients with a BMI < 50, 92% achieve a BMI < 35; 83% achieve these same results when starting with a BMI > 50. In addition, the resolution of comorbidities is exceptional after BPD/DS. Medications can be discontinued in 92% of diabetics, continuous positive

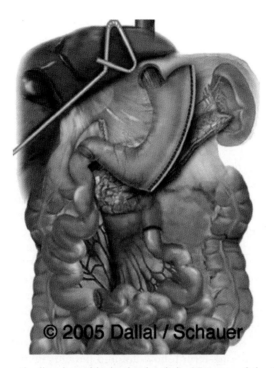

Fig. 3. Biliopancreatic diversion with duodenal switch. (*Courtesy of* the Cleveland Clinic Foundation, Cleveland, Ohio; with permission.)

airway pressure can be discontinued in 90% of those with sleep apnea, and the prevalence of those with a cardiac risk index greater than 5 is decreased by 86% [39]. Given the excellent weight loss seen in BPD/DS, especially given the consistency of results in patients with a BMI >50, it is a more attractive operative for the super obese population, especially if the risks associated with performing this operation due to a large abdominal incision can be ameliorated by performing the operation by a minimally invasive approach.

Malabsorptive procedures such as the BPD/DS have the advantage of providing excellent weight loss with fewer patient-related factors influencing weight loss. The preservation of the pylorus in these patients means they are less likely to experience the dumping syndrome when eating sweets, which may influence the surgeon's decision in offering this as a choice of operation; however, the overall flexibility in diet is what makes this option more attractive for some patients. Despite the decreased absorption, the gastric reservoir is large enough to eventually allow the patient to consume larger amounts of foods that may be detrimental to weight loss, especially those high in fat content. This consumption carries an increased risk and frequency of abdominal bloating and foul-smelling stool and gas which may ultimately alter patient satisfaction.

Long-term complications are mostly related to the short common channel and absorption and include the potential for protein malnutrition and deficiency of fat soluble vitamins and minerals and may place the individual at risk for metabolic bone disease. In Marceau's study of long-term results, 10% of patients presented with hypoalbuminemia, 5% were hospitalized at least once for malnutrition, and 0.7% required revision owing to malnutrition. Commonly seen was the risk of anemia, decreased vitamin A, increased vitamin D, and decreased calcium levels, with 20% of patients having below normal levels and 1.3% having serious deficiencies. The incidence of kidney stones was also significantly increased after surgery [39].

Despite a lack of studies prospectively comparing BPD/DS with other weight loss operations, BPD/DS appears to be a considerably effective operation for patients who are super obese (BMI > 50) when compared with the other procedures and is associated with a significant reduction in comorbidities related to obesity, especially diabetes. Because the stomach remains intact, surveillance continues to be possible, making BPD/DS a good choice for patients who may be at risk for developing gastric pathology. Nevertheless, as is true in RYGB, the ampulla will not be readily accessible to endoscopy and ERCP. Even with operative access, ERCP would be difficult and may not be possible. Patients who are considered at too high an operative risk to undergo this operation, patients who are a concern for being noncompliant with long-term follow-up, and patients taking required daily dietary supplements may be more suitable for one of the less invasive, less aggressive procedures.

Laparoscopic sleeve gastrectomy

Laparoscopic sleeve gastrectomy is one of the newer, purely restrictive procedures being performed as a primary weight loss operation and can be compared with the gastric segment of BPD/DS (Fig. 4). Sleeve gastrectomy is an embodiment of the Magenstrasse and Mill procedure (MM), which was designed to imitate the VBG by creating a long gastric tube but without a foreign body, eliminating the risk of erosion. Sleeve gastrectomy differs from MM by the resection of the defunctionalized fundus, which is left intact in MM. The MM has been performed most commonly in the United Kingdom where 60% EBWL has been reported [40,41]. Because of the similarity between these two operations, weight loss results are expected to be comparable. Currently, sleeve gastrectomy represents about 2% of the weight loss operations being performed in the United States [42].

Sleeve gastrectomy is commonly performed laparoscopically by dividing the vasculature along the greater curve to the angle of His to facilitate complete resection of the gastric fundus. Division of the stomach then begins 6 to 10 cm proximal to the pylorus, leaving an antral remnant volume of 150 to

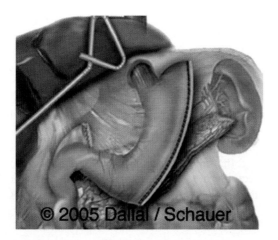

Fig. 4. Sleeve gastrectomy. (*Courtesy of* the Cleveland Clinic Foundation, Cleveland, Ohio; with permission.)

200 mL to facilitate gastric emptying. The gastric tube is then fashioned by placing a 32 to 60 F bougie along the lesser curve and stapling out the fundus to the angle of His. When the sleeve gastrectomy is designed as a definitive procedure, the bougie size can be varied to a smaller caliber to produce a smaller volume gastric tube in an effort to optimize weight loss. It is generally accepted that some reinforcement of the staple line must be performed by oversewing, using buttressing material, or applying a fibrin sealant [42].

Using the sleeve gastrectomy component as a bridge to a more definitive weight loss operation was first described by Chu in higher risk, super morbidly obese patients [43]. Because it is a technically easier operation laparoscopically than the BPD/DS or RYGB, its performance may allow the patient to have a safer operation, lose weight, and then undergo a second more definitive procedure under more favorable circumstances. Most commonly the second procedure is a BPD/DS, but it could also be easily converted to a RYGB or LAGB. Given the prior experience in bariatric surgery with stapled gastroplasties, it was assumed that these operations, while initially effective for weight loss, would ultimately fail to maintain this loss; therefore, the weight loss curves of these patients were closely monitored, and when maximal weight loss was achieved as evidenced by a prolonged plateau and the beginning of weight regain, the patient would undergo the second stage of the procedure. A subset of the super obese population who never underwent the second stage of the procedure were able to successfully maintain weight loss. In a multicenter study of sleeve gastrectomy performed on 163 patients, the percentages of EBWL at 1 and 2 years postoperatively were 59.45% and 61.52%, respectively [44]. In another study by Lee and colleagues [45] in 2007, 216 patients with 2 year follow-up data demonstrated an EBWL of 59% $\pm$ 17 with a preoperative mean

BMI of $49 \pm 11 \text{ kg/m}^2$. At the First International Consensus Summit for sleeve gastrectomy in New York in October of 2007, 87 surgeons completed questionnaires regarding the sleeve gastrectomy; 93.8% of them performed sleeve gastrectomy as a primary weight loss procedure, achieving $56.3\% \pm 21.6$ EBWL at 3 years.

Comorbidities also improve after sleeve gastrectomy. In one report of 193 patients who underwent sleeve gastrectomy, type II diabetes resolved in 66% of patients, improvement occurred in 20%, hypertension resolved in 88%, and sleep apnea resolved in 87% [46]. Other 5 year data presented by Crookes showed that 23 of 49 diabetic patients has resolution of disease after sleeve gastrectomy and another 11 reduced their medications [47,48]. Sleeve gastrectomy is also indicated for patients with a low preoperative BMI who might not normally be considered for a more aggressive operation. In one study from Korea, patients with a preoperative BMI <35 maintained an EBWL of 85% 3 years after surgery, and diabetes resolved in all patients [49].

Complications of sleeve gastrectomy can be related to the staple line and include leaks, which can be difficult to manage and have been reported in up to 5.52% of cases [44], bleeding, and strictures. Metabolic complications of sleeve gastrectomy should be rare owing to the preservation of the continuity of gastrointestinal tract, allowing for relatively normal absorption of nutrients, yet most surgeons treat patients with postoperative supplements [42].

Because it is a purely restrictive operation similar to LAGB, studies have compared sleeve gastrectomy with band surgery. These studies suggest that sleeve gastrectomy might have an advantage in producing better weight loss in the first few years after surgery. Himpens and colleagues [50] prospectively randomized 80 patients to sleeve gastrectomy or LAGB. At 1 and 3 years postoperatively, the LAGB patients had an EBWL of 41.4% and 48%, respectively, whereas sleeve gastrectomy patients had an EBWL of 57.7% and 66%, respectively.

Although more studies are needed to evaluate long-term data, it is clear that there are advantages to sleeve gastrectomy as a bridge operation and that it may be an acceptable definitive weight loss procedure. It is a technically easier operation to perform than the RYGB or BPD/DS, offering patients a greater chance of success with a minimally invasive operation, and it is performed with lower morbidity due to the absence of two additional anastomoses. Weight loss seems to be better with sleeve gastrectomy versus LAGB in the short term and up to 3 years after surgery. It also has the advantage of being able to be converted to other operations easily owing to the success in weight loss, allowing the second operation to be performed at a lower initial BMI. In addition, absorption is unchanged; therefore, minimal risk of nutritional deficiencies and dumping syndrome is incurred. Sleeve gastrectomy has the advantage of no foreign bodies, eliminating the risk of complications requiring future operations due to slip, prolapse, erosion, or device malfunction or infection, and it may be used as a preferred operation in patients who are at risk for these complications. Disadvantages include irreversible resection of normal gastric tissue and the lack of long-term data, especially given the negative history of gastroplasties in bariatric surgery, and the complications of staple lines, including leak and fistula formation that can be difficult to manage.

Summary

Choosing the right operation for weight loss continues to be a challenging and subjective process. In experienced hands, most operations have the ability to be successful in providing a given patient meaningful weight loss and impart better health through loss of adiposity, amelioration of comorbidities, and improvement of overall quality of life. Surgeons should have a thorough understanding of all operations available regardless of their desire to perform a given procedure to be able to give patients reasonable informed consent regarding what operation might be right for them and to answer questions posed from a population with access to seemingly limitless quantities of information from the Internet, television, support groups, and acquaintances. Novel treatments for obesity are also on the horizon, including endoluminal sleeves, endoluminal restrictive mechanisms, intragastric balloons, gastric pacing, and variations of current procedures that target metabolic diseases. The future availability of these procedures may further complicate the decision-making process for patients and surgeons.

A thorough understanding of the patient's medical history, his or her expectations from surgery, and the information garnered from mental health professionals and dietitians will help the practitioner guide the patient to the operation that meets his or her needs, is of an acceptable operative risk, and gives them the best chance for success.

References

[1] Mokdad AH, Ford ES, Bowman BA, et al. Prevalence of obesity, diabetes, and obesity-related health risk factors, 2001. JAMA 2003;289(1):76–9.
[2] Pastor PN, Makuc DM, Reuben C, et al. Chartbook on trends in the health of Americans, health, United States, 2002. Hyattsville (MD): National Center for Health Statistics; 2002.
[3] Flegal KM, Carroll MD, Kuczmarski RJ, et al. Overweight and obesity in the United States: prevalence and trends, 1960–1994. Int J Obes 1998;22:39–47.
[4] Flegal KM, Carroll MD, Ogden CL, et al. Prevalence and trends in obesity among US adults, 1999–2000. JAMA 2002;288:1723–7.
[5] Mokdad AH, Bowman BA, Ford ES, et al. The continuing epidemics of obesity and diabetes in the United States. JAMA 2001;286(10):1195–200.
[6] National Institute of Diabetes and Digestive and Kidney Diseases. Diabetes prevention program meeting summary. Bethesda, MD; August 2001. Diabetes Mellitus Interagency Coordinating Committee.
[7] Brown CD, Higgins M, Donato KA, et al. Body mass index and prevalence of hypertension and dyslipidemia. Obes Res 2000;8(9):605–19.

[8] Calle EE, Rodriguez C, Walker-Thurmond K, et al. Overweight, obesity, and mortality from cancer in a prospectively studied cohort of U.S. adults. N Engl J Med 2003;348(17): 1625–38.

[9] Huang Z, Hankinson SE, Colditz GA, et al. Dual effects of weight and weight gain on breast cancer risk. JAMA 1997;278:1407–11.

[10] Clinical guidelines on the identification, evaluation, and treatment of overweight and obesity in adults—the evidence report. National Institutes of Health. Obes Res 1998;6(Suppl 2): 51S–209S.

[11] Fontaine KR, Redden DT, Wang C, et al. Years of life lost due to obesity. JAMA 2003; 289(2):187–93.

[12] Colditz GA. Economic costs of obesity. Am J Clin Nutr 1992;55:503–7.

[13] Gastrointestinal surgery for severe obesity: National Institutes of Health consensus development conference statement. Am J Clin Nutr 1992;55:615S–9S.

[14] Buchwald H. Consensus conference statement, bariatric surgery for morbid obesity: health implications for patients, health professionals, and third-party payers. Surg Obes Relat Dis 2005;1:317–8.

[15] Bueter M, Thalheimer A, Lager C, et al. Who benefits from gastric banding. Obes Surg 2007; 17:1608–13.

[16] Lindroos AK, Lissner L, Sjostrom L. Weight change in relation to intake of sugar and sweet foods before and after weight reducing gastric surgery. Int J Obes Relat Metab Disord 1996; 20:634–43.

[17] Lemont D, Moorehead M, Parish M, et al. Suggestions for the presurgical psychological assessment of bariatric surgery candidates. American Society for Bariatric Surgery; 2004.

[18] Buchwald H. A bariatric surgery algorithm. Obes Surg 2002;12:733–46.

[19] Mason SE, Ito C. Gastric bypass in obesity. Surg Clin North Am 1967;47:1345–51.

[20] Sugerman H, Starkey J, Birkenhauer R. A randomized prospective trial of gastric bypass versus vertical banded gastroplasty for morbid obesity and their effects on sweets versus non-sweets eaters. Ann Surg 1987;205:613–20.

[21] Hudson SM, Dixon JB, O'Brien PE. Sweet eating is not a predictor of outcome after Lap-Band placement. Can we finally bury the myth? Obes Surg 2002;12:789–94.

[22] Brolin RE, Kenler HA, Gorman JH, et al. Long-limb gastric bypass: a five-year prospective randomized study. Ann Surg 1992;215:123–43.

[23] Buchwald H, Avidor Y, Braunwald E, et al. Bariatric surgery: a systematic review and meta-analysis. JAMA 2004;292:1724–37.

[24] Rubino F, Gagner M. Potential of surgery for curing type 2 diabetes mellitus. Ann Surg 2002;236(5):554–9.

[25] Sjostrom L, Narbro K, Sjostrom C, et al. Effects of bariatric surgery on mortality in Swedish obese subjects. N Engl J Med 2007;357:741–52.

[26] Sjostrom L, Lindroos AK, Peltonen M, et al. Lifestyle, diabetes, and cardiovascular risk factors 10 years after bariatric surgery. N Engl J Med 2004;351(26):2683–93.

[27] Lutfi R, Torquati A, Sekhar N, et al. Predictors of success after laparoscopic gastric bypass: a multivariate analysis of socioeconomic factors. Surg Endosc 2006;20:864–7.

[28] Belachew M, Legrand MJ, Defechereux TH, et al. Laparoscopic adjustable silicone gastric banding in the treatment of morbid obesity: a preliminary report. Surg Endosc 1994;8: 1354–6.

[29] Favretti F, O'Brien P, Dixon J. Patient management after Lap-Band placement. Am J Surg 2002;184(6):S38–41.

[30] Dixon J, O'Brien P, Playfair J, et al. Adjustable gastric banding and conventional therapy for type 2 diabetes: a randomized controlled trial. JAMA 2008;299(3):341–3.

[31] Cunneen S, Phillips E, Fielding G, et al. Studies of Swedish adjustable gastric band and Lap-Band: systematic review and meta-analysis. Surg Obes Relat Dis 2008;4(2):174–85.

[32] Chevallier J, Paita M, Rodde-Dunet M, et al. A nationwide survey on the role of center activity and patients' behavior. Ann Surg 2007;246(6):1034–9.

[33] Ren C, Horgan S, Ponce J. US experience with the Lap-Band system. Am J Surg 2002; 184(6B):46S–50S.

[34] Angrisani L, Di Lorenzo N, Favretti F, et al. The Italian group for Lap-Band: predictive value of initial body mass index for weight loss after 5 years of follow-up. Surg Endosc 2004;18(10):1524–7.

[35] Biagini J, Karam L. Ten years experience with laparoscopic adjustable gastric banding. Obes Surg 2008;18:573–7.

[36] Scopinaro N, Gianetta E, Civalleri D, et al. Biliopancreatic bypass for obesity. II. Initial experience in man. Br J Surg 1979;66:618–20.

[37] Hess DW, Hess DS. Biliopancreatic diversion with a duodenal switch. Obes Surg 1998;8: 267–82.

[38] Marceau P, Biron S, Bouroque R, et al. Biliopancreatic diversion with a new type of gastrectomy. Obes Surg 1993;3:29–35.

[39] Marceau P, Biron S, Hould F, et al. Duodenal switch: long-term results. Obes Surg 2007;17: 1421–30.

[40] Carmichael AR, Sue-Ling HM, Johnston D. Quality of life after the Magenstrasse and Mill procedure for morbid obesity. Obes Surg 2001;11:708–15.

[41] Johnston D, Dachtler J, Sue-Ling HM, et al. The Magenstrasse and Mill operation for morbid obesity. Obes Surg 2003;13:10–6.

[42] Deitel M, Crosby R, Gagner M. The first international consensus summit for sleeve gastrectomy. Obes Surg 2008.

[43] Chu CA, Gagner M, Quinn T, et al. Two-stage laparoscopic biliopancreatic diversion with duodenal switch: an alternative approach to super-super morbid obesity [abstract]. Surg Endosc 2002;16:S069.

[44] Nocca D. A prospective multicenter study of 163 sleeve gastrectomies: results at 1 and 2 years. Obes Surg 2008;18:560–5.

[45] Lee CM, Cirangle PT, Jossart GH. Vertical gastrectomy for morbid obesity in 216 patients: report of two-year results. Surg Endosc 2007;21(10):1810–6.

[46] Silecchia G, Boru C, Pecchia A, et al. Effectiveness of laparoscopic sleeve gastrectomy (first stage of biliopancreatic diversion with duodenal switch) on comorbidities in super-obese high-risk patients. Obes Surg 2006;16:1138–44.

[47] Almogy G, Crookes PF, Anthone GJ. Longitudinal gastrectomy as a treatment for the high-risk super-obese patient. Obes Surg 2004;14:492–7.

[48] Hamoui N, Anthone GJ, Kaufman HS, et al. Sleeve gastrectomy in the high-risk patient. Obes Surg 2006;16:1445–9.

[49] Moon Han SM, Kim WW, Oh JH. Results of laparoscopic sleeve gastrectomy at 1 year in morbidly obese Korean patients. Obes Surg 2005;15:1469–75.

[50] Himpens J, Dapri G, Cadiere GB. A prospective randomized study between laparoscopic gastric banding and laparoscopic isolated sleeve gastrectomy: results after 1 and 3 years. Obes Surg 2006;16(11):1450–6.

ELSEVIER
SAUNDERS

SURGICAL
CLINICS OF
NORTH AMERICA

Surg Clin N Am 88 (2008) 1009–1018

Minimally Invasive Resection of Gastrointestinal Stromal Tumors

Chirag Dholakia, MD[a], Jon Gould, MD, FACS[b],*

[a]Department of Surgery, University of Wisconsin School of Medicine and Public Health,
600 Highland Avenue, Madison, WI 53792, USA
[b]Department of Surgery, University of Wisconsin School of Medicine and Public Health,
H4/726 Clinical Science Center, 600 Highland Avenue, Madison, WI 53792, USA

Gastrointestinal stromal tumors (GISTs) are rare neoplasms, with an annual incidence of approximately 4 per million persons [1]. Historically, these tumors were classified as leiomyomas, leiomyosarcomas, and leiomyoblastomas because of a mistaken belief that they originated from smooth muscle in the bowel wall. The advent of electron microscopy and immunohistochemistry led to the realization that these tumors originate from pleuropotentail cells known as the interstitial cells of Cajal (ICCs). ICCs are located in and around the myenteric plexus and are believed to function as intestinal pacemaker cells that regulate intestinal motility. ICCs are found throughout the gastrointestinal (GI) tract [2]. The majority (approximately 95%) of GIST tumors express the CD117 antigen (KIT), a proto-oncogene product. CD34 is a commonly expressed human progenitor cell antigen also found in many GISTs.

GIST tumors can be found throughout the GI tract, but the stomach is the site of origin for more than 50% of these tumors [3]. Often, GISTs are asymptomatic and discovered incidentally during procedures, such as endoscopy or CT scanning, done for other reasons. The most common symptoms related to GISTs depend somewhat on their site of origin but include bleeding/anemia and abdominal pain [4,5].

It is difficult to determine whether or not an isolated primary GIST is malignant or benign. It is more appropriate to speak in terms of "malignant potential" with these tumors. The morphologic features demonstrated most predictive of recurrence or metastases are tumor size and mitotic rate. The site of origin also is relevant when discussing prognosis. Unfortunately,

---

* Corresponding author.
E-mail address: gould@surgery.wisc.edu (J. Gould).

doi:10.1016/j.suc.2008.05.006

GISTs are unpredictable and occasionally small tumors or tumors with a low mitotic index can recur or metastasize. Several classification schemes for determining the malignant potential of a GIST are proposed. The system used most commonly was developed during a consensus GIST workshop convened by the National Institutes of Health in 2001 [6]. According to this classification scheme, tumors are classified as very low risk, low risk, intermediate risk, or high risk for aggressive behavior depending on size and mitotic index (Table 1).

Historically, treatment of nonmetastatic GISTs has been surgical. DeMatteo and colleagues [7] demonstrated that the status of the microscopic margin of resection did not affect survival. Lymph node metastasis are extremely rare for GISTs, and routine lymphadenectomy is not warranted. These factors have provided oncologic justification for minimally invasive resection techniques with gross margins for GISTs. Minimally invasive resection provides certain advantages to patients in terms of morbidity and recovery. A variety of endoscopic, laparoscopic, and hybrid techniques are described for surgically excising GISTs in different anatomic locations.

Evaluation of GISTs before resection is somewhat dependant on the site of origin. The goals of the preoperative evaluation are to confirm the diagnosis of GIST (or at least increase the certainty of this diagnosis as much as possible before resection), to evaluate for resectability of the primary lesion, and to determine if metastatic disease is present. Endoscopic ultrasound (EUS) is a highly sensitive and accurate means of evaluating GISTs [8]. When coupled with ultrasound-guided fine needle aspiration (FNA), the sensitivity, specificity, and diagnostic accuracy are demonstrated as good when compared with surgically resected specimens [9]. Cells attained on EUS-FNA can be analyzed for cytology and tumor markers, securely differentiating these lesions from other tumors before surgery in many cases [10].

Esophagus

GISTs may occur anywhere in the tubular GI tract, even in extra-GI locations, such as the retroperitoneum, omentum, or mesentery. Of the

Table 1
Risk stratification for gastrointestinal stromal tumors

	Size	Mitotic count
Very low risk	<2 cm	<5/50 HPF
Low risk	2–5 cm	<5/50 HPF
Intermediate risk	<5 cm	6–10/50 HPF
	5–10 cm	<5/50 HPF
High risk	>5 cm	>5/50 HPF
	>10 cm	Any mitotic rate
	Any size	>10/50 HPF

Abbreviation: HPF, high power field.

potential sites for these tumors in the GI tract, the esophagus is among the least common locations, with an overall incidence of approximately 5% in large series [11]. Esophageal GISTs typically are located in the mid to distal third of the esophagus, and usually are small. Larger tumors may lead to dysphagia as a presenting symptom. These neoplasms usually are found incidentally on barium swallow studies, echocardiograms, CT scans, or on upper endoscopy. On endoscopy, esophageal GISTs appear as smooth, submucosal lesions. EUS and EUS-FNA can help differentiate esophageal GISTs from other esophageal tumors and masses. Blum and colleagues [12] recently reported their experience with the treatment of four patients who had submucosal lesions of the esophagus over a 4-year period. All lesions were biopsied with EUS-FNA performed before resection. Immunohistochemistry analysis of all four FNA aspirates was consistent with GIST in each specimen. At a median follow-up of 33 months, all four patients were alive; however, two of four patients had experienced a local recurrence. These investigators recommend esophagectomy rather than enucleation and believed that in selected patients, preoperative targeted therapy with imatinib may improve resectability. In their published manuscript, Blum's group reviewed the literature and found seven single case reports of esophageal GIST. Of these seven tumors resected by enucleation or esophagectomy, none had recurred after a median follow-up of 3 years. Few published reports of minimally invasive resection of esophageal GISTs exist. Ertem and colleagues [13] reported a thoracoscopic enucleation of an 8.5-cm esophageal GIST. The case went well and follow-up was limited to the 8 days after surgery. Given recent advances in minimally invasive esophagectomy and in thoracoscopy, it seems reasonable for experienced esophageal surgeons to consider a minimally invasive approach to an esophageal GIST.

Stomach

In large clinical series, the stomach is the site of origin for GISTs in approximately 40% to 60% of cases, making gastric GISTs far more common than GISTs originating from other sites [3,7]. Most lesions of the stomach are asymptomatic and discovered incidentally. Acute GI bleeding or chronic iron deficiency anemia is common among lesions with a symptomatic presentation [4]. EUS and EUS-FNA are useful tests for confirming the diagnosis of a gastric GIST preoperatively. On EUS, gastric GISTs appear as smooth submucosal lesions originating from the muscularis propria. EUS-guided FNA can help increase the diagnostic accuracy and preoperative certainty that the gastric lesion in question most likely is a GIST. CT scans before surgery can evaluate for metastatic disease. Based on the size and location of suspected GISTs, a variety of minimally invasive techniques can be used for resection.

Laparoscopic wedge, sleeve, or partial gastrectomy with grossly negative margins for amenable tumors is becoming the preferred approach. Yoshida and colleagues [14] first proposed laparoscopic wedge resection for gastric leiomyosarcomas in the mid 1990s. Between 1993 and 1997, this group performed 34 laparoscopic wedge gastric resections for lesions ranging from 8 to 60 mm. Over the 5-year follow-up period of the study, there were no recurrences [15].

Laparoscopic, stapled wedge gastric resections of greater and lesser curve lesions remote from the gastroesophageal (GE) junction and pylorus are relatively straightforward. During surgery, it is important to avoid manipulating the tumor, especially large lesions, because of the potential for tumor rupture. Intraoperative endoscopy is valuable for localizing the lesion and for confirming the integrity of staple lines after resection. For anterior lesions, seromuscular sutures proximal and distal to the lesion can help to elevate the anterior gastric wall for resection with an endoscopic linear stapler. Larger lesions can be resected with an energy source, such as an ultrasonic dissector or electrocautery. The gastrotomy then may be closed with a stapler or with sutures. Posterior lesions can be more difficult to resect. Techniques for posterior lesions include full mobilization of the greater curve, elevation, and cephalad rotation to expose the posterior stomach and then resection using techniques similar to those described previously for anterior lesions. An alternative technique involves the creation of an anterior gastrotomy over the endoscopically localized lesion. Sutures placed in the posterior gastric lumen proximal and distal to the lesion can be used to elevate the tumor through the gastrotomy, facilitating full-thickness resection with an intraluminal staple line. The anterior gastrotomy then can be closed with sutures or staples.

Endoluminal transgastric resection techniques also are described [16]. Balloon-tipped trocars can be placed directly through the anterior wall of the stomach. Combined endoscopic and laparoscopic techniques then are used to resect or, more commonly, enucleate lesions. These endoluminal gastric techniques are most appropriate for smaller lesions located in difficult locations, such as the pylorus and GE junction.

Case series documenting the feasibility and safety of laparoscopic gastric GIST resection have been published. Nguyen and colleagues [17] performed laparoscopic resection in 25 of 28 patients who had gastric GISTs. Three conversions were related to invasion into adjacent organs for a large (10-cm) lesion and proximity of the tumor to the GE junction in two cases. There were few complications and oncologic outcomes were not reported.

The outcomes after laparoscopic compared with open resection of gastric GISTs have been evaluated by a couple groups. Matthews and colleagues [18] reported their experience over 6 years in 33 patients who had gastric GISTs. Laparoscopic resections were performed in 21 and open resections in 12 patients. Tumor characteristics and demographics in each group were similar. There were no significant differences in mean operative time, blood loss, or perioperative complication rates based on surgical approach. The length of stay after laparoscopic resection was significantly shorter than after open resection (3.8 versus 6.2 days). Nishimura and colleagues [19] reviewed 67 cases of laparoscopic versus open resection of gastric GISTs over a 10-year period. Resection technique was chosen based on surgeon preference. Lesions in each group were similar in size, gastric location, and oncologic risk classification determined after resection. Operative time and blood loss did not differ between techniques. Recurrences occurred in 1 of 39 laparoscopic cases and in 4 of 28 open cases. Although this difference in recurrence rate was not statistically significant, a high recurrence rate was noted for enucleation (less than full-thickness resection) for the open and laparoscopic techniques (one recurrence in three laparoscopic enucleations and two after six open enucleations). The investigators concluded that the laparoscopic approach was preferred and that tumor enucleation should be avoided because of a high recurrence rate.

Long-term oncologic outcomes after laparoscopic resection of gastric GISTs have been reported by Novitsky and colleagues [4]. Fifty consecutive patients underwent laparoscopic or laparoendoscopic resection of gastric GISTs over a 10-year period. At a mean follow-up of 36 months, 92% of patients were disease free. Patient age, tumor size, mitotic index, tumor ulceration, and necrosis were statistically associated with recurrence. These investigators believed that the observed disease-free survival rate was comparable to that seen in series of open resection of gastric GISTs and that the laparoscopic method of resection should be the preferred approach.

Several published series specifically address resection of GE junction submucosal tumors. Song and coworkers [20] successfully performed laparoscopic wedge gastrectomies in 10 patients who had submucosal tumors located within 3 cm of the GE junction. Five of these tumors were addressed with exogastric (traditional) wedge resections. The remaining five tumors were resected using transgastric resection techniques. Transgastric resection in this series involved full-thickness excision through an anterior gastrotomy. The lesions were grasped, everted through the gastrotomy, and excised with an endoscopic stapler. There were no complications, no cases of narrowed GE junction after resection, and no recurrences at a mean 10 months' follow-up. Hiki's group [21] reported their experience with a novel technique described as laparoscopic endoscopic cooperative surgery (LECS). Seven patients, four who had GE junction submucosal tumors, underwent resection using this technique. In LECS, the mucosal and submucosal layers around the tumor are circumferentially dissected endoscopically. Next, the seromuscular stomach is dissected laparoscopically from the outside on the three-fourths cut line around the tumor. The submucosal tumor then is exteriorized and resected with a standard laparoscopic stapling device. There were no complications, and gross margins were clear. Walsh and colleagues [22] resected 14 lesions in 13 patients using combined endoscopic/laparoscopic endoluminal techniques. Resections in this series were not full thickness. These tumors ranged in size from 1.5 to 7 cm. Eight tumors were located at the GE junction. There was no operative morbidity or mortality in this series. All 14 tumors lacked any evidence of mitotic activity on final pathology. At a mean 16 months' follow-up, there were no recurrences. The long-term oncologic adequacy of less than full-thickness resections of GISTs that prove to have a moderate or high risk of recurrence is unproved. Laparoscopic enucleation of suspected GISTs is a technique that should be used with caution for this reason. Minimally invasive resection of GISTs seems feasible, safe, and effective. Morbidity and recovery may be decreased compared with standard open techniques, likely without affecting oncologic outcomes. A variety of techniques may be required to excise these tumors safely depending on size and location.

Duodenum

The duodenum is a rare primary site for GISTs (approximately 3%–5% in large series). A common presentation for duodenal GISTs is upper GI bleeding with hematemesis, melena, or chronic anemia. Many duodenal GISTs are discovered during upper endoscopy conducted to evaluate the source of bleeding. Many different surgical procedures have been described for duodenal GISTs, including pancreaticoduodenectomy, pancreas-sparing duodenectomy, segmental duodenectomy, and local resection based on the site of the tumor. Currently, there is controversy over the use of limited duodenal resection versus pancreaticoduodenectomy. Given the oncologic behavior of GISTs, extended resection with lymphadenectomy seems overly aggressive. Goh and colleagues [23] compared their experience in 22 patients who had local resection versus pancreaticoduodenectomy. Recurrence rates for duodenal GISTs in this series did not differ with either technique. All recurrences were distant, and size of the primary tumor was the only demonstrated predictor of recurrence.

Limited resection has been evaluated in many case reports revealing technical feasibility [24,25], even when the pancreatic head is involved [26]. Although laparoscopic duodenal and pancreatic head resections are described, published case reports of minimally invasive resection of duodenal GISTs do not exist at the time of this writing.

Small bowel

The jejunum and ileum is the most common nongastric site for GISTs in large series [3,7]. Common presenting symptoms include GI bleeding, abdominal pain, and small bowel obstruction. Many small bowel GISTs are asymptomatic and discovered incidentally during the course of an operation or a diagnostic evaluation being performed for another indication.

DeMatteo and colleagues [27] recently demonstrated that small bowel GISTs had a higher rate of recurrence than tumors of similar size and mitotic index originating from other GI tract sites. The predominant morphology of small bowel GISTs (paraganglioma-like with skeinoid fibers) tends to be different from that of gastric stromal tumors (predominantly epithelioid), perhaps partly accounting for small bowel GISTs having a worse prognosis than GISTs that originate elsewhere [3,28]. The recurrence rate for small bowel GISTs is high after surgical resection. In one recently published series, that recurrence rate after resection for 85 small bowel GISTs was 51.8% after a median follow-up of 33.2 months [29]. Most of these recurrences were in the form of liver metastasis. Published series of minimally invasive resection of small bowel GISTs are rare. Nguyen and colleagues [17] successfully resected 15 small bowel GISTs using laparoscopic techniques with intracorporeal or extracorporeal anastomosis. Two cases were converted to laparotomy and there were few complications. Oncologic outcomes were not determined after these resections. In 1998, Kok and colleagues [30] reported a case of a laparoscopic resection of a bleeding small bowel leiomyoma. Napolitano and colleagues [31] resected a small bowel GIST laparoscopically and reported that at 1 year postoperatively, their patient was disease free. Small bowel GISTs may be amenable to a technically successful and safe laparoscopic resection in some cases. The oncologic outcomes of this approach have yet to be determined. As for gastric GISTs, minimal manipulation and careful handling of the tumor during excision are critical.

Colon and other intra-abdominal nongastrointestinal sites

The colon is a rare site for primary GISTs. Approximately 5% of GISTs originate from the colon [7]. If the colon is involved, it often is invaded by an adjacent small bowel GIST. Primary colonic GISTs are fairly aggressive and often have metastasized at the time of diagnosis [32,33]. Extra-GI GIST tumors are rare. These tumors are histologically and immunophenotypically similar to their GI counterparts but have an aggressive course more akin to small intestinal than gastric stromal tumors [34–36]. Published reports of minimally invasive resection for colonic and extra-GI GISTs do not exist at the time of this writing.

Targeted adjuvant therapy

The discovery that mutations in the CD117 (KIT) gene caused increased KIT protein function, which drives the oncogenesis of most GISTs, was reported in 1998 [37]. Only 2 years later, imatinib mesylate (STI 571, Gleevec, Novartis Pharmaceuticals, Basel Switzerland), a potent inhibitor of KIT signaling, was first used in the care of a patient who had metastatic GIST [38]. This patient exhibited a dramatic response, and clinical trials ensued. Prospective trials have shown that approximately 50% of patients who have metastatic disease have a response to imatinib [39]. Although imatinib halts progression of disease in the majority of patients who have metastatic GIST, complete responses are rare. For this reason, imatinib should be considered an oncostatic rather than a cytotoxic agent. Stopping imatinib is associated with an increased risk for disease progression. Unfortunately, half the patients treated with imatinib for metastatic disease become resistant to this therapy within 2 years. The most common mechanism of acquired resistance is secondary KIT mutation [40]. In addition to treating metastatic disease, imatinib has been used before surgery in an attempt to shrink large tumors or tumors in precarious locations [41]. The role of imatinib as a precursor to surgical resection has yet to be defined.

Oncologic outcomes and surveillance

Many investigators have established that the risk factors for recurrence of GISTs include size, mitotic index, and tumor site of origin [1,3,4,7,27,29]. After the resection of primary GISTs, recurrence-free survival at 1, 2, and 5 years is 83%, 75%, and 63%, respectively, and is dependant on the risk factors described previously [27]. The first recurrence typically is in the abdomen with metastases to lung and bone sometimes developing later. The initial site of recurrence involves the liver in 65%, the peritoneal surfaces in 50%, and both in approximately 20% of cases [7,42]. Although there is no proof that earlier detection of recurrent GIST improves survival, targeted therapy can halt the progression of disease in most patients. It thus seems reasonable to perform routine postoperative surveillance. Most GIST recurrences occur within the first 3 to 5 years. The National Comprehensive Cancer Network guidelines recommend CT scans of the abdomen and pelvis with intravenous contrast every 3 to 6 months during this interval and yearly afterward [43].

Summary

GISTs are rare tumors. The stomach is the most common site of origin for these neoplasms. Fortunately, the prognosis is good for gastric GISTs with favorable morphology when completely resected. Most gastric GISTs are amenable to minimally invasive resection techniques, likely without compromising the oncologic outcomes. A variety of techniques can be used depending on the size and anatomic location of gastric GISTs to achieve a safe and complete resection. For gastric GISTs, minimally invasive resection techniques likely are associated with lower morbidity and quicker recovery than open techniques and are the approach of choice for most tumors.

References

[1] Miettinen M, Sarlomo-Rikala M, Lasota J. Gastrointestinal stromal tumors: recent advances in understanding of their biology. Hum Pathol 1999;30:1213–20.

[2] Kindblom LG, Remotti HE, Aldenborg F, et al. Gastrointestinal pacemaker cell tumor (GIPACT): gastrointestinal stromal tumors show phenotypic characteristics of the interstitial cells of Cajal. Am J Pathol 1998;152:1259–69.

[3] Emory TS, Sobin LH, Lukes L, et al. Prognosis of gastrointestinal smooth muscle cell (stromal) tumors: dependence on anatomic site. Am J Pathol 1999;23:82–7.

[4] Novitsky YW, Kercher KW, Sing RF, et al. Long-term outcomes of laparoscopic resection of gastric gastrointestinal stromal tumors. Ann Surg 2006;243:738–47.

[5] Nguyen SQ, Divino CM, Wang JL, et al. Laparoscopic management of gastrointestinal stromal tumors. Surg Endosc 2006;20:713–6.

[6] Fletcher CD, Berman JJ, Corless C, et al. Diagnosis of gastrointestinal Stromal tumors: a consensus approach. Hum Pathol 2002;33(5):459–65.

[7] DeMatteo RP, Lewis JJ, Leung D, et al. Two hundred gastrointestinal stromal tumors—recurrence patterns and prognostic factors for survival. Ann Surg 2000;231(1):51–8.

[8] Boyce GA, Sivak MV, Rosch T, et al. Evaluation of submucosal upper gastrointestinal tract lesions with ultrasound. Gastrointest Endosc 1991;37:449–54.

[9] Akahosi K, Sumida Y, Matsui N, et al. Preoperative diagnosis of gastrointestinal stromal tumor by endoscopic ultrasound guided fine needle aspiration. World J Gastroenterol 2007;13(14):2077–82.

[10] Rader AE, Avery A, Wait CL, et al. Fine-needle aspiration biopsy diagnosis of gastrointestinal stromal tumors using morphology, immunocytochemistry, and mutational analysis of c-kit. Cancer 2001;93(4):269–75.

[11] Miettinen M, Sarlomo-Rikala M, Sobin LH, et al. Esophageal stromal tumors: a clinicopathologic, immunohistochemical and molecular genetic study of 17 cases and comparison with esophageal leiomyomas and leiomyosarcomas. Am J Surg Pathol 2000;24:211–22.

[12] Blum MG, Bilimora KY, Wayne JD, et al. Surgical considerations for the management and resection of esophageal gastrointestinal stromal tumors. Ann Thorac Surg 2007;84(5): 1717–23.

[13] Ertem M, Baca B, Doğusoy G, et al. Thoracoscopic enucleation of a giant submucosal tumor of the esophagus. Surg Laparosc Endosc Percutan Tech 2004;14(2):87–90.

[14] Yoshida M, Otani Y, Ohgami M, et al. Surgical management of gastric leiomyosarcoma: evaluation of the propriety of laparoscopic wedge resection. World J Surg 1997;21(4):440–3.

[15] Otani Y, Ohgami M, Igarashi N, et al. Laparoscopic wedge resection of gastric submucosal tumors. Surg Laparosc Endosc Percutan Tech 2000;10(1):19–23.

[16] Rosen M, Heniford BT. Endoluminal gastric surgery: the modern era of minimally invasive surgery. Surg Clin North Am 2005;85:989–1007.

[17] Nguyen SQ, Divino CM, Wang JL, et al. Laparoscopic management of gastrointestinal tumors. Surg Endosc 2006;20:713–6.

[18] Matthews BD, Walsh RM, Kercher KW, et al. Laparoscopic vs. open resection of gastric stromal tumors. Surg Endosc 2002;16:803–7.

[19] Nishimura J, Nakajima K, Omori T, et al. Surgical strategy for gastric gastrointestinal tumors: laparoscopic vs. open resection. Surg Endosc 2007;21(6):875–8.

[20] Song KY, Kim SN, Park CH. Tailored approach of laparoscopic wedge resection for treatment of submucosal tumor near the esophagogastric junction. Surg Endosc 2007;21(12):2272–6.

[21] Hiki N, Yamamoto Y, Fukunaga T, et al. Laparoscopic and endoscopic cooperative surgery for gastrointestinal stromal tumor dissection. Surg Endosc 2007;22:729–35.

[22] Walsh R, Ponsky J, Brody F, et al. Combined endoscopic/laparoscopic intragastric resection of gastric stromal tumors. J Gastrointest Surg 2003;7:386–92.

[23] Goh BK, Chow PK, Kesavan S, et al. Outcome after surgical treatment of suspected gastrointestinal stromal tumors involving the duodenum: is limited resection appropriate? J Surg Oncol 2007;97:388–91.

[24] Goh BK, Chow PK, Ong HS, et al. Gastrointestinal stromal tumor involving the second and third part of the duodenum: treatment by Roux-en-Y duodenojejeunostomy. J Surg Oncol 2005;91(4):273–5.

[25] De Nicola P, Di Bartolomeo N, Francomano F, et al. Segmental resection of the third and fourth portions of the duodenum after intestinal derotation for a GIST: a case report. Suppl Tumori 2005;4(3):S108–10.

[26] Sakamoto Y, Yamamoto J, Takahashi H, et al. Segmental resection of the third portion of the duodenum for a gastrointestinal stromal tumor: a case report. Jpn J Clin Oncol 2003;33: 364–6.

[27] DeMatteo RP, Gold JS, Saran L, et al. Tumor mitotic rate, size, and location independently predict recurrence after resection of primary gastrointestinal stromal tumor (GIST). Cancer 2007;112:608–15.

[28] Min KW. Small intestinal stromal tumors with skeinoid fibers. Clinicopathological, immunohistochemical and ultrastructural investigations. Am J Surg Pathol 1992;16:145–55.

[29] Wu TJ, Lee LY, Yeh CN, et al. Surgical treatment and prognostic analysis for gastrointestinal stromal tumors (GISTs) of the small intestine: before the era of imatinib mesylate. BMC Gastroenterol 2006;24:6–29.

[30] Kok KY, Mathew VV, Yapp SK. Laparoscopic-assisted bowel resection for a bleeding leiomyoma. Surg Endosc 1998;12:995–6.

[31] Napolitano L, Waku M, De Nicola P, et al. Surgical laparoscopic therapy of small bowel tumors: review of the literature and report of two cases. G Chir 2004;25:235–7.

[32] Tworek JA, Goldblum JR, Weiss SW, et al. Stromal tumors of the abdominal colon: a clinicopathologic study of 20 cases. Am J Surg Pathol 1999;23:937–45.

[33] Tworek JA, Goldblum JR, Weiss SW, et al. Stromal tumors of the anorectum: a clinicopathologic study of 22 cases. Am J Surg Pathol 1999;23:946–54.

[34] Miettinen M, Monihan JM, Sarlomo-Rikala M, et al. Gastrointestinal stromal tumors/smooth muscle tumors (GISTs) primary in the omentum and mesentery: clinicopathologic and immunohistochemical study of 26 cases. Am J Surg Pathol 1999;23:1109–18.

[35] Reith JD, Goldblum JR, Lytes RH, et al. Extragastrointestinal (soft tissue) stromal tumors: an analysis of 48 cases with emphasis on histologic predictors of outcome. Mod Pathol 2000; 13:577–85.

[36] Weiss SW, Goldblum JR. Extragastrointestinal stromal tumors. In: Weiss SW, Goldblum JR, editors. Enzinger and Weiss's soft tissue tumors. 4th edition. St. Louis (MO): Mosby; 2001. p. 749–68.

[37] Hirota S, Isozaki K, Moriyama Y, et al. Gain-of-function mutations of c-kit in human gastrointestinal stromal tumors. Science 1998;279:577–80.

[38] Joensuu H, Roberts PJ, Sarlomo-Rikala M, et al. Effect of the tyrosine kinase inhibitor STI571 in a patient with a metastatic gastrointestinal stromal tumor. N Engl J Med 2001; 344:1052–6.

[39] Gold JS, DeMatteo RP. Combined surgical and molecular therapy: the gastrointestinal stromal tumor model. Ann Surg 2006;244:176–84.

[40] Chen LL, Trent JC, Wu EF, et al. A missense mutation in KIT kinase domain 1 correlates with imatinib resistance in gastrointestinal stromal tumors. Cancer Res 2004;64:5913–9.

[41] Gronchi A, Fiore M, Miselli F, et al. Surgery of residual disease following molecular-targeting therapy with imatinib mesylate in advanced/metastatic GIST. Ann Surg 2007;245(3): 341–6.

[42] Crosby JA, Catton CN, Davis A, et al. Malignant gastrointestinal stromal tumors of the small intestine: a review of 50 cases from a prospective database. Ann Surg Oncol 2001;8: 50–9.

[43] Demetri GD, Benjamin R, Blanke CD, et al. Optimal management of patients with gastrointestinal stromal tumors (GIST): expansion and update of NCCN clinical practice guidelines. Journal of the National Comprehensive Cancer Network 2004;2(Suppl 1):1–26.

ELSEVIER
SAUNDERS

Surg Clin N Am 88 (2008) 1019–1031

SURGICAL
CLINICS OF
NORTH AMERICA

Choledocholithiasis, Endoscopic Retrograde Cholangiopancreatography, and Laparoscopic Common Bile Duct Exploration

Matthew Kroh, MD, Bipan Chand, MD*

*Department of General Surgery, Cleveland Clinic Lerner College of Medicine,
9500 Euclid Avenue, M61, Cleveland, OH 44106, USA*

The successful introduction of laparoscopic cholecystectomy by Muhe in 1985 ushered in a new era of management of gallbladder and biliary disease [1]. Several trials have borne out the advantages of laparoscopy, including shorter hospitalizations, quicker return to work, decreased complications, and less postoperative pain. Despite initial skepticism, the overwhelming success of laparoscopic cholecystectomy has become a platform for an ever-expanding body of minimally invasive procedures. As technology and instrumentation have improved, so have the complexity of operations that can be performed in a minimally invasive way. This evolution also is manifest in approaches to management of choledocholithiasis.

Before the laparoscopic era, intraoperative cholangiography was performed routinely and common bile duct stones diagnosed at this time were dealt with by open duct exploration. Routine intraoperative cholangiography currently is not a part of most laparoscopic surgeons' techniques. A selective approach to intraoperative cholangiography during laparoscopic cholecystectomy has been shown to be safe when the ductal anatomy is defined clearly and there is no laboratory or clinical evidence of common bile duct abnormalities [2]. Some investigators assert, however, that routine cholangiography should be performed for evaluation of occult stones and to improve techniques for laparoscopic common bile duct exploration if needed [3].

* Corresponding author.
E-mail address: chandb@ccf.org (B. Chand).

0039-6109/08/$ - see front matter © 2008 Elsevier Inc. All rights reserved.
doi:10.1016/j.suc.2008.05.004   *surgical.theclinics.com*

Significant advances in endoscopic techniques for stone removal also have occurred and are commonplace. Endoscopic retrograde cholangiopancreatography (ERCP) is a successful approach to stone clearance and proposed by many as appropriate for management of pre- and postoperatively discovered choledocholithiasis [4–13]. In addition to endoscopic sphincterotomy, an ever-widening array of endoscopic baskets, balloons, and lithotripsy devices exist for stone removal.

As experience has accrued and instrumentation improved, laparoscopic approaches to choledocholithiasis also have evolved. Such techniques include transcystic stone removal, laparoscopic choledochotomy with stone extraction, and transcystic stenting followed by postoperative ERCP. Some surgeons propose using intraoperative ERCP in combination with laparoscopy [14,15].

With the litany of advances in laparoscopy and endoscopy, much has improved regarding management of choledocholithiasis. Controversy exists, however, regarding which of the appropriate interventions should be used in different clinical scenarios. This article examines the different approaches currently available to remove common bile duct stones, with an examination of the literature supporting different approaches and the techniques involved.

Indications for preoperative endoscopic retrograde cholangiopancreatography

Before the advent of laparoscopy, preoperative clearance of common bile duct stones with ERCP before open exploration was uncommon. Several well-performed studies did not demonstrate any improvement in morbidity or mortality with preoperative endoscopic sphincterotomy [16–18]. One study demonstrated an increase in morbidity when preoperative ERCP with sphincterotomy was added to open cholecystectomy compared with cholecystectomy and open common bile duct exploration [18]. Largely based on these studies, preoperative ERCP with sphincterotomy was uncommon in the era of open cholecystectomy and it did not become more widespread until laparoscopic approaches to cholecystectomy appeared.

When laparoscopic cholecystectomy was introduced, preoperative ERCP was used frequently for patients suspected of having choledocholithiasis [19–23]. This strategy was in large part due to unfamiliarity of most surgeons with the advanced laparoscopic techniques necessary for common bile duct exploration coupled with the high success of endoscopic extraction, with rates of clearance approaching 90% [19–21,24]. Patients who presented with jaundice, elevated cholestatic liver function tests, a history of pancreatitis, or a dilated biliary system on radiographic imaging were considered candidates for preoperative ERCP. Even with these criteria, however, it is difficult to predict which patients have choledocholithiasis. The majority of patients who had these abnormalities did not have common bile duct stones at the time of ERCP. Using these selective criteria, a negative preoperative ERCP is performed in 40% to 70% of patients. Most of these abnormalities were caused by transient biliary obstruction secondary to stones that subsequently passed into the duodenum [18–21,25].

Performing ERCP has clinical and financial costs and must be weighed against the likelihood of successful extraction of stones that otherwise would result in significant disease manifestation. Complications, including postprocedural pancreatitis, bleeding, infections, and perforations, are not uncommon. ERCP has an overall complication rate of 10%, serious morbidity of 1.5%, and mortality rate of less than 0.5% [19–24,26]. A recent systemic analysis of prospective studies has shown that complications continue to occur at a relatively consistent rate and that the majority of events are of mild-to-moderate severity [27]. These rates are increased in high risk, elderly patients. Laparoscopic cholecystectomy has is shown, however, to have increased morbidity in older patients and those who have pre-existing medical risk factors [28].

Additionally, the financial cost of a diagnostic ERCP is substantial. Several studies have demonstrated increased direct costs, total hospital costs, and increased length of stay in patients undergoing ERCP with sphincterotomy compared with patients undergoing laparoscopic cholecystectomy with common bile duct exploration [29–31]. Liberman and colleagues [30] conducted a retrospective study of 76 patients undergoing transcystic laparoscopic common bile duct exploration or laparoscopic cholecystectomy plus ERCP for urgent and elective management of choledocholithiasis. They found that patients undergoing laparoscopic common bile exploration for common bile duct stones, in urgent and elective situations, have markedly decreased morbidity rates, length of hospital stay, and costs compared with patients undergoing laparoscopic cholecystectomy and endoscopic sphincterotomy. The cost of treatment for patients undergoing single-stage therapy was $14,732 compared with $21,125 for patients undergoing laparoscopic cholecystectomy and ERCP with endoscopic sphincterotomy ($P<.05$).

There are indications in which preoperative ERCP should be implemented. Preoperative endoscopic drainage should be used in acute cholangitis for decompression and amelioration of sepsis [4]. A randomized trial from Hong Kong found 34% morbidity and 10% mortality rates in 41 patients who underwent endoscopic decompression compared with 66% morbidity and 32% mortality rates in patients who underwent primary surgical therapy [32].

Severe gallstone pancreatitis is another indication for ERCP with endoscopic sphincterotomy and decompression [4]. A prospective randomized control trial of urgent ERCP with sphincterotomy versus conservative management in patients predicted to have severe gallstone pancreatitis demonstrated a mortality rate of 4% in patients undergoing ERCP with decompression versus 24% in the conservative group [17]. Patients were stratified by predicted severity of the attack, according to the modified Glasgow system. ERCP was done within 72 hours, and if common bile duct stones were identified, patients underwent sphincterotomy immediately to extract the stones. There were fewer complications in the patients who underwent ERCP than among those treated conventionally, the difference confined to those patients whose attacks were predicted to be severe compared with conventional treatment. Hospital stay also was shorter for patients who had severe attacks and who underwent ERCP and sphincterotomy than for those who received conservative treatment. Preoperative ERCP also should be considered if the diagnosis is uncertain as in cases of persistent, severe hyperbilirubinemia when stricture and neoplasm cannot be ruled out.

Two prospective randomized controlled trials have been performed to compare preoperative ERCP with sphincterotomy followed by laparoscopic cholecystectomy during the same hospital admission with single-stage laparoscopic management [4,33]. The results demonstrate equivalent success rates of duct clearance and patient morbidity for the two management options. A significantly shorter hospital stay was demonstrated with simultaneous laparoscopic cholecystectomy and common bile duct exploration. In one of these studies, Cuschieri and colleagues [4] conclude that in fit patients (American Society of Anesthesiologists physical status I and II), single-stage laparoscopic treatment is the better option, and preoperative ERCP with sphincterotomy should be confined to poor-risk patients, such as those who have cholangitis or severe pancreatitis.

Intraoperative techniques for stone removal

Laparoscopic cholecystectomy has replaced open cholecystectomy in most elective instances and surgeons have developed a significant experience with surgical techniques, including intraoperative cholangiography. As skills have improved, less reliance is placed on preoperative endoscopic sphincterotomy. Surgeons should learn techniques of laparoscopic common bile duct exploration to allow definitive management during one procedure. If successful, this also circumvents the known morbidity and cost of ERCP and sphincterotomy.

The first requirement for successful removal of common bile duct stones is a good cholangiogram that clearly identifies the biliary anatomy. Attention must be paid to evaluating the intra- and extrahepatic biliary tree, including anomalies, flow of contrast into the duodenum, and any filling defects. The technique of performing intraoperative cholangiography is important. Although accuracy of detecting common bile duct stones is high [34], anatomic variants of the biliary tree are common and have the possibility of being misread. It is imperative for surgeons to understand fluoroscopic appearances of filling defects that are secondary to stones and air bubbles or biliary strictures. Successful performance of intraoperative cholangiography by experienced surgeons occurs in greater than 95% of cases [35,36].

Routine cholangiography is used by surgeons in elective laparoscopic cholecystectomy to varying degrees, with published reports of its use ranging from 37% to 67% in two international surveys [37,38]. In addition to cholangiography, laparoscopic ultrasound is shown effective at identifying common bile duct stones [39]. Among patients who have choledocholithiasis, however, 10% to 12% are asymptomatic and do not have alterations in liver function tests [40,41]. If not used as part of routine cholecystectomy, cholangiography should be performed in the settings of elevated liver function tests, a history of gallstone pancreatitis, or a dilated biliary system on preoperative imaging. After performance of intraoperative cholangiography, stone architecture is important. Stones should be noted for their size, location, and number to plan for successful extraction. Ultimately, clearance depends on the stone characteristics, resources available to surgeons, and surgeon expertise.

Laparoscopic transcystic removal

Transcystic common bile duct stone extraction is shown highly effective and has the advantage of avoiding choledochotomy and subsequent suture repair [6–8,10,12,42]. Depending on stone characteristics and surgeon experience, most cases of choledocholithiasis can be managed via the cystic duct. In a study of 300 consecutive patients discovered to have choledocholithiasis, Nathanson and colleagues [43] were able to clear two thirds transcystically, with the remainder undergoing choledochotomy. After successfully obtaining a quality cholangiogram and interpreting it correctly, access to the cystic duct and biliary system must be evaluated. Placement of an additional 5 mm trocar or a separate stab incision for catheter placement may be beneficial for manipulation of instruments and better access to the ductotomy. If the ductotomy made for the cholangiogram is too small, this may need to be extended. Once the biliary system is accessed, the first maneuver is to flush the cholangiocatheter with saline. This often is successful for small stones, approximately 4 mm or less. A greater success rate can be achieved with prior administration of intravenous glucagon, which promotes relaxation of the sphincter of Oddi, and flushing with 1% lidocaine [44]. This sequence should be performed under real-time fluoroscopic imaging.

Failure of this technique should prompt re-evaluation of stone characteristics. Mobile stones that are small enough to retrieve through the cystic duct can be removed by insertion of a wire basket, with retrograde extraction. Often, however, transcystic duct techniques require dilation of the cystic duct with balloon dilators to allow for percutaneous access and retrieval of stones. The cystic duct usually can be dilated to 5 to 7 mm, always in a controlled manner, and never should be dilated larger than the diameter of the common bile duct. Larger stones may be crushed with a lithotripsy device before attempts at removal. After cystic duct dilation and fracture of large calculi, additional attempts at fluoroscopic wire basket stone removal are performed. Biliary balloon catheters also can be used during transcystic explorations. The major limitation of balloon use is the potential to drag stones into the common hepatic duct, making extraction more difficult from a transcystic approach. Caution should be used with attempts at ante-grade propulsion of stones into the duodenum with balloon catheters because injury, bleeding, and pancreatitis can occur at the sphincter of Oddi. If this technique is used, ampullary balloon dilatation ought to be performed first.

Some surgeons routinely use a choledochoscope via the cystic duct. A 3-mm scope can be advanced and allows for direct visualization, wire basket manipulation, and retrieval of stones. In experienced hands, this technique is successful in 80% to 90% of patients [45,46]. An additional advantage of the choledochoscope is postprocedural surveillance to ensure complete clear-ance of the biliary tree. A disadvantage of this technique is difficulty in examining and extracting stones from the proximal common bile duct.

Transcystic common bile duct exploration has proved efficacious, although technically demanding and often time consuming [5–7,23,25,42]. Availability of a laparoscopic cart with common bile duct exploration in-struments is helpful, as this equipment is not used routinely and decreases delays and frustration when common bile duct stones are encountered. Sur-gical equipment companies also have created self-contained, single-use kits that are widely available. Long-term outcome data examining transcystic laparoscopic common bile duct explorations have demonstrated low rates of retained stones without stricturing of the biliary system [47].

Laparoscopic choledochotomy

Failure of transcystic exploration necessitates a different approach. Lap-aroscopic choledochotomy and common bile duct exploration is an effective technique but requires advanced laparoscopic skills, including intracorpor-eal suturing. Studies have demonstrated success with extracting larger stones, from 10 to 15 mm, with an associated dilated common bile duct through this approach [6,8,25]. Choledochotomy also is likely more success-ful for retrieving stones that are impacted and require lithotripsy. Choledo-chotomy is contraindicated in the setting of a small caliber duct, as this is more likely to stricture after exploration.

Once an appropriate cholangiogram is performed and the stone charac-teristics and biliary anatomy are delineated, the bile duct is exposed anteri-orly by opening the peritoneum parallel to the duct. This is accomplished by dissecting from the cystic duct toward the common bile duct. Once the com-mon bile duct is exposed, its identity can be confirmed by needle aspiration of bile. Alternatively, intraoperative ultrasound can be used, which has the advantage of also imaging the common bile duct stones. Two stay sutures routinely are placed for traction, as in the open technique. A ductotomy is made with scissors anteriorly along the vertical axis, to avoid the vascular supply, and an opening created of 15 to 20 mm in length. This incision should be made only as long as the diameter of the largest stone. A catheter then is inserted through the lateral 5-mm trocar and the duct is irrigated. The authors prefer to use a 14-Fr red rubber catheter. Firm flushing at this point often clears the duct. A guide wire then is inserted and passed into the duodenum under fluoroscopy. A balloon catheter is fed over the guide wire and passed proximal and distal through the duct to clear the stones. Fluoroscopic imaging should be performed throughout these maneuvers. A choledochoscope then is advanced into the bile duct to confirm complete clearance of all stones and debris.

After choledochotomy, consideration is made as to whether or not a T tube should be placed. Some surgeons place them routinely, whereas others use a selective approach. If a selective approach is used, common bile duct size is the main determinant. An appropriately sized T tube, usually between 10 and 14 French, then is inserted into the common bile duct. The choledochotomy is closed with interrupted, absorbable sutures. A completion cholangiogram is performed through the T tube to confirm no filling defects and no leak from the choledochotomy. In experienced hands, success rates are high, with some reports of rates greater than 90% [48]. Morbidity rates in this large series were reported as 8% and mortality 1%. This technique is successful for larger stones in the setting of a dilated common bile duct but requires advanced laparoscopic skills. Failures of laparoscopic choledochotomy can be managed by conversion to laparotomy with common bile duct exploration or postoperative ERCP with sphincterotomy. Published reports consistently demonstrate excellent results of laparoscopic common bile duct exploration, by transcystic approach and choledochotomy. These results are, however, generally from larger centers with higher volumes and are performed by surgeons who have expertise in laparoscopy. There are few data that examine advanced laproscopic procedures performed by less experienced surgeons [13].

What role does endoscopic retrograde cholangiopancreatography play in stone removal?

Reports vary widely, but 5% to 18% of patients undergoing cholecystectomy for gallstones have common bile duct stones. Treatment options for these stones include pre-, intra-, or postoperative endoscopic ERCP or open or laparoscopic surgery. Two prospective, randomized studies exist that evaluated intraoperative laparoscopic techniques versus postoperative ERCP with sphincterotomy for management of common bile duct stones. Rhodes and colleagues [49] in 1998 identified 80 patients discovered during intraoperative cholangiography to have common bile duct stones. These patients then were randomized to laparoscopic common bile duct exploration or postoperative ERCP with sphincterotomy. Patients were excluded from this study if they had undergone preoperative sphincterotomy, cholangitis, or acute pancreatitis. Primary duct clearance in both treatment groups after the first attempt was 75%. Patients in the laparoscopic group who failed this initial attempt then underwent open exploration or postoperative ERCP. Those patients randomized to postoperative ERCP underwent repeat procedures as necessary for complete duct clearance. No significant differences existed in morbidity and mortality between the study groups. Hospital stay, however, was a median of 1 day (range 1–26) in the laparoscopic group compared with 3.5 days (range 1–11) in the ERCP group ($P = .0001$; 95% CI, 1–2).

The other prospective study was conducted by Nathanson and colleagues [43] and evaluated patients having laparoscopic cholecystectomy who had failed transcystic duct clearance of bile duct stones. In seven hospitals, after failed transcystic duct clearance, 86 patients were randomized intraoperatively to have laparoscopic choledochotomy or postoperative ERCP. Their exclusion criteria were prior ERCP, severe cholangitis or acute pancreatitis requiring immediate decompression, common bile duct diameter of less than 7-mm diameter, or if biliary-enteric bypass was required in addition to stone clearance. Total operative time was less than 11 minutes longer in the choledochotomy group (158.8 minutes), with slightly shorter hospital stays of 6.4 days versus 7.7 days. Bile leak occurred in 14.6% of those having choledochotomy. Similar rates of pancreatitis (7.3% versus 8.8%), retained stones (2.4% versus 4.4%), reoperation (7.3% versus 6.6%), and overall morbidity (17% versus 13%) were observed in the choledochotomy versus ERCP groups. The investigators recommend avoidance of choledochotomy in ducts less than 7 mm and in inflamed friable tissues that might hamper an adequate dissection. They advocate choledochotomy as a good choice for patients who have postsurgical anatomy that would impair endoscopic access or previously failed ERCP access or when long delays would occur for patient transfer to other locations for the ERCP.

In 2006, a Cochrane database review was conducted to evaluate management of common bile duct stones by four different approaches: ERCP versus open surgical bile duct clearance, preoperative ERCP versus laparoscopic bile duct clearance, postoperative ERCP versus laparoscopic bile duct clearance, and ERCP versus laparoscopic bile duct clearance in patients who had previous cholecystectomy [50]. Included for analysis were 13 trials that randomized a total of 1351 patients. Eight trials (n = 760) compared ERCP with open surgical clearance, three (n = 425) compared preoperative ERCP with laparoscopic clearance, and two (n = 166) compared postoperative ERCP with laparoscopic clearance. There were no trials of ERCP versus laparoscopic clearance in patients who did not have an intact gallbladder. These studies conclude that in the era of open cholecystectomy, open common bile duct exploration was superior to ERCP in achieving common bile duct stone clearance. In the laparoscopic era, no significant difference between laparoscopic and ERCP clearance of common bile duct stones is clear. Additionally, they found that the use of ERCP necessitates an increased number of procedures per patient. Large and multiple stones found during laparoscopy may require multiple endoscopic procedures over a long course of time, with attendant risks, and may be dealt with best at the time of operation [19–23].

Intraoperative endoscopic retrograde cholangiopancreatography

Intraoperative ERCP is an effective method for dealing with common bile duct stones, especially stones found in the common hepatic or intrahepatic system [14,51]. The logistics of arranging this technique, however, limit its application. This requires the transport of endoscopic equipment, including fluoroscopy, into the operating room, and the presence of an endoscopist skilled in ERCP. Supine positioning of patients for laparoscopic surgery does make ERCP more difficult. This approach is dependent on many variables but results from certain centers have shown clearance rates of greater than 90% with minimal morbidity [51,52]. Intraoperative ERCP and sphincterotomy with simultaneous laparoscopic cholecystectomy also did not increase length of stay compared with laparoscopic cholecystectomy alone.

Some investigators have suggested antegrade transcystic passage of a sphincterotome to the ampulla guided by endoscopic visualization from the duodenum [15]. Once properly positioned, the sphincterotome cuts the sphincter under endoscopic direction, releasing stones into the duodenum. Another method involves laparoscopic transcystic passage of a guide wire into the duodenum, traversing the obstructing stone and sphincter. Once passed, an endoscopist grasps the wire with a snare, pulling the wire out through the working channel, through the patient's mouth. A sphincterotome then is advanced over the wire through the working channel in the usual manner. Stones then can be removed endoscopically using a basket or balloon catheter. Known commonly as the "rendezvous technique," this combined, simultaneous endoscopic and laparoscopic approach is feasible and successful although requiring significant coordination of equipment and additional personnel.

Postoperative endoscopic retrograde cholangiopancreatography

The decision to defer common bile duct stones discovered during laparoscopy to postoperative management is made by a surgeon intraoperatively. Postoperative ERCP is highly successful and the majority of stones can be dealt with endoscopically [28]. Many stones discovered in the operating room, however, turn out to be asymptomatic and routine postoperative ERCP for all common bile duct stones adds additional morbidity and mortality in addition to expense and prolonged hospital stay. A prospective, randomized study by Chang and colleagues [53] examined a series of patients who had gallstone pancreatitis and were at high risk for persistent common bile duct stones. Their criteria included common bile duct greater than 8 mm or elevated bilirubin or amylase. Patients were randomized to routine preoperative ERCP followed by laparoscopic cholecystectomy or laparoscopic cholecystectomy with selective postoperative ERCP and sphincterotomy only if a common bile duct stone was present on intraoperative cholangiogram. They found that in patients who had gallstone pancreatitis, selective postoperative ERCP and stone extraction is associated with a shorter hospital stay, less cost, no increase in combined treatment failure rate, and significant reduction in ERCP use compared with routine preoperative ERCP.

Martin and colleagues [50] in their review of two randomized trials comparing single stage laparoscopic therapy with postoperative ERCP found that clearance rates are equal with no significant difference in morbidity and mortality. Laparoscopic trials reported shorter hospital stays, however, and insufficient data were reported for cost analysis. Postoperative ERCP is a successful technique and a reasonable option in circumstances where definitive surgical therapy, laparoscopic or open, is unavailable.

Laparoscopic transcystic drainage and postoperative endoscopic retrograde cholangiopancreatography

Retained common bile duct stones left in place after laparoscopic cholecystectomy have the potential to create complications including jaundice, cholangitis, and obstruction leading to cystic duct stump leaks. With this strategy, a surgeon is relying on the successful endoscopic management of these stones. An alternative has been suggested to more safely bridge the time from surgery to endoscopic therapy and avoid these untoward complications. One such technique is laparoscopic transcystic drainage followed by postoperative ERCP. After unsuccessful laparoscopic management of choledocholithiasis, a tube is placed transcystically into the common bile duct. After securing the cystic duct to the tube, it is externalized in a fashion similar to a T tube. Left to gravity drainage, this provides decompression of the biliary system. A wire then can be passed under fluoroscopy through this drain and into the duodenum. This facilitates endoscopic access, allowing the duct to be swept free of stones. Once the duct is cleared, the drain is capped and removed in 3 to 4 weeks, after the tract has matured.

Transcystic stenting and postoperative endoscopic retrograde cholangiopancreatography

Similar to the technique described previously, Rhodes and colleagues [9] initially described transcystic stenting and postoperative ERCP. After detection of choledocholithiasis, a 7-Fr, 5-cm biliary stent is passed over a guide wire under fluoroscopic view. This is advanced through the biliary tree and partially into the duodenum, stenting the ampulla. Further endoscopic therapy can be performed on an elective basis, as normal biliary drainage is restored. This serves as an aide for endoscopists to identify and perform procedures, including sphincterotomy, and allows for continued internal drainage.

Summary

Choledocholithiasis is a common problem, present in 10% to 15% of patients undergoing laparoscopic cholecystectomy. As technology and experience have improved, the management of common bile duct stones has changed dramatically. Several of the approaches to managing choledocholithiasis are summarized in this article. Although few randomized trials exist, results of studies from the past 15 years have shown that single-procedure laparoscopic common bile duct exploration is safe and effective, especially when approached by a transcystic technique. Published reports consistently demonstrate excellent results of laparoscopic transcystic common bile duct exploration, with low morbidity and clearance rates of 80% to 90%. In more experienced hands, laparoscopic choledochotomy and stone extraction also are shown effective. Other techniques exist, including pre-, intra-, and postoperative ERCP and open common bile duct exploration. These approaches should be used as indicated by a particular clinical scenario. Individual surgeons must be aware of their capabilities to perform the safest successful operation and judicious use of available endoscopic techniques.

References

[1] Litynski GS. Erich Muhe and the rejection of laparoscopic cholecystectomy (1985): a surgeon ahead of his time. JSLS 1998;2(4):341–6.
[2] Robinson BL, Donahue JH, Gunes S, et al. Selective operative cholangiography. Appropriate management for laparoscopic cholecystectomy. Arch Surg 1995;130(6):625–30 [discussion: 630–1].
[3] Berci G. Biliary ductal anatomy and anomalies. The role of intraoperative cholangiography during laparoscopic cholecystectomy. Surg Clin North Am 1992;72(5):1069–75.
[4] Cuschieri A, Lezoche E, Morino M, et al. E.A.E.S. multicenter prospective randomized trial comparing two-stage vs single-stage management of patients with gallstone disease and ductal calculi. Surg Endosc 1999;13(10):952–7.
[5] Stoker ME. Common bile duct exploration in the era of laparoscopic surgery. Arch Surg 1995;130(3):265–8 [discussion: 268–9].
[6] Petelin JB. Laparoscopic approach to common duct pathology. Am J Surg 1993;165(4): 487–91.
[7] Carroll BJ, Phillips EH, Phillips R, et al. Update on transcystic exploration of the bile duct. Surg Laparosc Endosc 1996;6(6):453–8.
[8] Hunter JG, Soper NJ. Laparoscopic management of bile duct stones. Surg Clin North Am 1992;72(5):1077–97.
[9] Rhodes M, Nathanson L, O'Rourke N, et al. Laparoscopic exploration of the common bile duct: lessons learned from 129 consecutive cases. Br J Surg 1995;82(5):666–8.
[10] Petelin JB. Laparoscopic approach to common duct pathology. Surg Laparosc Endosc 1991; 1(1):33–41.

[11] Sackier JM, Berci G, Paz-Partlow M. Laparoscopic trancystic choledocholithotomy as an adjunct to laparoscopic cholecystectomy. Am Surg 1991;57(5):323–6.

[12] Phillips EH, Carroll BJ, Pearlstein AR, et al. Laparoscopic choledochoscopy and extraction of common bile duct stones. World J Surg 1993;17(1):22–8.

[13] Phillips EH, Toouli J, Pitt HA, et al. Treatment of common bile duct stones discovered during cholecystectomy. J Gastrointest Surg 2008;12:624–8.

[14] Deslandres E, Ganger M, Pomp A, et al. Intraoperative endoscopic sphincterotomy for common bile duct stones during laparoscopic cholecystectomy. Gastrointest Endosc 1993;39(1): 54–8.

[15] Curet MJ, Pitcher DE, Martin DT, et al. Laparoscopic antegrade sphincterotomy. A new technique for the management of complex choledocholithiasis. Ann Surg 1995;221(2):149–55.

[16] Heinerman PM, Boeckl O, Pimpl W. Selective ERCP and preoperative stone removal in bile duct surgery. Ann Surg 1989;209(3):267–72.

[17] Neoptolemos JP, Carr-Locke DL, London NJ, et al. Controlled trial of urgent endoscopic retrograde cholangiopancreatography and endoscopic sphincterotomy versus conservative treatment for acute pancreatitis due to gallstones. Lancet 1988;2(8618):979–83.

[18] Stain SC, Cohen H, Tsuishoysha M, et al. Choledocholithiasis. Endoscopic sphincterotomy or common bile duct exploration. Ann Surg 1991;213(6):627–33 [discussion: 633–4].

[19] Ponsky JL. Endoscopic management of common bile duct stones. World J Surg 1992;16(6): 1060–5.

[20] DeIorio AV Jr, Vitale GC, Reynolds M, et al. Acute biliary pancreatitis. The roles of laparoscopic cholecystectomy and endoscopic retrograde cholangiopancreatography. Surg Endosc 1995;9(4):392–6.

[21] Cotton PB. Endoscopic retrograde cholangiopancreatography and laparoscopic cholecystectomy. Am J Surg 1993;165(4):474–8.

[22] Davis WZ, Cotton PB, Arias R, et al. ERCP and sphincterotomy in the context of laparoscopic cholecystectomy: academic and community practice patterns and results. Am J Gastroenterol 1997;92(4):597–601.

[23] Cotton PB. Endoscopic management of bile duct stones; (apples and oranges). Gut 1984; 25(6):587–97.

[24] Cotton PB, Lehman G, Vennes J, et al. Endoscopic sphincterotomy complications and their management: an attempt at consensus. Gastrointest Endosc 1991;37(3):383–93.

[25] Cuschieri A, Croce E, Faggioni A, et al. EAES ductal stone study. preliminary findings of multi-center prospective randomized trial comparing two-stage vs single-stage management. Surg Endosc 1996;10(12):1130–5.

[26] Perissat J, Huibregtse K, Keane FB, et al. Management of bile duct stones in the era of laparoscopic cholecystectomy. Br J Surg 1994;81(6):799–810.

[27] Andriulli A, Loperfido S, Napolitano G, et al. Incidence rates of post-ERCP complications: a systematic survey of prospective studies. Am J Gastroenterol 2007;102(8):1781–8.

[28] Franceschi D, Brandt C, Margolin D, et al. The management of common bile duct stones in patients undergoing laparoscopic cholecystectomy. Am Surg 1993;59(8):525–32.

[29] Schroeppel TJ, Lambert PJ, Mathiason MA, et al. An economic analysis of hospital charges for choledocholithiasis by different treatment strategies. Am Surg 2007;73(5):472–7.

[30] Liberman MA, Phillips EH, Carroll BJ, et al. Cost-effective management of complicated choledocholithiasis: laparoscopic transcystic duct exploration or endoscopic sphincterotomy. J Am Coll Surg 1996;182(6):488–94.

[31] Poulose BK, Speroff T, Holzman MD. Optimizing choledocholithiasis management: a cost-effectiveness analysis. Arch Surg 2007;142(1):43–8 [discussion: 49].

[32] Lai EC, Mok FP, Tan ES, et al. Endoscopic biliary drainage for severe acute cholangitis. N Engl J Med 1992;326(24):1582–6.

[33] Sgourakis G, Karaliotas K. Laparoscopic common bile duct exploration and cholecystectomy versus endoscopic stone extraction and laparoscopic cholecystectomy for choledocholithiasis. A prospective randomized study. Minerva Chir 2002;57(4):467–74.

[34] Kitahama A, Kerstein MD, Overby JL, et al. Routine intraoperative cholangiogram. Surg Gynecol Obstet 1986;162(4):317–22.

[35] Petelin JB. Laparoscopic common bile duct exploration. Surg Endosc 2003;17(11):1705–15.

[36] Corbitt JD Jr, Leonetti LA. One thousand and six consecutive laparoscopic intraoperative cholangiograms. JSLS 1997;1(1):13–6.

[37] Dias MM, Martin CJ, Cox MR. Pattern of management of common bile duct stones in the laparoscopic era: a NSW survey. ANZ J Surg 2002;72(3):181–5.

[38] Gigot J, Etienne J, Aerts R, et al. The dramatic reality of biliary tract injury during laparoscopic cholecystectomy. An anonymous multicenter Belgian survey of 65 patients. Surg Endosc 1997;11(12):1171–8.

[39] Catheline JM, Turner R, Paries J. Laparoscopic ultrasonography is a complement to cholangiography for the detection of choledocholithiasis at laparoscopic cholecystectomy. Br J Surg 2002;89(10):1235–9.

[40] Murisona MS, Gartell PC, McGinn FP. Does selective peroperative cholangiography result in missed common bile duct stones? J R Coll Surg Edinb 1993;38(4):220–4.

[41] Rosseland AR, Glomsaker TB. Asymptomatic common bile duct stones. Eur J Gastroenterol Hepatol 2000;12(11):1171–3.

[42] Hunter JG. Laparoscopic transcystic common bile duct exploration. Am J Surg 1992;163(1): 53–6 [discussion: 57–8].

[43] Nathanson LK, O'Rourke NA, Martin IJ, et al. Postoperative ERCP versus laparoscopic choledochotomy for clearance of selected bile duct calculi: a randomized trial. Ann Surg 2005;242(2):188–92.

[44] McFarland RJ, Corbett CR, Taylor P, et al. The relaxant action of hymecromone and lignocaine on induced spasm of the bile duct sphincter. Br J Clin Pharmacol 1984;17(6):766–8.

[45] Topal B, Aerts R, Penninckx F. Laparoscopic common bile duct stone clearance with flexible choledochoscopy. Surg Endosc 2007;21(12):2317–21.

[46] Rojas-Ortega S, Arizpe-Bravo D, Martin Lopez ER, et al. Transcystic common bile duct exploration in the management of patients with choledocholithiasis. J Gastrointest Surg 2003; 7(4):492–6.

[47] Paganini AM, Guerrieri M, Sarnari J, et al. Thirteen years' experience with laparoscopic transcystic common bile duct exploration for stones. Effectiveness and long-term results. Surg Endosc 2007;21(1):34–40.

[48] Berthou J, Dron B, Charbonneau P, et al. Evaluation of laparoscopic treatment of common bile duct stones in a prospective series of 505 patients: indications and results. Surg Endosc 2007;21(11):1970–4.

[49] Rhodes M, Sussman L, Cohen L, et al. Randomised trial of laparoscopic exploration of common bile duct versus postoperative endoscopic retrograde cholangiography for common bile duct stones. Lancet 1998;351(9097):159–61.

[50] Martin DJ, Vernon DR, Toouli J. Surgical versus endoscopic treatment of bile duct stones. Cochrane Database Syst Rev 2006;(2):CD003327.

[51] Enochsson L, Lindberg B, Swahn F, et al. Intraoperative endoscopic retrograde cholangiopancreatography (ERCP) to remove common bile duct stones during routine laparoscopic cholecystectomy does not prolong hospitalization: a 2-year experience. Surg Endosc 2004; 18(3):367–71.

[52] Cox MR, Wilson TG, Toouli J. Peroperative endoscopic sphincterotomy during laparoscopic cholecystectomy for choledocholithiasis. Br J Surg 1995;82(2):257–9.

[53] Chang L, Lo S, Stabile BE, et al. Preoperative versus postoperative endoscopic retrograde cholangiopancreatography in mild to moderate gallstone pancreatitis: a prospective randomized trial. Ann Surg 2000;231(1):82–7.

ELSEVIER
SAUNDERS

SURGICAL
CLINICS OF
NORTH AMERICA

Surg Clin N Am 88 (2008) 1033–1046

Current Trends in Laparoscopic Solid Organ Surgery: Spleen, Adrenal, Pancreas, and Liver

Lora Melman, MD[a], Brent D. Matthews, MD[b],*

[a]Institute for Minimally Invasive Surgery, Department of Surgery, Washington University
School of Medicine, 660 South Euclid Avenue, Box 8109, St. Louis, MO 63110, USA
[b]Section of Minimally Invasive Surgery, Washington University School of Medicine,
660 South Euclid Avenue, Box 8109, St. Louis, MO 63110, USA

Laparoscopy has become a widely accepted technical platform in nearly all areas of surgery since its introduction with laparoscopic cholecystectomy in the late 1980s. The laparoscopic approach is now commonly used in colorectal, gastrointestinal, solid organ, and obesity surgery and is preferred by surgeons and patients owing to decreased pain, reduced perioperative morbidity, and an earlier return to self-reliance. Laparoscopic procedures in general have higher initial startup costs owing to the need to acquire specialized equipment but have been shown to successfully reduce perioperative recovery time, which, in the end, translates to reduced hospital costs with a positive impact on patient satisfaction. In a recent study of 508 laparoscopic cholecystectomies completed as outpatient surgery, 66% of patients were satisfied with a same-day discharge, whereas 32% of patients would have preferred to stay in the hospital longer [1]. In a similar study of 100 patients, average hospital costs were significantly reduced in the group of patients discharged the same day as their operation in a comparison with patients staying overnight. None of the patients in either group required readmission to the hospital after 30 days [2].

The laparoscopic era has been rapidly advancing, with continuous effort toward expanding the scope of procedures as well as enhancing cosmesis with even smaller incisions (needlescopic, 2–3 mm) in attempts to further reduce perioperative pain and analgesic requirements while maintaining similar outcomes for patients undergoing these procedures. In two recent

* Corresponding author.
E-mail address: matthewsbr@wustl.edu (B.D. Matthews).

trials comparing laparoscopic cholecystectomy with needlescopic cholecystectomy, needlescopic cholecystectomy was associated with less postoperative pain; however, the lower profile (2–3 mm) instruments were more flexible and therefore intermittently unable to provide adequate retraction [3,4]. When compared with traditional open procedures, an additional benefit of laparoscopy is the decreased immunologic insult. In fact, the physiologic stress response has been shown by several investigators to be lower in patients undergoing laparoscopic versus open abdominal surgery for many procedures including cholecystectomy, colon resection, gastric banding, hernia repair, hysterectomy, and fundoplication [5–7]. This decreased stress is a key component in the trend toward decreased morbidity with laparoscopy versus conventional open techniques regardless of the specific procedure. The realm of laparoscopy for solid organ surgery is still expanding and has been somewhat slower to evolve due to factors involving lower case volume and the refinement of technologies specific to these specialized operations in terms of hemostasis, exposure, parenchymal dissection, and adjunctive modalities such as intraoperative ultrasound [8]. This article reviews the latest trends in laparoscopic surgery with regard to splenectomy, adrenalectomy, and liver and pancreas surgery.

Spleen

Since its introduction in 1991 by Delaitre and Maignien, laparoscopic splenectomy has been increasingly used with excellent results for benign splenic disease. Controversy exists regarding minimally invasive techniques to manage lymphoproliferative, myeloproliferative, and malignant hematologic diseases involving the spleen, with perioperative complications most often related to patient comorbidities. Considerations for operative planning should include the type of splenic disease, spleen size, and patient comorbidities. General contraindications to laparoscopic splenectomy include portal hypertension, coagulopathy, and ascites [9]. A recent outcomes study by Kercher and colleagues [10] describes laparoscopic splenectomy to reverse thrombocytopenia in patients with hepatitis C cirrhosis and portal hypertension to allow patients to complete interferon therapy. This indication remains controversial because the technical difficulties and potential morbidity of laparoscopic splenectomy in patients with portal hypertension require expertise in laparoscopic solid organ surgery. In benign disease such as idiopathic thrombocytopenic purpura, laparoscopic splenectomy reliably relieves thrombocytopenia in patients with minimal perioperative morbidity. Other benign diseases managed with laparoscopic splenectomy include hereditary spherocytosis, thalassemia, idiopathic autoimmune hemolytic anemia, Felty's syndrome, Gaucher's disease, and splenic cysts [11]. Laparoscopic splenectomy for splenic abscess and trauma has been reported in several small case series [12,13], but the technical difficulties and success of nonoperative interventions have made these indications uncommon.

In patients with hematologic malignancy, splenectomy is indicated for marked leukopenia to allow for continued chemotherapy, to decrease transfusion requirements for anemia due to splenic sequestration, or to relieve symptoms of splenomegaly. Spleen size often poses a challenge to laparoscopic manipulation and retraction for hilar exposure and organ removal. Although no specific size criteria have been established, the authors agree that spleens that measure greater than 22 cm in craniocaudal length and 19 cm in width or spleens greater than 1600 g in weight should be managed with a hand-assist approach [14]. Additionally, the initiation of the hand-assisted approach from the beginning of the operative procedure may reduce intraoperative morbidity and operative time. It is helpful to obtain preoperative transaxial imaging via abdominal CT to calculate the craniocaudal and transverse dimensions of the spleen as well as an estimated weight based on volume.

Patient positioning is an important consideration in operative planning. The lateral approach has become almost universally accepted because it enhances exposure of the splenic hilum as well as the dorsal splenic ligaments. The anterior approach, used in the evolution of this technique, is now typically reserved for normal-sized spleens when a concomitant procedure such as laparoscopic distal pancreatectomy is planned. The lateral position may inhibit abdominal exploration for accessory spleens which are present in as many as 30% of patients with hematologic disease [15]. In patients who experience recurrent thrombocytopenia after laparoscopic splenectomy for idiopathic thrombocytopenic purpura and in whom an accessory spleen is localized by postoperative imaging, laparoscopic accessory splenectomy can be performed [16].

Portal or splenic vein thrombosis (PSVT) is a rare but recognized complication after laparoscopic splenectomy and is more common in patients with myeloproliferative disorders (eg, idiopathic thrombocytopenic purpura). PSVT outcomes range from spontaneous recovery to overt bowel necrosis depending on the volume of the thrombus and extent to which it obstructs flow from the mesenteric veins. Recent studies demonstrate an incidence as high as 55% when patients are screened postoperatively with contrast-enhanced abdominal CT scans [17]. The typical presentation of an acute PSVT is nonspecific with symptoms ranging from abdominal pain, diarrhea, and nausea to fever and dyspnea. Recognition of PSVT can be difficult and is often a diagnosis of exclusion after pancreatitis, pneumonia, sepsis, and pulmonary embolism have been ruled out. Duplex ultrasonography is highly sensitive for the diagnosis and monitoring of PSVT. Treatment options range from systemic anticoagulation with or without selective transcatheter thrombolysis to laparotomy for resection of ischemic bowel [18].

Adrenal

First introduced by Gagner and colleagues in 1992 for the management of Cushing's syndrome and pheochromocytoma, laparoscopic adrenalectomy has gained acceptance for the management of aldosteronomas, Cushing's syndrome, pheochromocytomas, and adrenal incidentalomas. Laparoscopic adrenalectomy results in fewer perioperative complications, decreased post-operative pain and hospital stay, and more effective use of health care expenditures [19,20]. It has been reported to be less morbid, more cost effective, and to allow patients to recover faster when compared with an open approach [21,22].

Controversy remains regarding laparoscopic adrenalectomy for large tumors and malignant or potentially malignant adrenal lesions. The most critical component of laparoscopic adrenalectomy is patient selection. A surgeon should be capable of coordinating the diagnostic evaluation of an incidental adrenal mass to determine whether it is a functional or non-functional tumor. The diagnostic evaluation of an adrenal incidentaloma requires a biochemical evaluation for hormonal activity. The most cost-effective evaluation of an adrenal incidentaloma includes a serum potassium, low-dose dexamethasone suppression test, and plasma metanephrines. If a patient is hypokalemic, plasma aldosterone and renin levels should be determined. A plasma aldosterone/renin activity ratio greater than 30 with a plasma aldosterone concentration greater than 5 nmol/L (20 ng/dL) suggests autonomous aldosterone activity. The finding of elevated plasma metanephrines has a sensitivity of 99% and specificity of 89% for pheochromocytoma. A low-dose overnight dexamethasone suppression test is used to screen for hypercortisolism. After the patient is given 1 mg of dexamethasone at 11 PM the night before an 8 AM serum cortisol blood sample, a normal individual will exhibit a suppressed serum cortisol level to less than 139 nmol/L (5 ug/dL). Failure of suppression suggests exogenous production of cortisol and is further evaluated by a high-dose dexamethasone suppression test to differentiate between Cushing's syndrome and pituitary tumors [23]. Radiographic imaging complements the biochemical evaluation and is discussed later.

The discovery of an incidental adrenal mass has become increasingly more common with the routine use of CT scans for diagnostic evaluations of abdominal pain, cancer screening, and other unrelated complaints. Based on autopsy studies, an adrenal mass is present in about 3% of people aged more than 50 years, making it one of the most common solid tumors. Although most adrenal masses are of no consequence, approximately 1 in 4000 is malignant [23]. Clinically inapparent adrenal masses, so-called "incidentalomas," are typically discovered on a work-up for unrelated conditions. The differential diagnosis includes benign lesions such as an adrenal adenoma, adrenal cyst, pheochromocytoma, myelolipoma, ganglioneuroma, or hematoma but must also include malignant lesions such as adrenal cortical carcinoma, malignant pheochromocytoma, or metastatic disease from a nonadrenal primary source. Adrenalectomy is warranted for all lesions suspected to be adrenal cortical carcinomas and for nonmalignant masses that are metabolically active. If a unilateral incidentaloma is found to be biochemically active, laparoscopic adrenalectomy is the treatment of choice after appropriate preoperative preparation such as alpha blockade for pheochromocytoma to prevent perioperative hypertensive crisis. Adrenal tumors considered to be adrenal cortical cancer should be resected in an open procedure due to the high rate of local recurrence and the need for aggressive, wide surgical margins.

In patients with a nonfunctioning adrenal mass, the size of the incidentaloma is the major determinant of which therapy is indicated. A lesion greater than 6 cm in size should be resected because 25% will be adrenal cortical carcinomas. In contrast, greater than 98% of incidentalomas less than 4 cm are benign. If an adrenal incidentaloma is less than 4 cm and deemed low risk by imaging criteria, there is no absolute indication for resection [23]. Six percent of adrenal lesions between 4 and 6 cm are malignant; therefore, laparoscopic adrenalectomy is recommended in appropriate surgical candidates. Nevertheless, repeat CT scan and nonoperative observation is an option in high-risk surgical candidates. Imaging characteristics that suggest anything other than a benign adenoma or rapid growth on repeat imaging at 6- to 12-month intervals should be managed with laparoscopic adrenalectomy.

The most common radiologic imaging for an adrenal mass is CT or MRI. Benign adrenal adenomas appear as a homogenous smooth mass and typically have an attenuation value less than 10 Hounsfield units. On MRI, adenomas have an intensity similar to liver on T2-weighted imaging. T2-weighted MRI for pheochromocytomas, on the other hand, classically shows an area of increased uptake of labeled noradrenaline analogues ^{123}I and ^{131}I-meta-iodobenzylguanidine [24]. The utility of fine-needle aspiration (FNA) has not been defined. Positron emission tomography scans have replaced the need for FNA except in rare situations of patients with a history of malignancy and an isolated adrenal mass who would not be appropriate surgical candidates for laparoscopic adrenalectomy. The complications of adrenal FNA, such as pneumothorax, bleeding, and hypertensive crisis, need to be considered before these procedures [23].

Surgical resection offers the only known cure for pheochromocytoma. The laparoscopic approach to this disease has been controversial in the past owing to concerns of excessive catecholamine release associated with pneumoperitoneum and laparoscopic manipulation. Even with appropriate preoperative alpha or beta blockade, intraoperative hypertension is common in both open and laparoscopic resection of pheochromocytoma. Several recent studies have shown laparoscopic adrenalectomy to be safe even for large tumors, with intraoperative hypertension occurring in 58% to 67% of patients compared with approximately 75% of open cases. In fact, laparoscopic tumor manipulation has been shown to cause less of a catecholamine surge when compared with open surgery, with 8.6- and 17.4-fold plasma increases in norepinephrine and epinephrine levels, respectively, during laparoscopic resection as compared with 13.7- and 34.2-fold increases with open resection [21].

The use of flexible laparoscopic ultrasound probes has proven to be helpful in cases of laparoscopic adrenalectomy. It can serve as a way to restore the haptic sense that is inherently reduced in laparoscopic surgery. Several investigators have endorsed their use intraoperatively to identify the adrenal gland and adrenal vein, to determine the laparoscopic respectability of large adrenal tumors, and to define the line of transection in cases in which only a partial adrenalectomy is performed [25,26]. Although laparoscopic ultrasound adds to overall hospital and procedural charges, if used selectively it has been shown to increase operative efficiency [27].

Pancreas

Over the past 20 years, minimally invasive techniques have become increasingly employed for the treatment of pancreatic disease. The role of laparoscopy in the staging and evaluation of pancreatic cancer has been evaluated extensively. It is currently used to avoid the potential morbidity of an unnecessary laparotomy in patients with occult metastatic disease not detectable on preoperative imaging [28]. Despite the potential impact of avoiding an unnecessary laparotomy in as many as 40% of patients, it remains controversial whether laparoscopic staging for pancreas cancer should be recommended routinely. Palliative endoscopic procedures to relieve biliary obstruction are reliable and effective. Laparoscopic gastrojejunostomy is an option in patients with duodenal obstruction due to unresectable periampullary tumors recognized either on preoperative imaging or during laparoscopic staging [29]. Laparoscopy can also be used to perform neurolytic celiac plexus block for chronic pain related to retroperitoneal invasion of tumor mass. The diagnostic accuracy of laparoscopy is dependent on the extent of intra-abdominal exploration directed toward the detection of vascular invasion or occult deep hepatic metastasis. The feasibility and reproducibility of diagnostic staging laparoscopy for pancreatic cancer requires further evaluation. Cost-effectiveness data for this technique are limited. Laparoscopic ultrasound and peritoneal cytology are adjuncts that increase the diagnostic accuracy of preoperative staging, and their current role in the evaluation of these patients is being defined.

Besides palliative laparoscopic procedures in patients with unresectable pancreatic cancer, laparoscopic enteric drainage of pancreatic pseudocysts was one of the first therapeutic procedures for pancreatic disease [30]. The traditional mantra to drain pancreatic pseudocysts larger than 6 cm or those persisting after 6 weeks was based on studies reporting serious morbidity due to rupture, abscess formation, or hemorrhage in up to 40% of untreated patients [31]. This disease, once treated uniformly with open surgery, is now routinely addressed with laparoscopic or endoscopic modalities. Percutaneous drainage has also been described but has become unpopular owing to the associated high failure rate, risk of infection, and increased incidence of pancreatic fistula when compared with surgical treatment. External drainage is currently used for palliation or as a temporizing measure in critically ill patients until a definitive surgical procedure can be tolerated [32–34]. Laparoscopic pancreatic cystgastrostomy and pancreatic cystjejunostomy are feasible depending on whether the pancreatic pseudocyst extends through the gastrocolic omentum or the paracolic gutter. The cyst can be localized with its borders demarcated by endoscopic ultrasound. The enteric-pancreatic cyst anastomosis is completed with an endoscopic linear stapler or intracorporeal suturing. In 106 cases, Palanivelu and colleagues [35] reported only one symptomatic failure requiring reoperation after a mean follow-up of 54 months after laparoscopic cystgastrostomy (n = 90), cystjejunostomy (n = 8), and laparoscopic external drainage (n = 8). Although endoscopic internal drainage using a flexible endoscope and placement of multiple stents transgastric into the pancreatic pseudocyst is performed regularly, the authors have witnessed a primary success rate of only 35% for this procedure compared with almost 90% for laparoscopic pancreatic cystgastrostomy (Brent D. Matthews, unpublished data, 2008). Primary endoscopic failures in our study were typically salvaged by open pancreatic cystgastrostomy. A review of recently published series demonstrates that both laparoscopic and endoscopic modalities are safe, with mortality rates of less than 1% compared with around 6% with open surgery. Complication rates are between 4% and 12% with minimally invasive techniques versus 24% with the traditional open approach [31,36,37]. Further case-control studies need to be done to compare long-term success rates in the minimally invasive approaches to traditional open surgery.

There are several obstacles to developing standardized and reproducible techniques for laparoscopic pancreas resection. These obstacles include a relatively low volume of patients requiring pancreas resection, the need for combined surgical expertise in minimally invasive and pancreas surgery, a lack of enabling technologies for vascular dissection and control, loss of tactile feedback with laparoscopic surgery, lack of reliable methods for managing the pancreatic stump to minimize pancreatic leak or fistula, and a relatively high percentage of patients with malignancy, which dictates adherence to oncologic principles. Many of these barriers are being addressed as laparoscopic pancreatic surgery becomes more universal, and clinical trials are underway to specifically address these concerns. To date, minimally invasive techniques to perform enucleation of neuroendocrine tumors, distal pancreatectomy, and pancreaticoduodenectomy have been established. In 1996, Sussman and Gagner [38,39], published the first reports of a laparoscopic distal pancreatectomy for insulinoma and laparoscopic islet cell enucleation, respectively. Preoperative location tests combined with intraoperative ultrasound and manual palpation via a hand port mimics techniques used for open surgery and allows for correct localization and identification of insulinomas in greater than 90% of cases [40]. Insulinomas in the body or tail of the pancreas without malignant features are amendable to laparoscopic enucleation or distal pancreatectomy with or without splenic preservation [41].

Laparoscopic pancreas resection is gaining ground as experience mounts in high-volume centers with these technically challenging operations. Mabrut and colleagues to date have published the largest series of patients undergoing laparoscopic pancreatic resection. Their experience includes a total of 127 patients, with 21 patients converted to an open procedure and 107 patients who successfully underwent laparoscopic pancreatic resections including 21 enucleations, 58 distal pancreatectomies, 24 distal splenopancreatectomies, and 3 pancreatoduodenal resections. Indications for resection included benign and malignant pathologies, and the median follow-up was 14 months. No mortality was reported; the postoperative complication rate was 39%, which was not significantly different than in patients at their institution who were converted to an open procedure; and the median hospital stay was 7 days versus 11 days in the converted patients. All surgical margins from malignant etiologies were negative on final pathology, but 23% of patients presented with recurrence at a median of 15 months postoperatively [42].

Teh and colleagues recently compared 12 patients who underwent laparoscopic distal pancreatectomy with 16 patients who underwent open distal pancreatectomy for benign disease and found that the mean hospital stay (10.6 versus 4.5 days, respectively) and total perioperative complications (9 versus 2 events, respectively) were significantly reduced. Park and Heniford published a series of 23 patients undergoing laparoscopic distal pancreatectomy for both malignant and benign disease, demonstrating the feasibility of this approach for centers with the appropriate clinical volume and expertise. They reported a mean operative time of 3.7 hours with a mean blood loss of 270 mL and mean postoperative stay of 4.1 days for laparoscopic distal pancreatectomy compared with a mean operative time of 4.7 hours, mean blood loss of 879 mL, and mean postoperative stay of 15 days in a series of open distal pancreatectomies published by Lillemoe and colleagues. Furthermore, they observed no perioperative mortality and reported a complication rate of 16%, which contrasts with a mortality rate of 0.9% and complication rate of 31% in the open series [43,44].

Based on a review of the published literature, laparoscopic distal pancreatectomy is the most common minimally invasive surgical procedure performed worldwide for pancreatic disease [45]. Instrumentation such as the ultrasonic coagulating shears and bipolar vessel sealers efficiently control bleeding from small vessels along the inferior and posterior borders of the pancreas, making spleen-preserving procedures feasible. The most common technique is prograde laparoscopic distal pancreatectomy performed by transecting the pancreatic body first and then moving distally toward the spleen. An alternative technique consists of a retrograde pancreatectomy with initial mobilization of the pancreatic body and dissection of the inferior margin of the gland to isolate the splenic vein with subsequent dissection of the splenic vein and artery away from the pancreas to complete a spleen-preserving laparoscopic distal pancreatectomy [46]. The major challenge for laparoscopic and even open distal pancreatectomy remains the management of the pancreatic stump. Case series using ultrasonic coagulating shears or bipolar vessel sealers with or without suture ligation of the pancreatic stump or fibrin sealant have been unreliable in preventing pancreatic leakage. Endoscopic linear staplers facilitate pancreatic transection; however, a leak rate of approximately 25% has been reported from a pooled analysis after stapled distal pancreatectomy [47]. The authors reported a 55% reduction in the leak rate after distal pancreatectomy using a 4.8-mm endoscopic linear stapler (US Surgical, Norwalk, Connecticut) and bioabsorbable mesh to reinforce the staple line (SeamGuard, W.L. Gore, Flagstaff, Arizona) placed over the stapler before firing [48]. We initiated this trial to evaluate a method to decrease the incidence of pancreatic fistula while facilitating a minimally invasive technique. A prospective randomized trial is ongoing to evaluate this methodology.

Liver

Liver surgery in general is technically demanding and typically performed for malignant disease. The best results with major hepatic resections are achieved at high-volume tertiary centers. Laparoscopic liver procedures initially consisted of liver biopsy, tumor staging, and fenestration of nonparasitic liver cysts [43]. More recently, longitudinal outcomes studies evaluating laparoscopic liver resection for benign and malignant disease have been reported [43,44,49–52], prompting interest in this technique. Nevertheless, laparoscopic liver resection has not yet become mainstream due to the level of specialized training required, the difficulties with mobilizing a large organ in the relatively confined space of the pneumoperitoneum, concerns over hemorrhage control, the fear of gas embolization into the hepatic venous system, and the uncertainty of the ability to perform adequate oncologic resections [44]. Limited hepatic resections involving the left lateral section or frontal segments of the liver have been shown by several groups to be feasible [53–56] and afford the patient the benefits associated with laparoscopic surgery, such as decreased postoperative pain and an earlier return to baseline function. Large prospective randomized trials comparing laparoscopic with open liver resection for malignant disease have not been completed, and the long-term oncologic efficacy of a minimally invasive approach is unestablished.

Solitary liver cysts are found in about 1% of adults at autopsy, with only a handful becoming large enough to produce symptoms of abdominal pain. Diagnosis is frequently made incidentally during abdominal imaging for an unrelated condition. Treatment is indicated in symptomatic patients, who may present with abdominal pain, nausea, vomiting, early satiety, fatigue, or jaundice. Percutaneous aspiration almost universally fails, although injection of sclerosants may decrease the recurrence rate to less than 20% [57]. Definitive treatment consists of unroofing the cyst, allowing it to drain into the peritoneal cavity. Lin and colleagues [58] first described this technique in 1968 as an open operation, but laparoscopic fenestration has become commonplace since the 1990s for simple nonparasitic liver cysts. Fluid aspirated from the cyst should be sent for Gram stain and cytologic evaluation, and a biopsy of the cyst wall should be sent to evaluate for malignancy. The cyst wall is then typically resected with ultrasonic coagulating shears, leaving the remaining portion of the cyst marsupialized to drain into the peritoneal cavity. Additional hemostasis at the cyst-liver interface can be achieved with intracorporeal suturing. Any bile leakage should be identified and ligated to prevent a postoperative biloma. Neoplastic cysts of the liver are rare and include biliary cystadenomas and cystadenocarcinomas. It is believed that cystadenomas can undergo malignant transformation; therefore, resection via enucleation or formal hepatic resection is mandatory for any neoplastic cyst of the liver [57].

A variety of existing technologies have been successfully employed in laparoscopic liver resection for mobilization and retraction, vascular control, parenchymal dissection/transection, and visualization of oncologic margins. Use of a hand-assist port is helpful for mobilization, retraction, and hemorrhage control. Some investigators report routine clamping of the portal vasculature to minimize hemorrhage during parenchymal dissection [56], whereas others use manual direct compression via the hand-assist port [53]. Ultrasonic coagulating technology is useful during transection of the parenchyma because it does not give off a plume that would obscure the laparoscopic field and has minimal thermal impact on surrounding tissues. Dissection can also be undertaken with a saline-linked cautery device (Tissue Link; Salient Surgical Technologies, Dover, New Hampshire), which has been shown to be effective at cutting tissue as well as sealing small vessels and bile ductules. The argon beam coagulator is also effective for surface hemostasis, although this device contributes to increased intra-abdominal pressure, and careful venting of laparoscopic ports during activation of the argon beam is important to minimize transduction of gas emboli into the hepatic venous system. Fibrin glue can also be employed as a topical hemostatic agent. Laparoscopic ultrasound has a key role in defining the appropriate surgical margins for resection of malignant disease and can also be used to detect smaller lesions (<1 cm) not previously seen on axial imaging [59].

Koffron and colleagues have presented the largest series of minimally invasive hepatic resections, including 110 segmentectomies, 63 bisegmentectomies, 47 left hepatectomies (segments 2–4), 64 right hepatectomies (segments 5–8), 8 extended right hepatectomies (segments 4–8), and 8 caudate lobe resections. Cases were completed using a range of laparoscopic platforms ranging from pure laparoscopic resection (241 patients) to hand-assisted laparoscopic resection (32 patients) to a laparoscopic-assisted open resection hybrid technique (27 patients). These cases were compared contemporaneously with 100 case-matched open hepatic resections at the same institution. Indications for resection were cysts (n = 70), hemangioma (n = 37), focal nodular hyperplasia (n = 23), adenoma (n = 47), liver donor right lobectomy (n = 20), hepatocellular carcinoma (n = 43), and metastatic lesions (n = 60). Perioperative outcome measures were favorable in the minimally invasive cases with respect to blood loss, transfusion requirements, and hospital length of stay. Postoperative biliary leak rates and local malignancy recurrence rates at a mean of 45 months postoperatively were comparable with that in open resection [55]. Hospital costs were also analyzed and found to be lower both in operating room and total hospital costs, suggesting an incentive benefit, particularly for high-volume institutions, to support this trend in care. A report by Buell and colleagues [53] also showed significant reductions with respect to operative blood loss, operative time, and hospital length of stay in a series of 17 patients undergoing hand-assisted laparoscopic liver resection versus the traditional open approach for both benign and malignant indications.

Summary

Future directions in the expanding frontier of minimally invasive solid surgery, in particular laparoscopic liver and pancreas surgery, involve further integration of technology and information systems with the surgeon's skill. The evolution of surgical technique must ultimately address the issue of training surgeons in an era of rapidly advancing technology. Current surgical robots and simulators have the capability to superimpose patient-specific imaging onto the operative field to allow for preoperative planning and rehearsal of surgical maneuvers. Future operating rooms may incorporate the use of automated scrub assistants and instruments that can actively sense and send feedback to allow the surgeon to "feel" the tissue even if the patient is many miles away. It remains to be seen which technologies will emerge that will allow us to maximize operative care for the best clinical outcome while conserving financial resources [60].

References

[1] Richardson WS, Furhman GS, Burch E, et al. Outpatient laparoscopic cholecystectomy: outcomes of 847 planned procedures. Surg Endosc 2001;15:193–5.

[2] Bringman S, Anderberg B, Heikkinen T, et al. Outpatient laparoscopic cholecystectomy: a prospective study with 100 consecutive patients. Ambul Surg 2001;9:83–6.

[3] Look M, Chew SP, Tan YC, et al. Postoperative pain in needlescopic versus conventional laparoscopic cholecystectomy: a prospective randomised trial. J R Coll Surg Edinb 2001; 46:138–42.

[4] Cheah WK, Lenzi JE, So JB, et al. Randomized trial of needlescopic versus laparoscopic cholecystectomy. Br J Surg 2001;88:45–7.

[5] Fuchs KH. Minimally invasive surgery. Endoscopy 2002;34(2):154–9.

[6] Sido B, Teklote JR, Hartel M, et al. Inflammatory response after abdominal surgery. Best Pract Res Clin Anaesthesiol 2004;18(3):439–54.

[7] Zengin K, Taskin M, Sakoglu N, et al. Systemic inflammatory response after laparoscopic and open application of adjustable banding for morbidly obese patients. Obes Surg 2002; 12:276–9.

[8] Kolecki R, Schirmer B. Intraoperative and laparoscopic ultrasound. Surg Clin North Am 1998;78(2):251–71.

[9] Burch M, Misra M, Phillips EH. Splenic malignancy: a minimally invasive approach. Cancer J 2005;11(1):36–42.

[10] Kercher KW, Carbonell AM, Heniford BT, et al. Laparoscopic splenectomy reverses thrombocytopenia in patients with hepatitis C cirrhosis and portal hypertension. J Gastrointest Surg 2004;8(1):120–6.

[11] Walsh RM, Brody F, Brown N. Laparoscopic splenectomy for lymphoproliferative disease. Surg Endosc 2004;18:272–5.

[12] Mostafa G, Matthews BD, Sing R, et al. Elective laparoscopic splenectomy for grade III splenic injury in an athlete. Surg Laparosc Endosc Percutan Tech 2002;12(4):283–6.

[13] Carbonell AM, Kercher KW, Matthews BD, et al. Laparoscopic splenectomy for splenic abscess. Surg Laparosc Endosc Percutan Tech 2004;14(5):289–91.

[14] Kercher KW, Matthews BD, Walsh RM, et al. Laparoscopic splenectomy for massive splenomegaly. Am J Surg 2002;183:192–6.

[15] Matteotti R, Assalia A, Pomp A. Splenectomy. In: Assalia A, Gagner M, Schein M, editors. Controversies in laparoscopic surgery. New York: Springer; 2006. p. 299–311.

[16] Szold A, Kamat M, Nadu A, et al. Laparoscopic accessory splenectomy for recurrent idiopathic thrombocytopenic purpura and hemolytic anemia. Surg Endosc 2000;14:761–3.

[17] Ikeda M, Sekimoto M, Takiguchi S, et al. High incidence of thrombosis of the portal venous system after laparoscopic splenectomy: a prospective study with contrast-enhanced CT scan. Ann Surg 2005;241(2):208–16.

[18] Kercher KW, Sing RF, Watson KW, et al. Transhepatic thrombolysis in acute portal vein thrombosis after laparoscopic splenectomy. Surg Laparosc Endosc Percutan Tech 2002; 12(2):131–6.

[19] Brunt LM. The positive impact of laparoscopic adrenalectomy on complications of adrenal surgery. Surg Endosc 2002;16:252–7.

[20] Brunt LM. Minimal access adrenal surgery. Surg Endosc 2006;20:351–61.

[21] Kercher KW, Novitsky YW, Park AP, et al. Laparoscopic curative resection of pheochromocytomas. Ann Surg 2005;241(6):919–28.

[22] Assalia A, Gagner M. Adrenalectomy. In: Controversies in laparoscopic surgery. Berlin Heidelberg: Springer; 2006. p. 315–56.

[23] NIH state-of-the-science statement on management of the clinically inapparent adrenal mass ("incidentaloma"). NIH Consens State Sci Statements 2002;19(2):1–23.

[24] Ilias I, Sahdev A, Reznek R, et al. The optimal imaging of adrenal tumours: a comparison of different methods. Endocr Relat Cancer 2007;14:587–99.

[25] Heniford BT, Iannitti DA, Hale J, et al. The role of intraoperative ultrasonography during laparoscopic adrenalectomy. Surgery 1997;122(6):1068–74.

[26] Assalia A, Gagner M. Laparoscopic adrenalectomy. Br J Surg 2004;91:1259–74.

[27] Brunt LM, Bennett HF, Teefy SA, et al. Laparoscopic ultrasound imaging of adrenal tumors during laparoscopic adrenalectomy. Am J Surg 1999;178:490–4.

[28] D'Angelica M, Fong Y, Weber S, et al. The role of staging laparoscopy in hepatobiliary malignancy: prospective analysis of 401 cases. Ann Surg Oncol 2003;10:183–9.

[29] Stefanidis D, Grove KD, Schwesinger WH, et al. The current role of staging laparoscopy for adenocarcinoma of the pancreas: a review. Ann Oncol 2006;17:189–99.

[30] Underwood RA, Soper NJ. Current status of laparoscopic surgery of the pancreas. J Hepatobiliary Pancreat Surg 1999;6:154–64.

[31] Bergman S, Melvin WS. Operative and nonoperative management of pancreatic pseudocysts. Surg Clin North Am 2007;87:1447–60.

[32] Criado E, DeStefano AA, Weiner TM, et al. Long-term results of percutaneous catheter drainage of pancreatic pseudocysts. Surg Gynecol Obstet 1992;175:293–8.

[33] Lang EK, Paolini RM, Pottmeyer A. The efficacy of palliative and definitive percutaneous versus surgical drainage of pancreatic abscesses and pseudocysts: a prospective study of 85 patients. South Med J 1991;84(1):55–64.

[34] Adams DB, Anderson MC. Percutaneous catheter drainage compared with internal drainage in the management of pancreatic pseudocyst. Ann Surg 1992;215(6):571–6.

[35] Palanivelu C, Senthilnathan P, Madhankumar MV, et al. Management of pancreatic pseudocyst in the era of laparoscopic surgery: experience from a tertiary centre. Surg Endosc 2007;21:2262–7.

[36] Aljarabah M, Ammori BJ. Laparoscopic and endoscopic approaches for drainage of pancreatic pseudocysts: a systematic review of published series. Surg Endosc 2007;21:1936–44.

[37] Gumaste VV, Pitchumoni CS. Pancreatic pseudocyst. Gastroenterologist 1996;4(1):33–43.

[38] Sussman LA, Christie R, Whittle DE, et al. Laparoscopic excision of distal pancreas including insulinoma. ANZ J Surg 1996;66:414–6.

[39] Gagner M, Pomp A, Hererra MF. Early experience with laparoscopic resections of islet cell tumors. Surgery 1996;120:1051–4.

[40] Ayav A, Bresler L, Brunaud L, et al. Laparoscopic approach for solitary insulinoma: a multicentre study. Langenbecks Arch Surg 2005;390:134–40.

[41] Toniato A, Meduri F, Foletto M, et al. Laparoscopic treatment of benign insulinomas localized in the body and tail of the pancreas: a single-center experience. World J Surg 2006;30:1916–9.

[42] Mabrut J, Fernandez-Cruz L, Azagra JS, et al. Laparoscopic pancreatic resection: results of a multicenter European study of 127 patients. Surgery 2005;137(6):597–605.

[43] Morino M, Morra I, Rosso E, et al. Laparoscopic vs open hepatic resection. Surg Endosc 2003;17:1914–8.

[44] Jarnagin W, Fong Y. Liver surgery for solid tumors. In: Controversies in laparoscopic surgery. Berlin Heidelberg: Springer; 2006. p. 287–95.

[45] Pierce RA, Spitler JA, Hawkins WG, et al. Outcomes analysis of laparoscopic resection of pancreatic neoplasms. Surg Endosc 2007;21:579–86.

[46] Melotti G, Butturini G, Piccoli M, et al. Laparoscopic distal pancreatectomy: results on a consecutive series of 58 patients. Ann Surg 2007;246(1):77–82.

[47] Knaebel HP, Diener MK, Wente MN, et al. Systematic review and meta-analysis of technique for closure of the pancreatic remnant after distal pancreatectomy. Br J Surg 2005;92(5):539–46.

[48] Thaker RI, Matthews BD, Linehan DC, et al. Absorbable mesh reinforcement of a stapled pancreatic transection line reduces the leak rate with distal pancreatectomy. J Gastrointest Surg 2007;11:59–65.

[49] Fong Y, Jarnagin W, Conlon KC, et al. Hand-assisted laparoscopic liver resection: lessons from an initial experience. Arch Surg 2000;135(7):854–9.

[50] Berends FJ, Meijer S, Prevoo W, et al. Technical considerations in laparoscopic liver surgery. Surg Endosc 2001;15(8):794–8.

[51] Koffron A, Geller D, Gamblin TC, et al. Laparoscopic liver surgery: shifting the management of liver tumors. Hepatology 2006;44(6):1694–700.

[52] Buell JF, Koffron AJ, Thomas MJ, et al. Laparoscopic liver resection. J Am Coll Surg 2005;200(3):472–80.

[53] Buell JF, Thomas MJ, Doty TC, et al. An initial experience and evolution of laparoscopic hepatic resectional surgery. Surgery 2004;136(4):804–11.

[54] Aldrighetti L, Pulitano C, Catena M, et al. A prospective evaluation of laparoscopic versus open left lateral hepatic sectionectomy. J Gastrointest Surg 2008;12:457–62.

[55] Koffron AJ, Auffenberg G, Kung R, et al. Evaluation of 300 minimally invasive liver resections at a single institution: less is more. Ann Surg 2007;246(3):385–94.

[56] Lesurtel M, Cherqui D, Laurent A, et al. Laparoscopic versus open left lateral hepatic lobectomy: a case-control study. J Am Coll Surg 2003;196(2):236–42.
[57] Cowles RA, Mulholland MW. Solitary hepatic cysts. J Am Coll Surg 2000;191:311–21.
[58] Lin TY, Chen CC, Wang SM. Treatment of non-parasitic cystic disease of the liver: a new
approach to therapy with polycystic liver. Ann Surg 1968;168:921–7.
[59] Are C, Fong Y, Geller DA. Laparoscopic liver resections. Adv Surg 2005;39:57–75.
[60] Satava R. Future trends in the design and application of surgical robots. Semin Laparosc
Surg 2004;11(2):129–35.

ELSEVIER
SAUNDERS

SURGICAL
CLINICS OF
NORTH AMERICA

Surg Clin N Am 88 (2008) 1047–1072

Laparoscopic and Minimally Invasive Resection of Malignant Colorectal Disease

Matthew C. Koopmann, MD,
Charles P. Heise, MD, FACS*

*Department of Surgery, University of Wisconsin School of Medicine and Public Health,
600 Highland Avenue, Madison, WI 53792-7375, USA*

Minimally invasive approaches have revolutionized the practice of general surgery. Upper abdominal procedures, such as cholecystectomy, Nissen fundoplication, and gastric bypass, are now predominantly performed using laparoscopy. Potential short-term benefits of minimally invasive techniques include reduced hospital stays, recovery times [1], narcotic analgesia requirements [2], and short-term complications of laparotomy, such as ileus [3]. Potential long-term benefits include reduced incisional hernia rates and improved cosmesis [4].

The introduction of laparoscopy and other minimally invasive techniques to colorectal surgery has been a more gradual process. In particular, laparoscopy for the treatment of malignant colorectal disease was initially met with skepticism and controversy. Although much of this skepticism has been assuaged since 2002 by results of several large, multicenter, randomized controlled trials (RCTs) comparing laparoscopic and open colon cancer resections, questions remain regarding similar treatment of rectal cancer. This review, pertaining to minimally invasive colorectal cancer surgery, emphasizes the comparative outcomes, controversies, advances, and emerging technologies in the field.

Minimally invasive colon cancer surgery

Inflammatory and immunologic responses

The physiologic basis for the benefits ascribed to minimally invasive surgery resides in the theoretic reduction in inflammatory and immune responses

* Corresponding author.
E-mail address: heise@surgery.wisc.edu (C.P. Heise).

when compared with a conventional open approach. Several RCTs have demonstrated these effects using various surrogate markers of inflammation and immunity comparing laparoscopic and open colorectal resections. Leung and colleagues [5] compared laparoscopic-assisted and open resections for rectosigmoid carcinoma and noted a significant reduction in peak levels of the inflammatory cytokines, interleukin (IL)-1β and IL-6, and in the acute phase reactant, C-reactive protein, in the laparoscopic-assisted group. Similarly, in a slightly larger trial, reductions in peak IL-6 and C-reactive protein levels were noted in a laparoscopically resected colon cancer group [6]. In addition, Braga and colleagues [7] demonstrated improved lymphocyte proliferation and gut oxygen tension, along with a significant reduction in 30-day morbidity in patients who had benign and malignant colorectal disease after laparoscopic rather than open resections. Conversely, a series evaluating the immune response after laparoscopic and open resection for rectal cancer failed to show differences between these groups with respect to lymphocyte counts, immunoglobulins, and cytokine levels [8]. With this limited data, a reduction in inflammatory response and immunosuppression with a laparoscopic approach to colon cancer resection is suggested. These findings may provide early mechanistic insight underlying the reported advantages of laparoscopic over standard open surgery.

Randomized controlled trials

Initial reports on outcomes of laparoscopic colon cancer surgery arose from retrospective individual surgeon or institution series based on prospectively maintained databases [9–11]. These series assessed the feasibility of laparoscopic colon cancer resection with respect to safety and short-term oncologic outcomes. Subsequent large prospective, nonrandomized studies [12] and small, single-center RCTs [3,13–18] comparing laparoscopic to open colon cancer resections provided preliminary evidence that the results of a laparoscopic approach were comparable to conventional open resection. Since 2002 four large RCTs (>100 patients in each arm) have been published assessing the oncologic outcomes of laparoscopic compared with open colon cancer resection [1,19–21]. The design of each trial is discussed briefly and summarized in Table 1.

Barcelona trial

The study by Lacy and colleagues [19] from the University of Barcelona was a randomized, prospective single-center trial comparing laparoscopic-assisted versus open colectomy for right- and left-sided colon cancer (minimum 15 cm from the anal verge). Patients who had transverse colon cancer, obstructing lesions, T4 lesions, distant metastases, or prior colon surgery were excluded. Between 1993 and 1998 this trial recruited 442 eligible patients, 223 of whom were excluded, leaving 105 and 101 patients to complete the trial in the laparoscopic and open arms, respectively. This study was

Table 1
Large randomized controlled trials comparing laparoscopic and open colon cancer resections: study designs and patient demographics

	Barcelona [19]	COST [1]	COLOR [20]	CLASICC [21]
Accrual years	1993–1998	1994–2001	1997–2003	1996–2002
Study sites	Single-center	Multicenter	Multicenter	Multicenter
Surgery	Laparoscopic assisted	Laparoscopic assisted	Laparoscopic assisted	Laparoscopic assisted
Exclusion criteria	TC, DM, IO, PCS	TC, DM, IO, SMI, IBD, FP, P, OM	TC, SF, DM, IO, PCS, PM, BMI >30	TC, IO, PM, P
Primary endpoint	Cancer-related survival	Time to tumor recurrence	Cancer-free survival at 3 y	Margin positivity, operative mortality
Subjects (n)	L: 106 O: 102	L: 435 O: 428	L: 536 O: 546	L: 273 O: 140
Median follow-up (mo)	L: 44 O: 43	52.8	Long-term results not yet reported	49.5

Abbreviations: DM, distant metastases; FP, familial polyposis; IBD, inflammatory bowel disease; IO, intestinal obstruction; L, laparoscopic-assisted resections; NR, not reported; O, open resections; OM, other concurrent malignancy; P, pregnancy; PCS, prior colon surgery; PM, prior malignancy; SF, splenic flexure cancers; SMI, severe medical illness; TC, transverse colon cancers.

unique in that all patients who had stage II and III disease (both arms) received adjuvant chemotherapy. The median length of follow-up was 44 months for the laparoscopic group and 43 months for the open group. The primary endpoint was cancer-related survival.

Clinical Outcomes of Surgical Therapy trial

The National Cancer Institute–sponsored Clinical Outcomes of Surgical Therapy (COST) Study Group of the Laparoscopic Colectomy Trial [1] was a randomized, prospective multicenter trial conducted at 48 institutions within the United States and Canada designed to show noninferiority of laparoscopic-assisted colectomy to open colectomy for colon cancer. Patients who had colon adenocarcinoma established histologically at the time of surgery and who were free of "prohibitive abdominal adhesions" were included in the study. Patients who had advanced local disease or metastases, rectal or transverse colon cancers, acute bowel obstruction or perforation, severe medical illness, inflammatory bowel disease, familial polyposis syndromes, pregnancy, or concurrent or previous malignancies were excluded. Unlike the Barcelona trial, adjuvant chemotherapy was used at the treating physician's discretion. The study accrual period was between 1994 and 2001; 872 patients underwent randomization resulting in 435 and 428 patients analyzed in the laparoscopic and open arms, respectively. The median follow-up time was 4.4 years. The primary endpoint was time to tumor recurrence. Secondary endpoints included disease-free survival, overall survival, complications, recovery, and quality of life. Analysis was conducted by intention-to-treat principles, such that laparoscopic converted to open patients remained in the laparoscopic group.

Colon Cancer Laparoscopic or Open Resection trial

The Colon Cancer Laparoscopic or Open Resection (COLOR) trial [20] was a randomized, prospective, multicenter European trial designed to assess the safety and benefit of laparoscopic-assisted versus open resection for right- and left-sided colon cancers. Patients who had solitary colon adenocarcinoma above the peritoneal reflection were included. The COLOR trial was the only trial taking body habitus into consideration, wherein a body mass index (BMI) greater than 30 kg/m^2 resulted in exclusion. Additional exclusion criteria included transverse or splenic flexure cancers, synchronous or clinical T4 lesions, metastatic disease, intestinal obstruction, previous ipsilateral colon surgery, previous malignancy (except basal cell carcinoma of the skin or cervical carcinoma in situ), and contraindications to general anesthesia or prolonged pneumoperitoneum. The accrual period was between 1997 and 2003 and randomized 1248 patients. This resulted in 536 and 546 patients included for final analysis in the laparoscopic and open arms, respectively. The primary endpoint was cancer-free survival 3 years post resection (not yet reported). Secondary endpoints included morbidity and mortality, overall survival, resection margin status, local recurrence, port site and wound recurrence, metastases, and blood loss. Only short-term outcomes have been reported at the time of this writing.

United Kingdom Medical Research Council Conventional versus Laparoscopic-Assisted Surgery in Colon Cancer trial
The United Kingdom Medical Research Council Conventional versus Laparoscopic-Assisted Surgery in Colon Cancer (MRC CLASICC) trial [21] was a multicenter, randomized prospective trial comparing laparo-scopic-assisted versus open resection for colon and rectal cancers. Exclusion criteria included transverse colon cancer, presence of chronic cardiac or pul-monary disease, acute intestinal obstruction, malignant disease in the prior 5 years, synchronous lesions, pregnancy, and need for additional concomi-tant surgical interventions. The accrual period was between 1996 and 2002, during which 794 patients underwent randomization. This trial randomized subjects to laparoscopic or open surgery at a two-to-one ratio allowing for expected conversions, thus 526 and 268 patients were analyzed in the laparoscopic and open groups, respectively, according to intention-to-treat principles. Of these subjects, 273 and 140 underwent laparoscopic and open resection for colon cancer, respectively, with the remainder undergoing resection for rectal cancer. Median follow-up time was 36.8 months [22]. Primary short-term endpoints were resection margin status, proportion of Dukes' C2 tumors, and in-hospital mortality. Secondary short-term end-points were complication rates, quality of life, and transfusion requirements. Long-term endpoints were survival, recurrence, and quality of life at 3 and 5 years follow-up.

Oncologic outcomes

Survival
Although none of the four large RCTs used overall survival as a primary endpoint, the Barcelona trial [19] reported similar overall survival between laparoscopic (82%) and open groups (74%, $P = 0.14$) (Table 2). When assessing only stage III tumors, however, those resected laparoscopically demonstrated improved overall survival ($P = 0.02$). In their discussion, the investigators suggest that a reduction in immunosuppression associated with laparoscopy may have been responsible. This study subset included only 37 and 36 patients, however, who had stage III disease in the laparo-scopic and open groups, respectively. A recent 5-year update of the COST trial (median follow-up 7 years) [23] also revealed equivalent overall survival between the laparoscopic and open groups (74.6% versus 76.4%, $P = 0.93$). A subgroup analysis this time revealed, however, that subjects who had stage I tumors treated by open resection demonstrated an improved overall survival ($P = 0.04$). The authors of the COST update acknowledge that the stage-specific findings were identified on subgroup analysis and were not adequately powered to conclude. Furthermore, disease-free survival and

Table 2
Large randomized controlled trials and meta-analysis comparing laparoscopic to open colon cancer resections: patient-oriented and oncologic outcomes

	Barcelona [19]	COST [1–3]	COLOR [20]	CLASICC [21,22]	Bonjer [24][a]
Lymph nodes retrieved (median no.)	L: 11.1 O: 11.1	L: 12 O: 12	L: 10 O: 10	L: 12 O: 13.5	L: 11.8 O: 12.2
Positive margins (%)	NR	NR	L: 2 O: 2	L: 7 O: 5	L: 1.3 O: 2.1
OR time (minutes)	L: 142 O: 118[b]	L: 150 O: 95[b]	L: 145 O: 115[b]	L: 180 O: 135[b]	NR
Conversion rate (%)	11	21	17	25	19
Length of stay (days)	L: 5.2 O: 7.9[b]	L: 5 O: 6[b]	L: 8.2 O: 9.3[b]	L: 9 O: 9	NR
Morbidity (%)	L: 10.8 O: 28.7[b]	L: 21 O: 20	L: 21 O: 20	L: 26 O: 27	NR
Mortality (%)	L: 0.9 O: 2.9	L: 0.5 O: 1	L: 1 O: 2	L: 4 O: 5	L: 1.4 O: 1.6
Port site mets (%)	L: 0.9 O: 0	L: 0.9 O: 0.5	NR	L: 2.5 O: 0.6	NR
Local recurrence (%)	L: 6.6 O: 13.7	L: 2.3 O: 2.6	NR	L: 7.3 O: 6.0	L: 4.9 O: 6.5
Disease-free survival (%)	L: 83 O: 73	L: 69.2 O: 68.4	NR	L: NS O: NS	L: 75.8 O: 75.3
Overall survival (%)	L: 18 O: 26	L: 76.4 O: 74.6	NR	L: NS O: NS	L: 82.2 O: 83.5

[a] Meta-analysis of the four RCTs (796 patients laparoscopic-assisted arm; 740 patients in the open arm). Disease-free survival and overall survival are at 3 years' follow-up.
[b] $P < 0.05$.

Abbreviations: L, laparoscopic-assisted resections; Mets, metastases; NR, not reported; NS, no significant difference between groups, actual numbers not reported in trial; O, open resections; OR, operating room.

recurrence rates for stage I tumors were similar in the laparoscopic and open groups, suggesting that the differences noted in overall survival may not be cancer related. Finally, 3-year results from the MRC CLASICC trial [22] also revealed similar overall survival between laparoscopic and open resections (68.4% versus 66.7%, respectively; $P = 0.55$). This trial failed to show a difference between treatments according to stage using the Dukes' rather than TNM system.

The Barcelona trial used cancer-specific survival as its primary endpoint and noted a significant difference between the laparoscopic and open groups (91% and 79%, respectively, $P = 0.03$). Again, when stratified by stage, only stage III patients treated laparoscopically demonstrated improved cancer-specific survival when compared with the open group ($P = 0.006$). These findings are difficult to interpret because the Barcelona trial was the smallest of the four main RCTs, the only one that was single center, and the only one that has shown a survival advantage favoring laparoscopy (out of the three main RCTs that have reported long-term data). Furthermore, a meta-analysis [24] of the Barcelona, COST, COLOR, and MRC CLASICC trials, using all four RCT subjects before 2000 (796 in the laparoscopic arm and 740 open), revealed equivalent 3-year overall survival rates and no differences according to stage of disease.

Disease-free survival was the primary endpoint of the COLOR trial (not yet reported) and a secondary endpoint of the COST and MRC CLASICC trials. Disease-free survival was not significantly different between the laparoscopic and open groups in the COST [23] or MRC CLASICC trials (COST: 68.4% laparoscopic versus 69.2% open, $P = 0.94$, at 5-years; MRC CLASICC: 66.3% laparoscopic versus 67.7% open, $P = 0.70$, at 3-years) [22] or in the meta-analysis of the four main RCTs [24].

Recurrence

The COST trial [23] was the only trial to use recurrence as a primary endpoint. There were no differences between the laparoscopic and open groups for local (2.6% laparoscopic and 2.3% open, $P = 0.79$) or overall (distant and local; 21.8% laparoscopic and 19.4% open, $P = 0.25$) recurrence, with the most common sites of distant recurrence being liver and lung in both groups. In the MRC CLASICC trial [22], local (7.3% laparoscopic and 6.0% open, $P = 0.68$) and distant (11.3% laparoscopic and 12.5% open, $P = 0.91$) recurrence rates also were equivalent between groups. Finally, tumor recurrence also was similar between groups in the Barcelona trial (17% laparoscopic and 27% open, $P = 0.07$), further confirmed in the meta-analysis of the four main RCTs [24].

Surgical wound and port site recurrence

An initial controversy surrounding laparoscopic colon cancer surgery involved the possibility of port site recurrences. Concern for this complication was heightened by a 1994 report by Berends and colleagues [25] where a 21% incidence (3 cases of 14 total) of subcutaneous metastases was noted in this early series of laparoscopic colectomy. The possibility of surgical wound recurrence with laparoscopy was theorized as related to tumor cell seeding at the time of pneumoperitoneum. Anecdotal reports of port site recurrence eventually gave way to larger series demonstrating rates between 0% and 2.5%, similar to the abdominal wall recurrence rates established in open resection series (0%–3.3%) [26]. A prospective trial [27] comparing 57 laparoscopic resections to 52 open resections for colorectal carcinoma identified no port site recurrences in the laparoscopic group and three wound recurrences in the open group despite similar oncologic outcomes. Finally, in the large RCTs reporting long-term results [1,19,22], wound/port site recurrence rates ranged from 0.5% to 2.5% in the laparoscopic group, none of which was significantly different from that seen in the open groups. Given this data, port site recurrence should be considered equivalent to that of wound recurrence after open resection and should not be viewed as an increased risk associated with laparoscopy.

Resection margin

In one of the earliest randomized trials comparing laparoscopic to open colon cancer resection, Milsom and colleagues [16] reported clear surgical margins in all patients, suggesting that a satisfactory oncologic resection could be obtained laparoscopically. This has since been confirmed in larger studies, as would be expected with the equivalent local recurrence rates (discussed previously). The COST trial revealed similar median proximal and distal margins between the laparoscopic and open groups and a similar percentage of patients with tumor margins less than 5 cm (5% laparoscopic and 6% open). Similarly, the COLOR trial reported identical numbers (10) and percentages (2%) of patients who had positive margins in each group. Furthermore, the MRC CLASICC trial failed to show a difference in positive circumferential resection margins between laparoscopic (7%) and open (5%) groups ($P = 0.45$). Finally, meta-analysis [24] did not reveal significant differences in resection margins between laparoscopic and open approaches.

Lymph node retrieval

Although attention often is given to the adequacy of lymph node sampling during laparoscopic colon cancer resection, few early RCTs report lymph node numbers in their results. Milsom and colleagues [16] noted a slight but insignificant increase in the median number of nodes procured with open (25) versus laparoscopic resection (19). Equivalent lymph node retrieval was reported in all of the major RCTs, both in the total number of lymph nodes sampled (Barcelona, MRC CLASICC, and COST trials) and in the number of positive lymph nodes identified (COLOR trial).

Based on the previous summary, mainly from RCTs reporting on short- and long-term oncologic outcomes, along with margin and lymph node adequacy, there is strong evidence to confirm that a laparoscopic resection is oncologically equivalent to open for colon cancer.

Conversion rates

The conversion from laparoscopic to open procedure may be necessary for many reasons and likely reflects good judgment. Acceptable conversion rates largely are undefined, however. In addition, the effect that converting from a laparoscopic to an open procedure has on outcome is unknown. Early trials of laparoscopic colon cancer resection reported conversion rates between 5% and 45% [7,15,17]. By comparison, the conversion rates reported in the major RCTs were 11% (Barcelona), 21% (COST), 17% (COLOR), and 25% (MRC CLASICC). This resulted in an overall rate of 19% on meta-analysis [24]. Although these conversion rates may be higher than those reported in large series for benign and malignant disease (11.4%–14.3%) [11,28], this may reflect the difficulty involved with providing adequate oncologic resection. In the RCTs, the major reasons reported for conversion included tumor invasion into other organs or adjacent structures (Barcelona and COLOR) and excessive tumor fixation or uncertainty of tumor clearance (MRC CLASICC), indicating primarily oncologic reasons. Although there is some suggestion that conversion to an open procedure may result in worse perioperative outcomes [29], this has not been substantiated, and a subgroup comparison from the MRC CLASICC trial revealed equivalent perioperative outcomes between laparoscopic, open, and laparoscopic to open converted groups.

Operative time, hospital length of stay, and cost

With the increased technical demands required of a laparoscopic approach, significantly longer operative times are evident, a finding noted in all four major RCTs. Operative times for laparoscopic resections in these trials ranged from 142 to 180 minutes compared with 95135 open [1,19–21]. Conversely, a laparoscopic colectomy for colon cancer resulted in a shorter hospital stay compared with open resection, a difference that ranged from 1 to 2.4 days in the major RCTs, all statistically significant. The reduced length of stay associated with laparoscopic colectomy likely is multifactorial and includes an earlier tolerance of oral intake [19], shorter duration of parenteral narcotic requirements [1], and earlier return of GI function (first bowel movement) [20]. A shortened hospital stay after laparoscopic colectomy also may reflect bias, however, in the postoperative decision-making process, perhaps pushing the recovery phase of laparoscopically treated patients. This is possible given the implementation of recent fast-track protocols. When doing so, one randomized, blinded study [30] showed similar lengths of stay (2 days) after laparoscopic and open colectomy in a population of patients that had primarily malignant disease.

There has been great variability in the literature regarding cost issues for laparoscopic and open colectomy. Cost analyses were performed in two of the four main RCTs comparing laparoscopic and open resection of colon cancer. A 12-week cost analysis in the COLOR trial [31] revealed a significantly higher cost to the health care system in the laparoscopic (€9479) compared with the open group (€7235). This is primarily due to greater operative costs (including OR times) generated by laparoscopy (€3493 laparoscopic and €2322 open). When productivity loss was taken into account, the total cost to society was found similar between groups because of the faster recovery time noted in the laparoscopic group. A short-term cost-analysis conducted as part of the MRC CLASICC trial [32] found that operative costs were higher in the laparoscopic group (£1596 laparoscopic and £1327 open), hospital (nonoperative) costs were higher in the open group (£2517 laparoscopic and £2667 open), and total costs were similar between groups (£5587 laparoscopic and £5503 open) at 3 months postoperatively.

Operative mortality and complications

Reported operative mortality rates associated with laparoscopic colectomy for colon cancer are similar to those for open colectomy. This has been shown in each of the four major RCTs. In addition, the meta-analysis based on these trials reported mortality rates of 1.4% and 1.6% for laparoscopic and open colectomy, respectively ($P = $ NS). It seems, however, there may be less agreement with respect to morbidity. The Barcelona trial reported significantly less blood loss, duration of postoperative ileus, and overall morbidity in the laparoscopic group compared with the open group. These differences in complications seemed driven by a higher number of wound infections (18 open versus 8 laparoscopic) and cases of persistent ileus (nine open versus three laparoscopic) in the open group. These findings were not corroborated by the subsequent other RCTs, except that the COLOR trial confirmed lower blood loss in the laparoscopic group. In a report evaluating long-term complications, an updated Italian RCT [4] compared 190 laparoscopic colon cancer resections to 201 open resections and noted fewer complications in the laparoscopic group (13% laparoscopic and 30% open, $P = 0.02$), namely incisional hernias and bowel obstructions. Despite these reports it seems that overall, mortality and short-term complication rates associated with laparoscopic colectomy for colon cancer are equivalent to open procedures.

Quality of life

One purported benefit of laparoscopic surgery is an improved short-term quality of life as a result of shorter hospital stays, smaller incisions, reduced postoperative pain, and faster return to work and normal activities. Quality of life was examined in three of the four major RCTs comparing laparoscopic and open colectomy for colon cancer. The COST trial [33] examined short-term quality of life by comparing several quality-of-life scores for laparoscopic and open colectomies at four time points: preoperative and 2 days, 2 weeks, and 2 months postoperatively. This revealed that despite fewer days of parenteral and oral narcotic analgesic requirements in the laparoscopic group, only one outcome (single-item global rating scale) at one time point (2 weeks postoperative) was found significantly improved. The MRC CLASICC trial found equivalent function and quality-of-life scores in the laparoscopic and open groups at baseline and 2 weeks, 3 months, 6 months, 18 months, and 3 years postoperatively [21], although this analysis included rectal and colon cancer patients. In contrast, the COLOR trial, in a recent updated report [34] assessing health-related quality of life, noted a significant improvement in social and role function at 2 weeks, and social function alone at 4 weeks postoperatively in the laparoscopic group. They concluded that the laparoscopic approach resulted in an improved quality of life during the first postoperative month. Furthermore, Braga and colleagues [4], in an update of their RCT comparing laparoscopic and open colon cancer resection, reported a better quality of life at 12 months (based on the Short Form 36 Health Survey questionnaire) in the laparoscopic group. Overall, the results of the major RCTs show laparoscopic colectomy to have equivalent or mildly improved short-term quality of life when compared with open colectomy in patients who have colon cancer.

Minimally invasive rectal cancer surgery

Laparoscopic approaches for rectal cancer first were reported in the early 1990s [35] and generally are considered more technically challenging than laparoscopic colectomies. Many of the controversies revolving around laparoscopic colon cancer surgery apply to laparoscopic rectal cancer surgery: adequacy of resection margins and lymph node harvest, local recurrence rates, survival rates, safety, and cost. Although there are fewer large, multicenter RCTs evaluating minimally invasive rectal cancer surgery than for colon cancer, there still is a substantial body of literature examining these outcomes. The majority of these studies are prospective, nonrandomized, and without control groups (Table 3) [36–49], although several large studies [50–54] comparing laparoscopic and open resections suggest that laparoscopic rectal cancer surgery is safe, with favorable short-term patient-oriented and oncologic outcomes (Table 4).

Oncologic and patient-oriented outcomes

At the time of this writing there have been five prospective RCTs comparing laparoscopic-assisted and open resection for rectal cancer (see Table 4).

Table 3
Laparoscopic resection for rectal cancer: prospective series with at least 100 patients

Author	Procedures	Patients (n)	Follow-up (mos)	OR time (min)	Conversion (%)	LNs (mean)	Morbidity/ mortality (%)	Local recurrence (%)
Köckerling, et al [49]	APR	116	16	226	3.4	11.5	34.4/1.7	6
Scheidbach, et al [36]	AR, APR	380	24.8	208	6.1	13	37/1.6	6.6
Morino, et al [47]	AR	100	45.7	250	12	12.8	36/2	4.2
Delgado, et al [38]	AR, APR	220	18	178.5	20	13.8	26.3/1.3	5.3
Leroy, et al [46]	AR, APR	102	36	202	3	8	27/2	6
Law, et al [48]	AR, APR	100	NR	195	15	9	31/1	NR
Dulucq, et al [42]	AR	218	57	138	12	24.5	25.6/1	6.8
Bärlehner, et al [40]	AR, APR	194		174	1	25.4	20.1/0	4.1
Kim, et al [37]	AR	312	27	212	8	23	20.5/0.3	8
Tsang, et al [45]	AR	105	26.9	170.4	1.9	NR	25/0	4.8
Laurent, et al [39]	AR	200	NR	360	15.5	11	25/1	NR
Hasegawa, et al [43]	AR, APR	131	42	320	3.1	12	22.1/0	6
Bianchi, et al [44]	AR, APR	107	35.8	278	18.7	18	18.7/0	18.7

Abbreviations: APR, abdominoperineal resection; AR, anterior resection; LN, lymph nodes harvested; NR, not reported; OR, operating room.

Table 4
Prospective studies comparing laparoscopic and open resections for rectal cancer

Author	Accrual years	Pts (n)	Conversion (%)	LNs (mean)	Morbidity/ mortality (%)	Follow-up (mo)	Local recurrence (%)	Survival (%) Disease-free	Overall
Randomized controlled trials									
CLASICC [21,22]	1996–2002	L: 253 O: 128	34	NS	L: 40/NS O: 37/NS	36.8	L: 9.7 O: 10.1	L: NS O: NS	L: NSO: NS
Leung, et al [55]	1993–2002	L: 203 O: 200	23.2	L: 11.1 O: 12.1	L: 19.7/0.6 O: 22.5/2.4	L: 52.7 O: 49.2	L: 6.6 O: 4.4	L: 75.3 O: 78.3[b]	L: 77.2O: 76.5[b]
Braga, et al [58]	2007	L: 83 O: 85	7.2	L: 12.7 O: 13.6	L: 28.9/1 O: 40/1	53.6	L: 4 O: 5.2	L: NS O: NS	L: NSO: NS
Zhou, et al [87]	2001–2002	L: 82 O: 89	NR	NR	L: 6.1/0 O: 12.4[a]/0	NR	NR	NR	NR
Araujo, et al [88]	1997–2000	L: 13 O: 15	0	L: 5.5 O: 11.9[a]	L: 69/0 O: 46.7/0	47.2	L: 0 O: 13	NR	NR
Nonrandomized trials									
Bretagnol, et al [41]	2000–2003	L: 144 O: 83	14	L: 10 O: 12[a]	L: 34/1 O: NR	18	L: 1.4 O: NR	L: NS O: NS	L: NO: NS
Staudacher, et al [50]	1998–2005	L: 108 O: 79	12	L: 14.3 O: 15.3	L: 29.7/0 O: 27.8/0	27.6	L: 6.4 O: 5.0	L: 77.8 O: 76.0	NR
Lelong, et al [51]	2002–2004	L: 104 O: 68	14.5	L: 11 O: 9	L: 43.3/1 O: 48.5/2.9	NR	NR	NR	NR
Anthuber, et al [52]	1996–2002	L: 101 O: 334	10.9	L: 15.3 O: 21.9[a]	L: 30.7/0 O: 65.0[a]/1.5	NR	L: 2.0 O: NR	NR	NR
Morino, et al [53]	1994–2002	L: 98 O: 93	18.4	L: 12.4 O: 10.5	L: 24.4/1.0 O: 23.6/2.2	L: 46.3 O: 49.7	L: 3.2 O: 12.6[a]	L: 65.4 O: 58.9[b]	L: 80.0O: 68.9[b]
Law, et al [54]	2000–2004	L: 98 O: 167	12	L: 10 O: 11	L: 25.5/1 O: 29.3/2.4	21.2	L: 2.0 O: 3.0	L: NS O: NS	L: NSO: NS

[a] $P < 0.05$.
[b] Probability at 5 years.
Abbreviations: L, laparoscopic-assisted resections; LN, lymph nodes; NR, not reported; NS, no significant difference between groups, numbers not reported; O, open resections; Pts, patients.

A trial from Hong Kong [55] randomized 403 patients to laparoscopic-assisted (203 patients) or open (200 patients) resection for "rectosigmoid" cancer. This study demonstrated significantly improved short-term patient oriented outcomes in the laparoscopic group. These included reduced pain scores and analgesic requirements, shorter time to flatus and bowel movement, earlier resumption of normal diet and ambulation, and a shorter hospital stay. Patients receiving a laparoscopic resection returned to their usual routine activities, on average, 11.5 days sooner than those having an open resection ($P = 0.002$). Although the conversion rate was 23%, operative mortality, complications, and oncologic outcomes (including distal resection margin, number of lymph nodes, local recurrence, disease-free survival, and overall survival) were found equivalent between groups, although operative times were longer and total costs higher with laparoscopy.

The MRC CLASICC trial [21] included a subgroup of 253 patients assigned to laparoscopic resection and 128 patients assigned to open resection for rectal cancer. This comparison revealed similar rates of positive resection margins and numbers of lymph nodes harvested, although patients having laparoscopic low anterior resection had a slight but nonsignificant increase in circumferential margin positivity. Operative mortality, complication rates, and quality-of-life scores also were similar between groups, and those assigned to the laparoscopic group were discharged 2 days earlier than those in the open group (P value not reported). A conversion rate of 34% was reported in this trial. Subsequently, when results were analyzed according to actual treatment received, those having a laparoscopic converted to open resection demonstrated significantly higher complication rates compared with those having a laparoscopic or open resection (93% rate if conversion, 44% laparoscopic, and 51% open; $P = 0.002$). This may be secondary to factors associated with the conversion itself or more likely due to factors leading to conversion, because more locally advanced tumors were noted in those requiring conversion. A subsequent 3-year update of this trial [22] revealed equivalent oncologic and quality-of-life outcomes for the laparoscopic and open groups, even when stratified by low anterior (overall survival 74.6% laparoscopic and 66.7% open, $P = 0.17$) or abdominoperineal resection (overall survival 65.2% laparoscopic and 57.7% open, $P = 0.41$). In addition, the trend toward increased circumferential resection margin positivity seen in the laparoscopic low anterior resection group did not result in an increased rate of local recurrence (7.8% laparoscopic and 7.0% open, $P = 0.70$) and the administration of neoadjuvant chemoradiation and adjuvant chemotherapy was equivalent in both groups.

Overall, the published RCT reports to date give supportive evidence to suggest that laparoscopic rectal cancer surgery provides earlier postoperative recovery and allows comparable oncologic resections compared with an open approach. A meta-analysis [56] of all studies comparing laparoscopic and open resections for rectal cancer between 1993 and 2004 also supports these conclusions. Finally, the results of planned future multicenter

RCTs comparing laparoscopic and open rectal cancer surgery in Europe (COLOR II) [57] and North America (American College of Surgeons Oncology Group [ACOSOG] Z6051) will provide further clarity in regards to the short- and long-term patient-oriented and, especially, oncologic outcomes associated with this technique.

Quality-of-life and functional outcomes

The assessment of quality-of-life and functional outcomes between laparoscopic and open resections for rectal cancer are an ongoing area of controversy. In contrast to the MRC CLASICC trial, a RCT from Italy [58] reported an improved quality of life during the first year after resection using a laparoscopic approach. Despite this report, further evidence may suggest substandard functional outcomes after laparoscopic anterior resection, especially in men. A retrospective analysis [59] of 40 laparoscopic-assisted and 40 open rectal cancer resections in men and women noted higher rates of sexual dysfunction (impotence or impaired ejaculation), but not urinary dysfunction, in men in the laparoscopic group [47% (7/15) laparoscopic and 4.5% (1/22) open, $P = 0.004$]. An assessment of urinary and sexual function from the MRC CLASICC trial [60] revealed a trend toward altered sexual function in men after laparoscopic resection ($P = 0.068$). As there were more total mesorectal excisions (TMEs) in the laparoscopic group compared with open, and TME was an independent predictor of postoperative male sexual dysfunction (along with conversion to open procedure), the investigators suggest that the higher TME rate may be responsible for the noted trend. A Dutch prospective study of 38 patients undergoing laparoscopic rectal cancer resection reported worse sexual function but improved global quality-of-life scores at 1 year. This evidence suggests that many factors likely contribute to quality of life, some of which may be improved with a laparoscopic approach to rectal cancer resection.

Robotic surgery

Unlike other surgical subspecialties, such as urology, robotic surgery has been slow to enter the realm of colon and rectal surgery. In contrast to minimally invasive prostatectomy, where robotic surgery offers a distinct technical advantage over laparoscopy [61], most minimally invasive general surgery procedures can be performed with the same ease laparoscopically as with a robot, with much lower associated costs. Rectal surgery, like prostate surgery, however, may be well suited for robotics because of the difficulty of performing a laparoscopic resection and anastomosis within the pelvis. The potential technical advantages that robotic surgery may offer over laparoscopy include improved comfort for the operator because of the ergonomics of the operating console, improved visualization because of 3-D viewing, tremor filtering, and increased degrees of freedom, such as the wrist action used for suturing.

To date there are few reports of robotic rectal cancer surgery. A report from City of Hope National Medical Center [62] examined outcomes for 39 consecutive unselected patients who had primary rectal cancer undergoing robotic-assisted laparoscopic resection (22 low anterior, 11 intersphincteric, and 6 abdominoperineal). The splenic flexure, descending, and sigmoid colon were mobilized laparoscopically, followed by a TME using the da Vinci robotic system (Intuitive Surgical, Sunnyvale, California). The distal rectum was divided using a roticulating stapler. For anterior resections, the specimen was extracted through a 4-cm incision and an end-to-end anastomosis created with a circular stapler. For very low tumors, the specimen was extracted through the anus and a hand-sewn coloanal anastomosis was performed. For abdominoperineal resections, the specimen was removed through the perineal wound and a sigmoid colostomy was created. There were no deaths, with a 12.8% morbidity rate, and 2.6% conversion rate (1/39). Median operative time was 285 minutes and patients were discharged on the fourth postoperative day (range 2–22). All resection margins were negative with a median of 13 lymph nodes harvested. This early report suggests that robotic-assisted laparoscopic rectal cancer surgery may be safe and feasible, although at present still considered early in its development.

Local excision/transanal endoscopic microsurgery

When considering minimally invasive approaches for the treatment of rectal cancer, a transanal local approach also must be taken into consideration. Although most advocate that this approach is not sound oncologically for more advanced tumors, there may be a subgroup of favorable, early rectal cancers that can be approached with this methodology.

Local excision

There is evidence to suggest that the use of local excision for the treatment of rectal cancer has increased over the past decade [63]. A standard transanal excision seems beneficial when considering that this natural orifice approach leaves no visible scars, is only mildly uncomfortable with a minimal hospital stay, generally has minimal effect on rectal function, and potentially may avoid a permanent colostomy. Unfortunately, the shortcomings of this approach are that an oncologic lymphadenectomy is not part of the procedure and that this approach often is limited by lesion size and location, not to mention that actual resection can be difficult. Many retrospective series have suggested that recurrence after local excision is not trivial. Local recurrence rates after transanal excision of T1 tumors is reported between 5% and 23% [64–67]. More significantly, resection for T2 tumors seems less favorable, with local recurrence rates as high as 26% to 45% [65–67]. For this reason it is generally accepted that local therapy alone for T2 tumors is inappropriate. Unfortunately, there are no prospective, randomized trials comparing standard transanal excision to more radical surgery (low anterior resection or abdominoperineal resection), although comparative analyses suggest that even when considering only T1 tumors, recurrence is more likely after local excision [68,69]. Furthermore, a large cohort study from the National Cancer Database [63] revealed that local recurrence rates after local excision of T1 cancer was 12.5% versus 6.9% with radical resection and 22.1% versus 15.1% for T2 tumors. Therefore, when considering a local approach for rectal cancer, proper staging (with endorectal ultrasound or MRI scan) along with a careful patient discussion regarding alternatives, recurrence rates, and sphincter preservation issues should assist in the decision-making process before proceeding.

Transanal endoscopic microsurgery

Transanal endoscopic microsurgery (TEM) is a more recent technologic advance in the local treatment of limited rectal cancer. This approach was developed and first described by Buess and colleagues in 1985 [70]. The technique uses an operating rectoscope, stereoscopic viewing, and CO_2 rectal insufflation along with specially designed instrumentation to ideally visualize and excise the tumor within the distended rectum. As a result, this device allows optimal tumor margin assessment and clearance and the ability to reach more proximally located tumors. Although prospective, randomized trials are lacking between standard local excision and TEM for early rectal cancer, several case series suggest that TEM may have an advantage with respect to local recurrence rates. This seems more evident for T1 tumors where recurrence rates range from 0% to 26% (Table 5). When considering the smaller number of series reporting T2 tumors, however, it seems that recurrence remains high (9.5%–42.8%) (Table 6). In addition to using tumor depth to stratify risk for recurrence, there is evidence that optimal histopathology (lack of poor differentiation or lymphovascular invasion

Table 5

Series reporting transanal endoscopic microsurgery for local excision of pT1 rectal adenocarcinoma

Author	Patients (n)	Local recurrence (%)	Follow-up (months)
Winde, et al [72]	24	4.2	41
Smith, et al [89]	300	10	12
Mentges, et al [90]	52	3	29
Heintz, et al [91]	58	10.3	52
Lee, et al [92]	52	4.1	31
Palma, et al [93]	21	4.8	30
Floyd, et al [94]	53	7.5	34
Stipa, et al [95]	23	8.6	78
Bretagnol, et al [96]	31	9.7	33
Maslekar, et al [97]	27	0	40
Zacharakis, et al [98]	14	7.1	37
Whitehouse, et al [99]	23	26	34

Table 6
Series reporting transanal endoscopic microsurgery for local excision of pT2 rectal adenocarcinoma

Author	Patients (n)	Local recurrence (%)	Follow-up (months)
Smith, et al [89]	15	40	12
Lee, et al [92]	22	19.5	31
Stipa, et al [95]	21	9.5	78
Bretagnol, et al [96]	17	11.8	33
Zacharakis, et al [98]	11	42.8	37
Smith, et al [89]	20	35	45
Lee, et al [92]	9	22	34

and margins greater than 1 mm) is important in determining the appropriate use of TEM for T1 carcinoma [71].

Only one prospective, randomized study [72] has compared TEM to anterior resection for T1 rectal cancer, citing equivalent local recurrence rates (4.2%) and 5-year survival (96%) after a follow-up of 41 (TEM) and 46 (anterior resection) months. In contrast, a prospective, multicenter observational study revealed higher local recurrence rates (6% versus 2%, $P = 0.049$) but similar actuarial survival when comparing local to radical resection for pT1 tumors. Unfortunately, this report considered TEM and standard local excision approaches together within the local resection group [73]. Finally, Lezoche and colleagues [74] reported a prospective, randomized comparison of TEM versus laparoscopic TME for T2 cancer after neoadjuvant chemoradiation therapy. A local recurrence rate of 5.7% (2/35) was noted after TEM versus 2.8% after laparoscopic resection with a median follow-up period of 84 months.

It seems that the same advantages of using a standard local excision approach can be expected with TEM. Reports have demonstrated that TEM can be performed safely with minimal morbidity and without adverse effects on continence or quality of life [75,76]. Unfortunately, this technology carries with it a significant learning curve along with the added expense of a complex operating apparatus.

Chemoradiation therapy

Aside from radical excision, another treatment alternative involves the addition of chemoradiation therapy to local excision. An assessment of adjuvant chemoradiation after local excision of T2 rectal cancers was previously undertaken by the Cancer and Leukemia Group B [77]. This phase II study reported a 20% (10/51) recurrence rate with this approach. An alternative treatment method uses neoadjuvant chemoradiation followed by local excision. Borschitz and colleagues [78] reviewed several small published series that assessed this approach for T2 and T3 rectal cancer and noted that the extent of response to chemoradiation was a strong predictor of local recurrence, with absence of residual tumor (ypT0) being most favorable. When considering only T2 tumors from these combined series (local excision and TEM), a 7% (6/85) local recurrence rate was determined. Further assessment of neoadjuvant chemoradiotherapy followed by local excision is under way in a phase II trial for T2N0 rectal cancer by the ACOSOG (Z6041).

General considerations

Patient selection

None of the four major randomized trials comparing laparoscopic to open resection for colon cancer included patients who had transverse lesions, obstructing colon cancer, synchronous lesions, or metastatic disease. There have been smaller, uncontrolled studies, however, examining the use of laparoscopy in these patient groups. Resecting cancers of the transverse colon by laparoscopic means is perceived as more difficult than left- or right-sided resections because of the difficulty in ligation of the middle colic vessels and reduced visibility due to the greater omentum. A report [79] comparing 22 laparoscopic transverse colectomies (12 extended right colectomies, 9 transverse colectomies, and 1 extended left colectomy) to 285 "other" colectomies (sigmoid, right, left, and anterior resections) found that laparoscopic transverse colectomies had similar complications, conversion rates, and oncologic outcomes at 17 months' follow-up. Operative time was significantly longer in the transverse colectomy group compared with the laparoscopic "other" group, reflecting the increased difficulty with this operation. A major flaw of this study is the lack of an open comparison group. Regardless, at present there does not seem to be evidence to suggest that transverse colon cancers should not be approached laparoscopically in the hands of experienced minimally invasive colorectal surgeons.

Colonic obstruction is considered a relative contraindication to laparoscopic colectomy. This is likely because dilated bowel may prohibit adequate visualization and the ability to grasp and manipulate, not to mention the possibility of iatrogenic perforation. A recent report from Hong Kong [80], however, describes a series of seven consecutive patients treated with emergent laparoscopically assisted right hemicolectomy for obstructing right-sided colon cancer. There were no conversions and the lone complication was a death from a postoperative myocardial infarction. Adequate lymph nodes were harvested (mean 17) and the median time to return of bowel function was 5 days. An alternative approach as described in a series from Italy [81] used endoscopically placed self-expanding stents in 23 patients who had obstructing left or transverse colon cancer to facilitate an elective resection. In 19 of these patients, a laparoscopic resection was used after bowel preparation was completed. There were no major complications reported. Although there is little supporting evidence for routine practice, a laparoscopic approach for obstructing colon cancer may be feasible in the hands of experienced laparoscopists.

The advent of minimally invasive liver surgery also has created the possibility for simultaneous treatment of colorectal cancer with associated hepatic metastases. One group reported [82] the use of laparoscopic radio-frequency ablation of liver tumors in 16 patients performed concomitantly with various colorectal procedures, five of which included laparoscopic colorectal cancer resection. A case report from Hong Kong [83] described the simultaneous resection of a rectal cancer and a liver metastasis via a laparoscopic low anterior resection and laparoscopic left lateral segmentectomy. Although these reports show feasibility, they are far from entering routine practice.

Totally laparoscopic versus laparoscopic-assisted versus hand-assisted laparoscopic colectomy

The majority of key trials included in this review have used a laparoscopic-assisted approach to colectomy, in which the colon is mobilized intracorporeally (usually along with mesentery division) and the bowel resection and anastomosis occur outside of the abdomen after making a small incision. Totally laparoscopic colectomy involves intracorporeal mesenteric division and anastomosis with minimal incision for extraction only. An early prospective trial [84] comparing 34 totally laparoscopic colectomies to 63 laparoscopic-assisted procedures showed no benefit to the totally laparoscopic approach, as there were similar lengths of hospital stay and times to return of bowel function. The third approach, the hand-assisted laparoscopic colectomy (HALC), uses a hand port placed through a small (6–8 cm) incision allowing tactile feedback to complete dissection. A RCT [85] comparing only HALC to open colectomy for right-sided colon cancers showed the same benefits as the other laparoscopic approaches when compared with open (less narcotic use, faster recovery, and shorter hospital stay). The HALC still requires significantly longer operative times, however, than open colectomy, along with the added expense of the hand port. Currently, studies comparing HALC to laparoscopic-assisted resections specifically for colorectal cancer are lacking.

Learning curve/quality assurance

As with other technically challenging procedures, there is evidence that surgeon or hospital volume for laparoscopic colectomy affects outcomes. A prospective multicenter study [86] from Germany evaluating the quality of oncologic resection for patients having their procedure performed laparoscopically revealed a marked variability in the number of lymph nodes harvested by surgeons. They noted that the number of lymph nodes harvested increased over time, suggesting that larger case volumes might improve oncologic resection. To account for this learning curve, the major multicenter RCTs evaluating laparoscopic colon cancer resection required at least 20 prior laparoscopic-assisted colectomies for participating surgeons in each study. In addition, the MRC CLASICC trial [21] found that the conversion rate fell from 34% during year 1 to 16% in year 6, suggesting fewer conversions with increasing surgeon experience. An analysis of the centers participating in the COLOR trial revealed that high-volume centers had significantly lower conversion rates, median operative times, larger numbers of lymph nodes harvested, fewer complications, and shorter hospital stays when compared with low- and medium-volume centers. This may suggest that short-term outcomes are improved at centers performing high volumes of laparoscopic colon cancer surgery. There currently are no reports addressing long-term oncologic outcomes based on hospital or surgeon case volume.

Summary

Laparoscopic resection of colorectal cancer results in shorter hospital stays and equivalent short-term patient-oriented outcomes, long-term oncologic outcomes, and quality of life compared with open resection. This is at the expense of longer operative times and questionably higher health care costs. Because of their exclusion from RCTs, more evidence is required before laparoscopic colectomy may be offered routinely to patients who have transverse colon lesions and synchronous or obstructing colon cancers. Although earlier in its evolution, laparoscopic rectal cancer surgery may result in improved short-term patient-oriented outcomes and equivalent oncologic resections compared with the open approach. Ongoing multicenter RCTs will address oncologic comparisons and outcomes further. Transanal approaches, such as TEM, are additional adjuncts in select early rectal cancers, whereas robotic-assisted laparoscopic rectal surgery likely will evolve further in the future.

References

[1] A comparison of laparoscopically assisted and open colectomy for colon cancer. N Engl J Med 2004;350(20):2050–9.

[2] Schwenk W, Bohm B, Muller JM. Postoperative pain and fatigue after laparoscopic or conventional colorectal resections. A prospective randomized trial. Surg Endosc 1998; 12(9):1131–6.

[3] Schwenk W, Bohm B, Haase O, et al. Laparoscopic versus conventional colorectal resection: a prospective randomised study of postoperative ileus and early postoperative feeding. Langenbecks Arch Surg 1998;383(1):49–55.

[4] Braga M, Frasson M, Vignali A, et al. Laparoscopic vs. open colectomy in cancer patients: long-term complications, quality of life, and survival. Dis Colon Rectum 2005;48(12): 2217–23.

[5] Leung KL, Lai PB, Ho RL, et al. Systemic cytokine response after laparoscopic-assisted resection of rectosigmoid carcinoma: a prospective randomized trial. Ann Surg 2000; 231(4):506–11.

[6] Delgado S, Lacy AM, Filella X, et al. Acute phase response in laparoscopic and open colectomy in colon cancer: randomized study. Dis Colon Rectum 2001;44(5):638–46.

[7] Braga M, Vignali A, Gianotti L, et al. Laparoscopic versus open colorectal surgery: a randomized trial on short-term outcome. Ann Surg 2002;236(6):759–66.

[8] Hu JK, Zhou ZG, Chen ZX, et al. Comparative evaluation of immune response after laparoscopical and open total mesorectal excisions with anal sphincter preservation in patients with rectal cancer. World J Gastroenterol 2003;9(12):2690–4.

[9] Poulin EC, Mamazza J, Schlachta CM, et al. Laparoscopic resection does not adversely affect early survival curves in patients undergoing surgery for colorectal adenocarcinoma. Ann Surg 1999;229(4):487–92.

[10] Lumley J, Stitz R, Stevenson A, et al. Laparoscopic colorectal surgery for cancer: intermediate to long-term outcomes. Dis Colon Rectum 2002;45(7):867–72.

[11] Senagore AJ, Delaney CP. A critical analysis of laparoscopic colectomy at a single institution: lessons learned after 1000 cases. Am J Surg 2006;191(3):377–80.

[12] Law WL, Lee YM, Choi HK, et al. Impact of laparoscopic resection for colorectal cancer on operative outcomes and survival. Ann Surg 2007;245(1):1–7.

[13] Stage JG, Schulze S, Moller P, et al. Prospective randomized study of laparoscopic versus open colonic resection for adenocarcinoma. Br J Surg 1997;84(3):391–6.

[14] Hasegawa H, Kabeshima Y, Watanabe M, et al. Randomized controlled trial of laparoscopic versus open colectomy for advanced colorectal cancer. Surg Endosc 2003;17(4):636–40.

[15] Kaiser AM, Kang JC, Chan LS, et al. Laparoscopic-assisted vs. open colectomy for colon cancer: a prospective randomized trial. J Laparoendosc Adv Surg Tech A 2004;14(6):329–34.

[16] Milsom JW, Bohm B, Hammerhofer KA, et al. A prospective, randomized trial comparing laparoscopic versus conventional techniques in colorectal cancer surgery: a preliminary report. J Am Coll Surg 1998;187(1):46–54.

[17] Curet MJ, Putrakul K, Pitcher DE, et al. Laparoscopically assisted colon resection for colon carcinoma: perioperative results and long-term outcome. Surg Endosc 2000;14(11):1062–6.

[18] Tang CL, Eu KW, Tai BC, et al. Randomized clinical trial of the effect of open versus laparoscopically assisted colectomy on systemic immunity in patients with colorectal cancer. Br J Surg 2001;88(6):801–7.

[19] Lacy AM, Garcia-Valdecasas JC, Delgado S, et al. Laparoscopy-assisted colectomy versus open colectomy for treatment of non-metastatic colon cancer: a randomised trial. Lancet 2002;359(9325):2224–9.

[20] Veldkamp R, Kuhry E, Hop WC, et al. Laparoscopic surgery versus open surgery for colon cancer: short-term outcomes of a randomised trial. Lancet Oncol 2005;6(7):477–84.

[21] Guillou PJ, Quirke P, Thorpe H, et al. Short-term endpoints of conventional versus laparoscopic-assisted surgery in patients with colorectal cancer (MRC CLASICC trial): multicentre, randomised controlled trial. Lancet 2005;365(9472):1718–26.

[22] Jayne DG, Guillou PJ, Thorpe H, et al. Randomized trial of laparoscopic-assisted resection of colorectal carcinoma: 3-year results of the UK MRC CLASICC trial group. J Clin Oncol 2007;25(21):3061–8.

[23] Fleshman J, Sargent DJ, Green E, et al. Laparoscopic colectomy for cancer is not inferior to open surgery based on 5-year data from the COST study group trial. Ann Surg 2007;246(4): 655–62.

[24] Bonjer HJ, Hop WC, Nelson H, et al. Laparoscopically assisted vs open colectomy for colon cancer: a meta-analysis. Arch Surg 2007;142(3):298–303.

[25] Berends FJ, Kazemier G, Bonjer HJ, et al. Subcutaneous metastases after laparoscopic colectomy. Lancet 1994;344(8914):58.

[26] Stocchi L, Nelson H. Wound recurrences following laparoscopic-assisted colectomy for cancer. Arch Surg 2000;135(8):948–58.

[27] Hartley JE, Mehigan BJ, MacDonald AW, et al. Patterns of recurrence and survival after laparoscopic and conventional resections for colorectal carcinoma. Ann Surg 2000;232(2): 181–6.

[28] Le Moine MC, Fabre JM, Vacher C, et al. Factors and consequences of conversion in laparoscopic sigmoidectomy for diverticular disease. Br J Surg 2003;90(2):232–6.

[29] Belizon A, Sardinha CT, Sher ME. Converted laparoscopic colectomy: what are the consequences? Surg Endosc 2006;20(6):947–51.

[30] Basse L, Jakobsen DH, Bardram L, et al. Functional recovery after open versus laparoscopic colonic resection: a randomized, blinded study. Ann Surg 2005;241(3):416–23.

[31] Janson M, Bjorholt I, Carlsson P, et al. Randomized clinical trial of the costs of open and laparoscopic surgery for colonic cancer. Br J Surg 2004;91(4):409–17.

[32] Franks PJ, Bosanquet N, Thorpe H, et al. Short-term costs of conventional vs laparoscopic assisted surgery in patients with colorectal cancer (MRC CLASICC trial). Br J Cancer 2006; 95(1):6–12.

[33] Weeks JC, Nelson H, Gelber S, et al. Short-term quality-of-life outcomes following laparoscopic-assisted colectomy vs open colectomy for colon cancer: a randomized trial. JAMA 2002;287(3):321–8.

[34] Janson M, Lindholm E, Anderberg B, et al. Randomized trial of health-related quality of life after open and laparoscopic surgery for colon cancer. Surg Endosc 2007;21(5):747–53.

[35] Tate JJ, Kwok S, Dawson JW, et al. Prospective comparison of laparoscopic and conventional anterior resection. Br J Surg 1993;80(11):1396–8.

[36] Scheidbach H, Schneider C, Konradt J, et al. Laparoscopic abdominoperineal resection and anterior resection with curative intent for carcinoma of the rectum. Surg Endosc 2002;16(1): 7–13.

[37] Kim SH, Park IJ, Joh YG, et al. Laparoscopic resection for rectal cancer: a prospective analysis of thirty-month follow-up outcomes in 312 patients. Surg Endosc 2006;20(8): 1197–202.

[38] Delgado S, Momblan D, Salvador L, et al. Laparoscopic-assisted approach in rectal cancer patients: lessons learned from > 200 patients. Surg Endosc 2004;18(10):1457–62.

[39] Laurent C, Leblanc F, Gineste C, et al. Laparoscopic approach in surgical treatment of rectal cancer. Br J Surg 2007;94(12):1555–61.

[40] Bärlehner E, Benhidjeb T, Anders S, et al. Laparoscopic resection for rectal cancer: outcomes in 194 patients and review of the literature. Surg Endosc 2005;19(6):757–66.

[41] Bretagnol F, Lelong B, Laurent C, et al. The oncological safety of laparoscopic total mesorectal excision with sphincter preservation for rectal carcinoma. Surg Endosc 2005;19(7): 892–6.

[42] Dulucq JL, Wintringer P, Stabilini C, et al. Laparoscopic rectal resection with anal sphincter preservation for rectal cancer: long-term outcome. Surg Endosc 2005;19(11):1468–74.

[43] Hasegawa H, Ishii Y, Nishibori H, et al. Short- and midterm outcomes of laparoscopic surgery compared for 131 patients with rectal and rectosigmoid cancer. Surg Endosc 2007; 21(6):920–4.

[44] Bianchi PP, Rosati R, Bona S, et al. Laparoscopic surgery in rectal cancer: a prospective analysis of patient survival and outcomes. Dis Colon Rectum 2007;50(12):2047–53.

[45] Tsang WW, Chung CC, Kwok SY, et al. Laparoscopic sphincter-preserving total mesorectal excision with colonic J-pouch reconstruction: five-year results. Ann Surg 2006;243(3):353–8.

[46] Leroy J, Jamali F, Forbes L, et al. Laparoscopic total mesorectal excision (TME) for rectal cancer surgery: long-term outcomes. Surg Endosc 2004;18(2):281–9.

[47] Morino M, Parini U, Giraudo G, et al. Laparoscopic total mesorectal excision: a consecutive series of 100 patients. Ann Surg 2003;237(3):335–42.

[48] Law WL, Chu KW, Tung HM. Early outcomes of 100 patients with laparoscopic resection for rectal neoplasm. Surg Endosc 2004;18(11):1592–6.

[49] Köckerling F, Scheidbach H, Schneider C, et al. Laparoscopic abdominoperineal resection: early postoperative results of a prospective study involving 116 patients. The laparoscopic colorectal surgery study group. Dis Colon Rectum 2000;43(11):1503–11.

[50] Staudacher C, Vignali A, Saverio DP, et al. Laparoscopic vs. Open total mesorectal excision in unselected patients with rectal cancer: impact on early outcome. Dis Colon Rectum 2007; 50(9):1324–31.

[51] Lelong B, Bege T, Esterni B, et al. Short-term outcome after laparoscopic or open restorative mesorectal excision for rectal cancer: a comparative cohort study. Dis Colon Rectum 2007; 50(2):176–83.

[52] Anthuber M, Fuerst A, Elser F, et al. Outcome of laparoscopic surgery for rectal cancer in 101 patients. Dis Colon Rectum 2003;46(8):1047–53.

[53] Morino M, Allaix ME, Giraudo G, et al. Laparoscopic versus open surgery for extraperitoneal rectal cancer: a prospective comparative study. Surg Endosc 2005;19(11):1460–7.

[54] Law WL, Lee YM, Choi HK, et al. Laparoscopic and open anterior resection for upper and mid rectal cancer: an evaluation of outcomes. Dis Colon Rectum 2006;49(8):1108–15.

[55] Leung KL, Kwok SP, Lam SC, et al. Laparoscopic resection of rectosigmoid carcinoma: prospective randomised trial. Lancet 2004;363(9416):1187–92.

[56] Aziz O, Constantinides V, Tekkis PP, et al. Laparoscopic versus open surgery for rectal cancer: a meta-analysis. Ann Surg Oncol 2006;13(3):413–24.

[57] Bjoholt I, Janson M, Jonsson B, et al. Principles for the design of the economic evaluation of COLOR II: an international clinical trial in surgery comparing laparoscopic and open surgery in rectal cancer. Int J Technol Assess Health Care 2006;22(1):130–5.

[58] Braga M, Frasson M, Vignali A, et al. Laparoscopic resection in rectal cancer patients: outcome and cost-benefit analysis. Dis Colon Rectum 2007;50(4):464–71.

[59] Quah HM, Jayne DG, Eu KW, et al. Bladder and sexual dysfunction following laparoscopically assisted and conventional open mesorectal resection for cancer. Br J Surg 2002;89(12):1551–6.

[60] Jayne DG, Brown JM, Thorpe H, et al. Bladder and sexual function following resection for rectal cancer in a randomized clinical trial of laparoscopic versus open technique. Br J Surg 2005;92(9):1124–32.

[61] Menon M, Tewari A, Peabody JO, et al. Vattikuti Institute prostatectomy, a technique of robotic radical prostatectomy for management of localized carcinoma of the prostate: experience of over 1100 cases. Urol Clin North Am 2004;31(4):701–17.

[62] Hellan M, Anderson C, Ellenhorn JD, et al. Short-term outcomes after robotic-assisted total mesorectal excision for rectal cancer. Ann Surg Oncol 2007;14(11):3168–73.

[63] You YN, Baxter NN, Stewart A, et al. Is the increasing rate of local excision for stage I rectal cancer in the United States justified? a nationwide cohort study from the national cancer database. Ann Surg 2007;245(5):726–33.

[64] Madbouly KM, Remzi FH, Erkek BA, et al. Recurrence after transanal excision of T1 rectal cancer: should we be concerned? Dis Colon Rectum 2005;48(4):711–9.

[65] Paty PB, Nash GM, Baron P, et al. Long-term results of local excision for rectal cancer. Ann Surg 2002;236(4):522–9.

[66] Garcia-Aguilar J, Mellgren A, Sirivongs P, et al. Local excision of rectal cancer without adjuvant therapy: a word of caution. Ann Surg 2000;231(3):345–51.

[67] Varma MG, Rogers SJ, Schrock TR, et al. Local excision of rectal carcinoma. Arch Surg 1999;134(8):863–7.

[68] Mellgren A, Sirivongs P, Rothenberger DA, et al. Is local excision adequate therapy for early rectal cancer? Dis Colon Rectum 2000;43(8):1064–71.

[69] Bentrem DJ, Okabe S, Wong WD, et al. T1 adenocarcinoma of the rectum: transanal excision or radical surgery? Ann Surg 2005;242(4):472–7.

[70] Buess G, Theiss R, Gunther M, et al. Endoscopic surgery in the rectum. Endoscopy 1985; 17(1):31–5.

[71] Borschitz T, Heintz A, Junginger T. The influence of histopathologic criteria on the long-term prognosis of locally excised pT1 rectal carcinomas: results of local excision (transanal endoscopic microsurgery) and immediate reoperation. Dis Colon Rectum 2006;49(10):1492–506.

[72] Winde G, Nottberg H, Keller R, et al. Surgical cure for early rectal carcinomas (T1). Transanal endoscopic microsurgery vs. anterior resection. Dis Colon Rectum 1996;39(9):969–76.

[73] Ptok H, Marusch F, Meyer F, et al. Oncological outcome of local vs radical resection of low-risk pT1 rectal cancer. Arch Surg 2007;142(7):649–55.

[74] Lezoche G, Baldarelli M, Guerrieri M, et al. A prospective randomized study with a 5-year minimum follow-up evaluation of transanal endoscopic microsurgery versus laparoscopic total mesorectal excision after neoadjuvant therapy. Surg Endosc 2008;22:352–8.

[75] Kreissler-Haag D, Schuld J, Lindemann W, et al. Complications after transanal endoscopic microsurgical resection correlate with location of rectal neoplasms. Surg Endosc 2008;22: 612–6.

[76] Cataldo PA, O'Brien S, Osler T. Transanal endoscopic microsurgery: a prospective evaluation of functional results. Dis Colon Rectum 2005;48(7):1366–71.

[77] Steele GD Jr, Herndon JE, Bleday R, et al. Sphincter-sparing treatment for distal rectal adenocarcinoma. Ann Surg Oncol 1999;6(5):433–41.

[78] Borschitz T, Wachtlin D, Mohler M, et al. Neoadjuvant chemoradiation and local excision for T2-3 rectal cancer. Ann Surg Oncol 2007.

[79] Schlachta CM, Mamazza J, Poulin EC. Are transverse colon cancers suitable for laparoscopic resection? Surg Endosc 2007;21(3):396–9.

[80] Ng SS, Yiu RY, Li JC, et al. Emergency laparoscopically assisted right hemicolectomy for obstructing right-sided colon carcinoma. J Laparoendosc Adv Surg Tech A 2006;16(4): 350–4.

[81] Olmi S, Scaini A, Cesana G, et al. Acute colonic obstruction: endoscopic stenting and laparoscopic resection. Surg Endosc 2007;21(11):2100–4.

[82] Berber E, Senagore A, Remzi F, et al. Laparoscopic radiofrequency ablation of liver tumors combined with colorectal procedures. Surg Laparosc Endosc Percutan Tech 2004;14(4): 186–90.

[83] Leung KL, Lee JF, Yiu RY, et al. Simultaneous laparoscopic resection of rectal cancer and liver metastasis. J Laparoendosc Adv Surg Tech A 2006;16(5):486–8.

[84] Bernstein MA, Dawson JW, Reissman P, et al. Is complete laparoscopic colectomy superior to laparoscopic assisted colectomy? Am Surg 1996;62(6):507–11.

[85] Chung CC, Ng DC, Tsang WW, et al. Hand-assisted laparoscopic versus open right colectomy: a randomized controlled trial. Ann Surg 2007;246(5):728–33.

[86] Kockerling F, Reymond MA, Schneider C, et al. Prospective multicenter study of the quality of oncologic resections in patients undergoing laparoscopic colorectal surgery for cancer. The Laparoscopic Colorectal Surgery Study Group. Dis Colon Rectum 1998; 41(8):963–70.

[87] Zhou ZG, Hu M, Li Y, et al. Laparoscopic versus open total mesorectal excision with anal sphincter preservation for low rectal cancer. Surg Endosc 2004;18(8):1211–5.

[88] Araujo SE, da Silva eSousa AH Jr, de Campos FG, et al. Conventional approach x laparoscopic abdominoperineal resection for rectal cancer treatment after neoadjuvant chemoradiation: results of a prospective randomized trial. Rev Hosp Clin Fac Med Sao Paulo 2003;58(3):133–40.

[89] Smith LE, Ko ST, Saclarides T, et al. Transanal endoscopic microsurgery. Initial registry results. Dis Colon Rectum 1996;39(10 Suppl):S79–84.

[90] Mentges B, Buess G, Effinger G, et al. Indications and results of local treatment of rectal cancer. Br J Surg 1997;84(3):348–51.

[91] Heintz A, Morschel M, Junginger T. Comparison of results after transanal endoscopic microsurgery and radical resection for T1 carcinoma of the rectum. Surg Endosc 1998;12(9): 1145–8.

[92] Lee W, Lee D, Choi S, et al. Transanal endoscopic microsurgery and radical surgery for T1 and T2 rectal cancer. Surg Endosc 2003;17(8):1283–7.

[93] Palma P, Freudenberg S, Samel S, et al. Transanal endoscopic microsurgery: indications and results after 100 cases. Colorectal Dis 2004;6(5):350–5.

[94] Floyd ND, Saclarides TJ. Transanal endoscopic microsurgical resection of pT1 rectal tumors. Dis Colon Rectum 2006;49(2):164–8.

[95] Stipa F, Burza A, Lucandri G, et al. Outcomes for early rectal cancer managed with transanal endoscopic microsurgery: a 5-year follow-up study. Surg Endosc 2006;20(4):541–5.

[96] Bretagnol F, Merrie A, George B, et al. Local excision of rectal tumours by transanal endoscopic microsurgery. Br J Surg 2007;94(5):627–33.

[97] Maslekar S, Pillinger SH, Monson JR. Transanal endoscopic microsurgery for carcinoma of the rectum. Surg Endosc 2007;21(1):97–102.

[98] Zacharakis E, Freilich S, Rekhraj S, et al. Transanal endoscopic microsurgery for rectal tumors: the St. Mary's experience. Am J Surg 2007;194(5):694–8.

[99] Whitehouse PA, Armitage JN, Tilney HS, et al. Transanal endoscopic microsurgery: local recurrence rate following resection of rectal cancer. Colorectal Dis 2008;10(2):187–93.

ELSEVIER
SAUNDERS

SURGICAL
CLINICS OF
NORTH AMERICA

Surg Clin N Am 88 (2008) 1073–1081

Laparoscopic versus Open Inguinal Hernia Repair

Jon Gould, MD, FACS

University of Wisconsin School of Medicine and Public Health, Department of Surgery, H4/726 Clinical Science Center, 600 Highland Avenue, Madison, WI 53792, USA

Inguinal hernias are common, with a lifetime risk of 27% in men and 3% in women [1]. Today, inguinal hernia repair is one of the most common operations in general surgery, with a rate of 28 per 100,000 in the United States [2]. Despite more than 200 years of experience, the optimal surgical approach to inguinal hernia remains controversial. Surgeons and patients are faced with many options and decisions when it comes to inguinal hernias: repair or no repair, mesh or no mesh, what kind of mesh, open or laparoscopic, extraperitoneal or transabdominal, and so forth. Repair of inguinal hernias have a recurrence rate and long-term morbidity rate that is not inconsequential [3,4]. The search for the gold standard of repair continues.

To repair or not to repair

The initial decision facing surgeons and patients alike is, should this inguinal hernia be repaired? For many patients who have significant symptoms the answer is obviously yes. For others who have more mild or moderate symptoms, the answer may be less clear. A multicenter, prospective, randomized trial of watchful waiting versus elective repair of asymptomatic and minimally symptomatic inguinal hernias recently was published and has helped to provide some guidance [5]. For many years before the publication of this study, the usual recommendation to most patients of reasonable operative risk was to repair the hernia regardless of symptoms to prevent a hernia accident, such as incarceration or strangulation. This was in part related to a lack of knowledge regarding the natural history of untreated inguinal hernias. In the watchful waiting versus elective surgery trial, similar proportions of patients in each group had pain

---

E-mail address: gould@surgery.wisc.edu

doi:10.1016/j.suc.2008.05.008

sufficient to limit usual activities after 2 years. Patients assigned to watchful waiting who requested surgical repair (23%) most commonly reported increased pain as the reason for the crossover. These symptoms improved for most patients after hernia repair. Hernia accidents were rare in the watchful waiting group, at a rate of 1.8 per 1000 patient years. The authors of this study concluded, "a strategy of watchful waiting is a safe and acceptable option for men with asymptomatic or minimally symptomatic inguinal hernias." Subsequent studies also have demonstrated that a watchful waiting approach is cost effective [6] and that patients who ultimately undergo an operation because of symptoms after a period of watchful waiting do as well as those who proceed with immediate repair [7].

As a result of this trial, many surgeons and patients opt for the watchful waiting approach for relatively asymptomatic patients who have inguinal hernia. Several questions, however, have yet to be answered. Hernia accidents may be more common in elderly patients and the morbidity and mortality related to urgent repair may be higher than in younger patients [8]. Because the risk for hernia accident increases with the length of time that the hernia is present, a trial with an endpoint of 2 years may not be adequate to assess risks, particularly in the elderly. This trial did not examine risks with specific types of inguinal hernias. Evidence suggests that the rate of incarceration/strangulation, bowel resections, and emergency operations is high for femoral hernias [9]. Elderly patients who have femoral hernias may be better served by an operation for a minimally symptomatic hernia than by a watchful waiting approach for these reasons.

Mesh or sutured repair?

In the 1990s, it became apparent that the use of mesh in inguinal hernia repair could significantly reduce the incidence of recurrence and that patients may return to normal activities with less pain after open mesh–based repairs compared with nonmesh repairs [10]. A meta-analysis from the EU Hernia Trialists Collaboration compared mesh with sutured techniques in 58 trials comprising 11,174 patients [11]. Recurrence was less common after mesh repair (odds ratio [OR] 0.43). Recurrence rates were 4.9% for nonmesh and 2.0% for mesh repairs. A population-based study examining risk for recurrence 5 years or more after primary mesh (Lichtenstein repair) and sutured inguinal hernia repair in 13,674 patients found that recurrence after mesh repair was a quarter of that after sutured repair (hazard ratio 0.25) [12]. Today, the majority of inguinal hernia repairs, open or laparoscopic, are mesh-based and tension-free repairs.

Open inguinal hernia repair

Open nonmesh inguinal hernia repairs are used most commonly when mesh is contraindicated, such as with a contaminated field. The most commonly used techniques are the Bassini, McVay, and Shouldice repairs. The Bassini repair involves suturing the triple layer of internal oblique, transversus abdominus, and transversalis fascia to the iliopubic tract/inguinal ligament. McVay's repair is similar to the Bassini except that the triple layer is approximated to Cooper's ligament medially. The Shouldice repair is a three-layer reconstruction with running, continuous, nonabsorbable sutures. Recurrence rates for nonmesh-based repairs generally are lowest for the Shouldice technique [13].

In 1989, Lichtenstein and colleagues [14] reported their use of a prosthetic screen onlay technique for hernia repair, the tension-free hernioplasty, in 1000 patients who had minimal complications and a 0% recurrence rate after a follow-up of 1 to 5 years. Unlike others using mesh for repairs at the time, Lichtenstein was the first to advocate the routine use of mesh for all hernias. One of the most alluring aspects of the Lichtenstein repair is that it is easily taught with reproducible results in the hands of general surgeons [15]. Other open mesh–based techniques for inguinal hernia repair are described and involve the placement of a prosthesis ventral to the abdominal wall, dorsal to it, or both. The mesh plug hernioplasty [16], the Prolene Hernia System [17], and the Stoppa repair [18] are commonly used open mesh alternatives to the Lichtenstein repair. In their metanalysis, the EU Hernia Trialists Collaboration did not find a difference in recurrence or rates of persistent pain for open mesh hernia repair based on mesh placement technique [11]. The overall rate of recurrence for open mesh–based repairs (n = 4426) was 1.7%. Persistent pain was observed in 0.95% of open mesh hernia repairs (n = 999).

Laparoscopic inguinal repair

Transabdominal repair

Ger and colleagues [19] first performed laparoscopic inguinal hernia repair in 1982. This initial repair involved the simple closure of the internal ring with a stapler. In 1991, Arregui reported the transabdominal preperitoneal (TAPP) technique [20]. In a TAPP repair, the peritoneum is incised cephalad to the inguinal floor and the hernia defects are dissected. A piece of mesh is placed in the preperitoneal space, and the peritoneum is closed to isolate the mesh from the intra-abdominal viscera. Intraperitoneal onlay mesh (IPOM) placement of polypropylene mesh is advocated by a few investigators [21]. Concerns related to possible mesh erosion into the bowel and a higher recurrence rate than alternative laparoscopic techniques [22] has led most surgeons to abandon an IPOM approach.

Totally extraperitoneal repair

Totally extraperitoneal repair (TEP) was developed out of concern for possible complications related to intra-abdominal access required for TAPP [23]. This method allows for access to the preperitoneal space and avoids the need for a peritoneal incision. In an extraperitoneal laparoscopic repair, access to the preperitoneal space is achieved with a dissecting balloon, a laparoscope, or blunt dissection/carbon dioxide dissection while visualizing the dissection from the peritoneal cavity. A mesh prosthesis is inserted into the preperitoneal space. As in the TAPP repair, technical variations exist in fixation methods (tacks, no tacks, or fibrin glue) and mesh configuration (wrapped around cord or 3-D). Unlike in the TAPP method, closure of a peritoneal flap is not necessary in a TEP.

Totally extraperitoneal repair versus transabdominal preperitoneal

Compared to TEP, TAPP is easier to learn and may be associated with a shorter learning curve [24]. This is largely related to the small working space in TEP compared with TAPP repairs. In a review of the available literature comparing TAPP versus TEP repairs, no statistical difference in length of operation, length of stay, time to return to normal activity, or recurrence rates was found between the two techniques [25]. The reviewed studies did report higher rates of intra-abdominal injuries and port site hernias in TAPP repairs. In the EU Hernie Trialists Collaboration metanalysis, the rate of recurrence for laparoscopic hernia repair was 2.2% [11]. Chronic pain was reported in 0.65% of patients in this study after laparoscopic repair (n = 1004).

Laparoscopic versus open repair of inguinal hernias

Many prospective randomized clinical trials comparing various techniques of open and laparoscopic inguinal hernia repair have been published. In the United States, the most commonly cited and controversial trial is the Veterans Affairs cooperative trial [3]. In this trial, 1983 veterans underwent an open Lichtenstein or a laparoscopic inguinal hernia repair (TEP or TAPP, surgeon's preference). Two-year follow-up was completed in 85.5% of patients. The primary outcome was recurrence at 2 years. Recurrences were more common in the laparoscopic group than in the open group (10.1% versus 4.9%; OR 2.2; 95% CI, 1.5 to 3.2). Post hoc evaluation of the association between surgeon self-reported experience (number of cases previously performed) and recurrences revealed a significant relationship. Surgeons who had more than 250 prior laparoscopic inguinal hernia repairs had a recurrence rate less than 5%, significantly less than the recurrence rate for any other experience category. In this trial, the rate of complications was greater in laparoscopic than after open repair (39% versus 33.4%; OR 1.3, 95% CI, 1.1 to 1.3). The laparoscopic group had less pain at 1 day and at 2 weeks and returned to normal activity 1 day earlier than the open group. The investigators concluded that for primary unilateral hernias an open mesh repair was safer and associated with a lower recurrence rate. Critics of this trial point out that the average age of trial participants was high and the health-related quality of life was low compared with the general population.

The EU Hernia Trialists Collaboration metanalysis included 41 prospective randomized trials comparing laparoscopic to open inguinal hernia repair. All 41 trials had been published before July 2000, and 7294 patients were included (17 of these trials involving 3065 patients compared laparoscopic mesh to open nonmesh repairs). There was no significant difference in recurrence rates between laparoscopic and open mesh repairs (2.2% versus 1.7%; OR 1.26; 95% CI, 0.76 to 2.08) [11]. With regards to persisting pain, analysis of trials comparing laparoscopic with open mesh placement showed fewer reports after laparoscopic repair (OR 0.64; 95% CI, 0.52 to 0.78; $P < .001$).

Another metanalysis examining this issue was conducted and included 29 prospective randomized trials and 5588 patients [26]. Some 3017 hernias were repaired laparoscopically and 2972 were repaired using an open method. Six outcome variables were analyzed including operating time, time to discharge from hospital, return to normal activity and return to work, postoperative complications, and recurrence rate. For four of the six outcomes, the summary point estimates favored laparoscopic over open inguinal hernia repair. There was a significant reduction of 38% in the relative odds of postoperative complications (OR 0.62; 95% CI, 0.46 to 0.84) for laparoscopic repair. Laparoscopic patients returned to normal activity (4.73 days sooner; 95% CI, 3.51 to 5.96) and to work sooner (6.96 days; 95% CI, 5.34 to 8.58) than did patients who underwent open repair. Discharge from the hospital also was achieved sooner (3.43 hours; 95% CI, 0.35 to 6.5 hours). Compared to open hernia repair, laparoscopic repairs took longer (15.2 minutes longer; 95% CI, 7.78 to 22.63 minutes). The relative odds of short-term hernia recurrence were increased by 50% for laparoscopic hernia repair, although this result was not statistically significant (OR 1.51 of recurrence; 95% CI, 0.81 to 2.79).

A Cochrane review on laparoscopic versus open inguinal hernia repairs identified 41 published reports of eligible trials involving 7161 participants [27]. Sample sizes ranged from 38 to 994, with follow-up of 6 weeks to 36 months. Duration of operation was longer in the laparoscopic group. Operative complications were uncommon for both methods but more frequent in the laparoscopic group for visceral (overall 8/2315 versus 1/2599) and vascular (overall 7/2498 versus 5/2758) injuries. Length of hospital stay did not differ between groups, but return to usual activity was earlier for laparoscopic groups. The data available showed less persisting pain (290/2101 versus 459/2399) and less persisting numbness (102/1419 versus 217/1624) in the laparoscopic groups. In total, 86 recurrences were reported among 3138 allocated laparoscopic repair and 109 among 3504 allocated to open repair (OR 0.81; 95% CI, 0.61 to 1.08; $P = .16$).

Recurrent hernias

The optimal operative approach to a recurrent inguinal hernia likely depends on the technique used in the primary repair. Many surgeons consider a laparoscopic approach the optimal choice after a recurrent open mesh inguinal hernia repair. A recently published nationwide analysis provides some evidence to support this approach [28]. Over a 6-year period, 67,306 hernia operations were prospectively recorded in the Danish Hernia Database. There were 2117 reoperations (3.1%) and 187 re-reoperations (8.8%). The re-reoperation rate after primary Lichtenstein repair (n = 1124) was significantly reduced after laparoscopic operation for recurrence (1.3%; 95% CI, 0.4 to 3.0) compared with open repairs for recurrence (Lichtenstein 11.3%; 95% CI, 8.2 to 15.2; nonmesh 19.2%; 95% CI, 14.0 to 25.4; and non-Lichtenstein mesh 7.2%; 95% CI, 4.0 to 11.8). After primary non-mesh (n = 616), non-Lichtenstein mesh (n = 277), and laparoscopic repair (n = 100), there was no significant difference in re-reoperation rates between a laparoscopic repair and all open techniques of repair for recurrence.

A recent prospective randomized trial specifically evaluated the outcomes after laparoscopic or open repairs of recurrent inguinal hernias [29]. A total of 147 patients were randomized to TAPP or Lichtenstein repair. Operative time did not differ. Postoperative pain and time to return to work were less with laparoscopic repair. The re-recurrence rate 5 years after surgery was 18% for TAPP and 19% for Lichtenstein repair.

Bilateral inguinal hernias

Concurrent repair of bilateral hernias may best be accomplished laparoscopically. Long-term data demonstrate no difference in recurrence between bilateral open compared with bilateral laparoscopic inguinal hernia repair [30]. Perioperative pain has been demonstrated to be significantly less (at 24 hours, 72 hours, and 7 days) after laparoscopic bilateral TAPP compared with bilateral open Lichtenstein repair in a prospective randomized trial [31]. The median time to return to work also was significantly less for laparoscopic repair in this trial (16 versus 30 days; $P < .05$).

Cost

One criticism of laparoscopic inguinal hernia repair relates to increased operative cost compared with open repair. In a recently published issue of the *Surgical Clinics of North America*, 10 articles containing cost comparisons for laparoscopic and open inguinal hernia repair were reviewed, all favoring open repair [32]. When attempting to account for indirect cost savings, such as earlier return to work, the process becomes more complex. Increased operative costs may be justified if patients benefit to a significant degree. The Medical Research Council Laparoscopic Groin Hernia Trial Group performed a cost-utility analysis on a prospective randomized trial conducted in the United Kingdom comparing laparoscopic to open inguinal hernia repair [33]. Costs for laparoscopic repair were greater, mostly due to increased operating room time and the costs of disposable equipment. In this analysis, when quality-adjusted life-years (QALYs) were evaluated for each approach, laparoscopic repair was associated with slightly improved

QALYs up to 3 months post repair. The cost incurred to produce additional QALYs by a laparoscopic approach was high, but a sensitivity analysis suggested that if reusable equipment were used for laparoscopic hernia repair this approach would be economically viable.

In the United States, a similar study recently was published comparing treatment options for more than 1.5 million hernia patients from a cost utility perspective [34]. Four treatment strategies were modeled: laparoscopic repair, open mesh repair, open nonmesh repair, and expectant management. Compared with expectant management, the incremental cost per QALY gained was $605 for laparoscopic repair, $697 for open mesh repair, and $1711 for open nonmesh repair. In sensitivity analysis, the two major components that affect the cost-effectiveness ratio of the different types of repair were the ambulatory facility cost and the recurrence rate. The investigators concluded that from a societal perspective, laparoscopic repair can be a cost-effective treatment option for inguinal hernia repair.

Summary

For procedures, such as cholecystectomy and Nissen fundoplication, the laparoscopic approach was quickly adopted as the preferred technique within a few years of introduction. Almost 20 years after the first laparoscopic inguinal hernia repair, the optimal operative approach to inguinal hernia is still debatable. The evidence suggests that routine use of mesh for most inguinal hernias is important. Open mesh–based repairs probably are easier to learn and to teach than laparoscopic repairs. Although there is justifiable concern that laparoscopic inguinal hernia repairs may be associated with an increased recurrence rate, this may not be true for experienced laparoscopic hernia surgeons. For unilateral primary inguinal hernias, laparoscopic techniques are associated with a quicker recovery and perhaps less long-term pain and numbness. Direct costs of laparoscopic repairs are more than for open repairs, but this cost may be largely offset from a societal perspective with a quicker return to normal activity and to work. For recurrent and bilateral inguinal hernias, the laparoscopic approach to repair seems to have more obvious benefits and may be the technique of choice. The bottom line seems to be that experienced surgeons are capable of achieving durable results with minimal morbidity, regardless of whether or not a laparoscopic or an open mesh–based technique is used.

References

[1] Kingsnorth A, LeBlanc K. Hernias: inguinal and incisional. Lancet 2003;362:1561–71.
[2] Devlin HB. Trends in hernia surgery in the land of Astley Cooper. In: Soper NJ, editor. Problems in general surgery. vol. 12. Philadelphia: Lippincott-Raven; 1995. p. 85–92.
[3] Neumayer L, Giobbie-Hurder A, Jonasson O, et al. Open vs. laparoscopic mesh repair of inguinal hernias. N Engl J Med 2004;350(18):1819–27.

[4] Cunningham J, Temple WJ, Mitchell P, et al. Cooperative hernia study: pain in the post repair patient. Ann Surg 1996;224:598–602.

[5] Fitzgibbons RJ, Giobbie-Hurder A, Gibbs JO, et al. Watchful waiting vs. repair of inguinal hernia in minimally symptomatic men. JAMA 2006;295(3):285–92.

[6] Stroupe KT, Manheim LM, Luo P, et al. Tension-free repair versus watchful waiting for men with asymptomatic or minimally symptomatic inguinal hernias: a cost effectiveness analysis. J Am Coll Surg 2006;203(4):458–68.

[7] Thompson JS, Gibbs JO, Reda DJ, et al. Does delaying repair of an asymptomatic hernia have a penalty? Am J Surg 2008;195(1):89–93.

[8] Malek S, Torella F, Edwards PR. Emergency repair of groin herniae: outcome and implications for elective surgery waiting times. Int J Clin Pract 2004;58:207–9.

[9] Alimoglu O, Kaya B, Okan I, et al. Femoral hernia: a review of 83 cases. Hernia 2006;10(1): 70–3.

[10] Scott N, Go PM, Graham P, et al. Open mesh versus non-mesh for groin hernia repair [review]. Cochrane Database Syst Rev 2001;(3):CD002197.

[11] EU Hernia Trialists Collaboration. Repair of groin hernia with synthetic mesh, meta-analysis of randomized controlled trials. Ann Surg 2002;235:322–32.

[12] Bisgaard T, Bay-Nielsen M, Christensen IJ, et al. Risk of recurrence 5 years or more after primary Lichtenstein mesh and sutured inguinal hernia repair. Br J Surg 2007;94: 1038–40.

[13] Beets GL, Oosterhuis KJ, Go PM, et al. Longterm followup (12–15 years) of a randomized controlled trial comparing Bassini-Stetten, Shouldice, and high ligation with narrowing of the internal ring for primary inguinal hernia repair. J Am Coll Surg 1997;185(4): 352–7.

[14] Lichtenstein IL, Shulman AG, Amid PK, et al. The tension free hernioplasty. Am J Surg 1989;157:188–93.

[15] Shulman AG, Amid PK, Lichtenstein IL. A survey of non-expert surgeons using the open tension-free mesh patch repair for primary inguinal hernias. Int Surg 1995;80:35–6.

[16] Rutkow IM, Robbins AW. Mesh plug hernia repair: a follow-up report. Surgery 1995;117: 597.

[17] Vironen J, Nieminen J, Eklund A, et al. Randomized clinical trial of Lichtenstein patch or Prolene Hernia System for inguinal hernia repair. Br J Surg 2006;93(1):33–9.

[18] Stoppa RE. The treatment of complicated groin and incisional hernias. World J Surg 1989; 13:545–54.

[19] Ger R, Monroe K, Duvivier R, et al. Management of indirect inguinal hernias by laparoscopic closure of the neck of the sac. Am J Surg 1990;159:370–3.

[20] Arregui ME. Laparoscopic preperitoneal herniorrhaphy. Presented at the Society of American Endoscopic Surgeons Annual Meeting. Monterey, CA, April 18–21, 1991.

[21] Fitzgibbons RJ Jr, Camps J, Cornet DA, et al. Laparoscopic inguinal herniorrhaphy. Results of a multicenter trial. Ann Surg 1995;221(1):3–13.

[22] Sarli L, Pietra N, Choua O, et al. Laparoscopic hernia repair: a prospective comparison of TAPP and IPOM techniques. Surg Laparosc Endosc 1997;7(6):472–6.

[23] Soper NJ, Swanstrom LL, Eubanks WS. Mastery of endoscopic and laparoscopic surgery. Philadelphia: Lippincott Williams & Wilins; 2005. p. 49.

[24] Leibl BJ, Jager C, Kraft B, et al. Laparoscopic hernia repair: TAPP or/and TEP? Langenbecks Arch Surg 2005;390:77–82.

[25] Wake BL, McCormack K, Fraser C, et al. Transabdominal preperitoneal (TAPP) vs totally extraperitoneal (TEP) laparoscopic techniques for inguinal hernia repair. Cochrane Database Syst Rev 2005;(1):CD004703.

[26] Memon MA, Cooper NJ, Memon B, et al. Meta-analysis of randomized clinical trials comparing open and laparoscopic inguinal hernia repair. Br J Surg 2003;90(12):1479–92.

[27] McCormack K, Scott NW, Go PM, et al. Laparoscopic techniques versus open techniques for inguinal hernia repair. Cochrane Database Syst Rev 2003;(1):CD001785.

[28] Bisgaard T, Bay-Nielsen M, Kehlet H. Re-recurrence after operation for recurrent inguinal hernia. A nationwide 8-year follow-up study on the role of type of repair. Ann Surg 2008; 247(4):707–11.

[29] Eklund A, Rudberg C, Leijonmarck CE, et al. Recurrent inguinal hernia: randomized multicenter trial comparing laparoscopic and Lichtenstein repair. Surg Endosc 2007;21(4): 634–40.

[30] Kald A, Fridsten S, Nordin P, et al. Outcome of repair of bilateral groin hernias: a prospective evaluation of 1,487 patients. Eur J Surg 2002;168(3):150–3.

[31] Sarli L, Iusco DR, Sansebastiano G, et al. Simultaneous repair of bilateral inguinal hernias: a prospective, randomized study of open, tension-free versus laparoscopic approach. Surg Laparosc Endosc Percutan Tech 2001;11(4):262–7.

[32] Takata MC, Duh QY. Laparoscopic inguinal hernia repair. Surg Clin North Am 2008;88: 157–78.

[33] The MRC Laparoscopic Groin Hernia Trial Group. Cost-utility analysis of open versus laparoscopic groin hernia repair: results from a multicentre randomized clinical trial. Br J Surg 2001;88:653–61.

[34] Stylopoulos N, Gazelle GS, Rattner DW. A cost–utility analysis of treatment options for inguinal hernia in 1,513,008 adult patients. Surg Endosc 2003;17(2):180–9.

ELSEVIER
SAUNDERS

SURGICAL
CLINICS OF
NORTH AMERICA

Surg Clin N Am 88 (2008) 1083–1100

Laparoscopic Versus Open Ventral Hernia Repair

Judy Jin, MD[a], Michael J. Rosen, MD, FACS[a,b,*]

[a]Department of Surgery, University Hospitals Case Medical Center,
11100 Euclid Avenue, Cleveland OH 44106, USA
[b]Case Comprehensive Hernia Center, University Hospitals Case Medical Center,
11100 Euclid Avenue, Cleveland OH 44106, USA

The repair of ventral hernias remains one of the most common operations performed by general surgeons. Despite the frequency with which this procedure is performed, there is little agreement and extensive controversy as to the cause of most of the hernias, or the ideal approach to repair these problems. Most of this controversy is surrounding surgical lure, anecdotal experience, few well-designed trials, and rare long-term follow-up. This article attempts to identify and provide some clarification of these controversial issues in abdominal wall reconstruction after ventral herniation based on the available literature.

Causes of ventral hernia formation

Ventral herniation is a common long-term complication of abdominal surgery. The exact incidence of incisional hernia formation after laparotomy is unknown, but it is estimated to be between 10% and 50% [1–3]. Certain patient risk factors such as malnutrition, obesity, steroid use, type 2 diabetes, chronic obstructive pulmonary disease (COPD), and radiation therapy result in a predictably high incidence of ventral herniation [4]. Other molecular disorders and cellular derangements in hemostasis, inflammation, angiogenesis, and remodeling can impair wound healing and predispose patients to incisional hernia formation. Notably, collagen synthesis, particularly the ratio of type 1 to type 3 collagens, tends to be lower in patients who have ventral hernias [5]. In addition, some authors have linked the

* Corresponding author. Department of Surgery, University Hospitals Case Medical Center, 11100 Euclid Avenue, Cleveland OH 44106.
 E-mail address: michael.rosen@uhhospitals.org (M.J. Rosen).

0039-6109/08/$ - see front matter. Published by Elsevier Inc.
doi:10.1016/j.suc.2008.05.015
surgical.theclinics.com

high rate of hernia formation after abdominal aortic aneurysm repair to a defect in matrix metalloprotease [6–8]. Abnormally high levels of this enzyme not only predispose to weakening of the abdominal aorta, but also correlate with poor wound healing and high hernia formation. Furthermore, other investigators have described a syndrome of metastatic emphysema [9]. In patients who are chronic smokers with evidence of significant lung damage, the connective tissue disorder that affects the lung also affects the abdominal wall fascia and predisposes these patients to hernia formation. Although the exact mechanism of hernia formation is likely multifactorial in most patients, it remains one of the most common procedures performed by general surgeons in the United States, with approximately 200,000 ventral hernia repairs performed annually [10].

Types of repair

One of the initial controversies in ventral hernia repair was whether to repair defects primarily or routinely use a synthetic prosthesis. In the beginning, attempts at repairing ventral hernias involved simply reapproximating the fascial edges with either running or interrupted sutures. Understanding some of the underlying factors that lead to hernia formation and the associated tension on these repairs, it is thus not surprising that simple reapproximation of the edges of the defect (primary repair) has been associated with unacceptably high recurrence rates of up to 63% with long-term follow-up [11]. Recognizing these unsatisfactory results, the concept of tension-free hernia repair was introduced. Usher and colleagues [12] first described the use of synthetic polypropylene mesh in the incisional hernia repair in the 1950s. Over the next 50 years, the open approach to ventral hernia repair has undergone many modifications. Today, however, in all but the smallest ventral hernias, the principle of tension-free mesh reinforcement is still considered the gold standard of all hernia repairs [13]. Despite this near universal acceptance of mesh in ventral hernia repair, the ideal technique for placing that mesh remains heavily debated.

Open repair

One of the most pressing controversies of ventral hernia repair is whether to approach the problem in an open or laparoscopic fashion. For open ventral hernia repair, multiple techniques have been described for the use of tension-free mesh repair. The prosthetic can be placed superficial to the fascial closure (onlay), as a bridge secured to the fascial edges (inlay), or underneath the fascia (underlay) in either a retro-rectus, preperitoneal, or intraperitoneal position. The onlay repair carries the disadvantage of placing the prosthetic in a subcutaneous position, predisposing it to infectious complications associated with wound breakdown. The inlay repair has been associated with high failure rates secondary to mesh contraction, inadequate mesh tissue interface, and eventual mesh disruption from the fascial edges [14]. Currently, the gold standard for open ventral hernia repair according to the American Hernia Society is the Rives Stoppa Wantz retro-rectus repair. This technique involves placing a wide prosthetic mesh in either a retro-rectus or preperitoneal plane. The authors' preferred approach involves placing full-thickness transfascial fixation sutures with a Reverdin needle. In large series, consistently low recurrence rates of 0% to 14% were reported with long term follow up (Table 1). Although these techniques reduce hernia recurrence rates, they are not without pitfalls. Extensive tissue dissection and creation of new tissue planes can result in increased patient morbidity requiring prolonged hospital stay and increased incidence of seroma and wound infections, sometimes even requiring the removal of the infected prosthetic mesh. These drawbacks have led some surgeons to investigate minimally invasive ventral hernia repair using the same wide underlay principles of the Stoppa technique.

Laparoscopic repair

While laparoscopic cholecystectomy and laparoscopic colectomy were becoming more popular and acceptable in the surgical community, the idea of laparoscopic ventral hernia repairs also began to form. In 1993, LeBlanc and Booth [15] was the first to report laparoscopic repair of an incisional hernia. Over the years, the laparoscopic repair has become the preferred method of repair for some surgeons because of reports of decreased hospital stay, decreased complication rates, and lower recurrence rates. One major advantage of the laparoscopic approach is that it provides wide mesh overlap in an underlay position similar to the open retro-rectus repair, without the associated soft-tissue dissection. This reduction in tissue

Table 1
Outcome of retro-muscular open repair

Author	Year	#	Wound complication %	Mortality %	Follow-up	Recurrence %
Stoppa	1989	368	12	1.8	5.5 y	14.6
Rives	1992	258	7.7	0.8	–	6.2
Wantz	1991	30	0	0	–	0
McLanahan	1997	106	18	–	2 y	3.5
Schumpelick	1999	81	–	–	22 mo	5
Martin-Duce	2001	152	11	0	6 y	1.3
Petersen	2004	175	8	0	20 mo	9
Kingsnorth	2004	33	–	–	6 mo–6 y	3.3
Paajanen	2004	84	6	0	3 y	5
Burger	2004	60	10	0	10 y	32
Israelsson	2006	228	–	–	12–24 mo	7.3
Novitsky	2006	32	12	–	3 y	2.8
Totals		1607	9.3	0.3		7.5

trauma results in a predictable reduction in wound morbidity and mesh infections. Additionally, the laparoscopic approach provides a unique internal view of the entire abdominal wall, enabling the surgeon to identify remote small Swiss cheese-type defects. Although the laparoscopic technique provides many intuitive advantages, it still has certain technical challenges and internal controversies as to the best practice techniques that must be overcome to realize the aforementioned stated outcome advantages. Some of these controversial issues include the best approach to regain access to a multiple reoperative field safely, the ability to perform extensive adhesiolysis if required, and accurately sizing and placing a prosthetic mesh, which must be brought into the field and secured to the abdominal wall with sufficient overlap to invoke a long-term repair.

Gaining access to the reoperative abdomen can be achieved with an open cut down, Veress needle, or various optical viewing trocars. Although large studies have failed to find superiority of one approach over another, the authors prefer an open cut down technique. Regardless of one's access technique, the principle of placing one's trocars in a lateral abdominal position to provide adequate space for mesh placement and distance from the hernia to work on the anterior abdominal wall is critical. Safe adhesiolysis is paramount. The authors' approach involves sharp dissection with absolutely no use of electrocautery or other hemostatic devices such as ultrasonic dissectors or the Ligasure (ValleyLab, Boulder, Colorado). If bleeding is encountered, liberal use of metallic clips or immediate conversion to an open procedure is preferred over the potential consequences of a missed or delayed enterotomy.

Once the abdominal wall is freed of adhesions, the defect dimension and appropriately sized mesh must be ascertained. Obtaining an accurate measurement for the defect is paramount in ensuring adequate mesh and tissue overlap, thus minimizing postoperative recurrence. The most appropriate technique to measure the hernia defect remains controversial. The three common measurement techniques include the intracorporeal with pneumoperitoneum, extracorporeal with/without pneumoperitoneum, and extracorporeal desufflated. Extracorporeal measurements with/without pneumoperitoneum employ long spinal needles inserted intra-abdominally to mark the boundary of the hernia defect within the abdominal cavity. Measurements are then taken outside the peritoneal cavity based on the boundary outlined by the spinal needles. The intracorporeal measurements require measuring the defect with a ruler placed into the abdominal cavity. One of the conceptual problems with obtaining measurements extracorporeally is that the diameter of the circle on the skin is larger than the diameter of the inner circle of the peritoneal cavity. In fact, this is directly proportional to the size of the abdominal wall and degree of obesity. Obtaining falsely elevated measurements can create significant difficulties for the surgeon if the mesh is oversized in a large defect. In these circumstances, one can encounter more mesh than the abdominal cavity can accommodate, resulting in laxity of the mesh and bulging into the defect. Although these issues are not likely relevant in small hernia repairs, in large defects, this can result in substantial surgeon frustration and poor patient outcomes. A group of experienced laparoscopic surgeons recently systematically evaluated the significance of alternative measuring strategies in laparoscopic ventral hernia repairs [16]. They found that the extracorporeal method of measurements overestimates the hernia defects by 1.7 to 3.1 cm compared with the intracorporeal method.

Once the mesh is sized, it must be brought into the abdominal cavity. If large sheets of mesh are necessary, this can be a particularly challenging step in the operation. Some surgeons directly insert the mesh through either a 5 or 10 mm trocar site; sometimes a counter trocar site may be necessary to facilitate the introduction of the mesh [17]. Other alternatives include introducing the mesh through a 2 to 2.5 cm incision over the center of the hernia defects [18]. Opponents of this technique argue that taking the mesh through an area of compromised skin can predispose the patient to postoperative wound complications. Other authors have tried to reduce potential skin contamination further by placing the mesh in a sterile plastic sleeve for introduction into the abdominal cavity [19].

One of the most highly controversial areas of laparoscopic ventral hernia repair is the appropriate method of mesh fixation. The basic argument is whether spiral tack fixation is sufficient or whether transfascial fixation sutures are needed. Most surgeons would agree that transfascial fixation sutures might provide some benefit in terms of preventing mesh migration and hernia recurrence. These sutures, however, can be a site of significant early and long-term postoperative discomfort. It is believed that the suture site pain most likely is caused by tissue or nerve entrapment during the initial suture placement. Most of these pains resolve or can be managed with local anesthetic injections. Several experienced laparoscopic ventral hernia surgeons have advocated the routine use of transfascial fixation sutures [17,20,21]. These authors noted in their early experience a high incidence of recurrence when tacks alone were used. If one considers that a 5 mm spiral tack is typically only 3.8 mm in depth; most meshes are approximately 1 mm thick, and an appropriately placed tack typically has a 1 mm cuff on the visceral side, only 1.8 mm of tack is available to obtain purchase into the abdominal wall. In an obese patient who has preperitoneal fat, this rarely achieves reliable fascial purchase. Although most surgeons would agree that transfascial sutures are necessary, the exact number remains unknown. The authors' approach to this problem is based on the patient and the type of defect. In a Swiss cheese-type defect with adequate mesh overlap, a minimum of 4 sutures is probably sufficient. In an obese patient, or one who has a single large defect, significant forces are acting on the mesh, pushing it out into the defect; the authors typically put significantly more sutures, placed at 4 cm intervals. Further long-term studies will be necessary to clarify this issue.

Meshes available for use

Based on long-term follow-up, most surgeons agree that unprotected polypropylene or polyester mesh placed in an intraperitoneal position should be avoided because of the long-term risk of bowel erosion, fistula formation, and small bowel obstruction [22]. For extraperitoneal placement, such as a Stoppa repair, polypropylene or polyester mesh remains a popular choice. Other alternatives now include light-weight polypropylene mesh. In the case of laparoscopic and open intraperitoneal repair of ventral hernias, special attention is given to the choice of the mesh as to avoid mesh-related complications. Most synthetic mesh available for intraperitoneal usage contains one side that faces the viscera and attempts to reduce adhesion formation, and the other side to promote good tissue ingrowth into the abdominal wall. Although there is extensive comparative literature in animal models evaluating different meshes, little if any human data is available directly comparing the long-term outcomes of different meshes [23–30]. Based on this, most mesh selections are based on surgeon's experience and anecdotal evidence. Prospective studies comparing all of these meshes in terms of clinical outcomes are needed.

More recently, biologic scaffolds made of allograft or xenograft acellular dermis, porcine small intestine submucosa, or bovine pericardium have been introduced as another option for hernia repair. These biologic meshes are recommended for patients when active contamination is present or when the risk of synthetic mesh placement is too high. Because angiogenesis is a known aspect of biologic mesh remodeling, these materials have the potential to resist infections. These biologics once were thought to be capable of replacing native fascia, and liberal use of them to bridge the fascial edge has resulted in unacceptably high hernia recurrence rate. Recent study [31] has shown that these biologics are used best as reinforcements when the fascial edge has been brought back to the midline, either by using component separation or through staged repair. Given the expense of these products, the main indications have been in circumstances of contamination or infection. Whether these products have a role in routine ventral hernia repair remains unknown. With the explosion of these meshes onto the market and the minimal data that are available in evaluating these products, it is difficult to provide much guidance. There are, however, some distinct differences in the source material of these products, the way in which they are processed, and the unique handling characteristics that may have importance on their appropriate selection. There are few data to suggest that the source product, whether allogenic or xenogenic, plays a significant role in outcomes. One of the main differences in the processing of these materials is whether the proteins are cross- linked. Cross linking is a biochemical process that alters the composition of the graft. Some products are cross-linked heavily, while others fall throughout the spectrum of cross-linking. Again there is little evidence to suggest superiority of cross-linking to improve outcomes with biologic mesh. Proponents of cross-linking feel that the modifications enable the mesh to perform more like a synthetic mesh and resist long-term breakdown. Although this may provide long-term advantages in terms of reducing laxity and recurrence, it can also result in minimal graft incorporation and neovascularization. In the case of contaminated fields, this could potentially result in graft loss. Given the absolute lack of prospective comparative trials, the authors feel that this is only speculation, and no firm conclusions can be drawn.

Clinical outcomes of open versus laparoscopic ventral hernia repairs

A recent internet survey was conducted among practicing United States surgeons to identify current trends and opinions about incisional hernia repairs [32]. Most of the surgeons reported that they practice in either an academic or urban setting. Although 96% of the 207 surgeons who responded routinely performed laparoscopic cholecystecomies, only 10% of the surgeons performed laparoscopic incisional hernia repairs. Of those 90% of surgeons who did not perform laparoscopic ventral hernia repairs routinely, 82% indicated that they did not plan to learn how to perform laparoscopic ventral hernia repair. When asked why they had these beliefs, most felt the results of laparoscopic repair are not superior to a traditional open repair, and the risk of enterotomy, higher cost, and longer operative times do not make the procedure attractive to them. On the other hand, 85% of the surgeons who routinely perform laparoscopic repair would continue to perform more laparoscopic procedures. Lower recurrence rates and a lower incidence of postoperative complications were the most common reasons cited among surgeons performing laparoscopic ventral hernia repair. These polarizing opinions are not entirely surprising, given the overwhelming lack of well-designed comparative trials evaluating the outcomes of laparoscopic versus open ventral hernia repair.

Whether laparoscopic repair confers advantage over the open approach has been debated among general surgeons. Multiple retrospective studies have been completed looking at the short- and long-term results of these two approaches. Although laparoscopic repair was shown to have significant reduction in wound complications and mesh infections, all of these studies suffer from serious methodological flaws and thus limit the conclusion one can draw. Most of these studies had small numbers of patients, and the method of open repair varied based on each surgeon's preference. Here in Table 2, the authors evaluated eight larger comparative trials with at least 100 patients within the last 10 years [23–30]. Seven of these studies were conducted in the United States. Although polypropylene mesh was used most commonly for open repairs, various meshes were used for the laparoscopic repair. The operative time for the laparoscopic repair was slightly shorter than the open procedure, and similar intraoperative complication rates were reported. In most series, a significant reduction in the length of

Table 2
Comparative studies between open and laparoscopic ventral hernia repair

Author	Year	Study	Patient number		Mesh used		Operation time (min)		Percent intraoperative complications		LOS (days)		Percent postoperative complication %		Follow-up (Mo)		% Recurrence	
			Lap	Open	Lap	Open	Lap	Open	Lap	Open	Lap	Open	Lap %	Open %	Lap	Open	Lap	Open
Park	1998	Retrospective	56	49	ePTFE	PP	95.4	78.5	N/A	N/A	N/A	N/A	17.90	36.70	24	54	11%	35%
Ramshaw	1999	Retrospective	79	174	N/A	N/A	58	82	N/A	N/A	1.7	2.8	19	26.40	21	21	3%	21%
Wright	2002	Retrospective	86	90	N/A	N/A	131	102	2.30%	2.20%	1.5	2.5	25.60	40	N/A	N/A	1%	6%
Van't Riet	2002	Retrospective	25	76	PP	PP	120	110	8%	6.50%	4	5	52	39.50	16	19	16%	18%
Mc Geevy	2003	Prospective	65	71	ePTFE or polyester/collagen	PP	N/A	N/A	N/A	N/A	1.1	1.5	7.70	21.10	N/A	N/A	N/A	N/A
Lomanto	2006	Prospective	50	50	polyester/collagen	ePTFE	90.6	93.3	2%	2%	2.74	4.7	26	40	19.6	21	2%	10%
Bingener	2007	Prospective	127	233	ePTFE or PP/ ePTFE	PP	N/A	N/A	N/A	N/A	N/A	N/A	33.10	43.30	36	36	13%	9%
Olmi	2007	Prospective	85	85	polyester/collagen	PP	61	151	N/A	N/A	2.7	9.9	16.50	29.40	24	24	2%	4%
Total			573	828			93	103			2.3	4.4	24.7	34.6	23	29	7%	15%

Abbreviations: ePTFE, expanded polytetrafluoethylene; Lap, laparoscopic; LOS, length of stay; PP, polypropylene.

hospital stay and postoperative complications was observed. Long-term follow-up of these patients had shown a reduction in hernia recurrence rates with the laparoscopic approach. Of note, the study by Olmi and colleagues [30] was the only large prospective randomized comparative study performed to evaluate the two approaches. This study showed not only a shorter operative time in the laparoscopic group, but also a significantly lower mean length of hospital stay (2.7 days versus 9.9 days), reduced complication rate (16% versus 29%), and faster time of return to work (13 days versus 25 days). Although the surgical community has been slow to adopt the laparoscopic approach to ventral hernia repair, these results certainly underscore the importance of a well-designed prospective randomized trial to accurately identify the advantages of either a laparoscopic or an open approach to ventral hernia repair. Most importantly, these studies would help guide appropriate patient selection to identify those patients who would benefit most from each approach.

Other technical adjunct for ventral hernia repair

Although the routine use of synthetic mesh has reduced hernia recurrence rates significantly, certain situations preclude its usage. In the setting of removing an infected prosthetic mesh, active infection, or intraoperative contamination, most surgeons agree that the usage of permanent prosthetic mesh is contraindicated. In addition, a substantial replacement of the abdominal wall with prosthetic mesh has the potential to reduce the dynamic function of the abdominal wall, resulting in a stiff noncompliant wall with poor functional outcome. Other options for native tissue replacement of the abdominal wall include tensor fascia lata, gracilis, vastus lateralis, rectus femoris, or latissmus dorsi muscle flaps. These flaps have variable recurrence rates and donor site morbidity. To date, the most popular autologous tissue flap used is the abdominal wall component separation technique. First described by Ramirez and colleagues [33] in 1990, the procedure has multiple variations, but basically involves gaining access to the lateral abdominal wall musculature, transecting the external oblique aponeurosis 2 cm lateral to its insertion into the linea semilunaris, and separating the external oblique muscle from the internal oblique muscle in its avascular plane. The rectus abdominus complex then is advanced medially, creating a vascularized and innervated myofascial flap to cover the hernia defect. This technique allows for up to 10 cm of unilateral myofascial advancement at the umbilicus.

The open component separation technique can aid the surgeon in closing abdominal wall defects in complicated fields in a single stage without permanent mesh. One major drawback to this technique is the substantial lipocutaneous flap dissection that is necessary to gain access to the lateral abdominal wall musculature. These flaps can result in considerable devascularization of the abdominal wall and the dreaded complication of skin flap necrosis. The extensive dissection required to access the correct plane between external and internal oblique muscle can also result in seromas, hematomas, and increased incidence of wound infection postoperatively. The authors recently reported the initial experience of using a novel approach of minimally invasive component separation [34,35]. In this minimally invasive component separation technique, a 10 mm laparoscopic port site was first chosen just below the costal margin lateral to the rectus muscle (Fig. 1). After blunt dissection of the subcutaneous tissue was completed, the potential space between the internal and external oblique was created using a bilateral laparoscopic inguinal balloon dissector (Fig. 2). A structural balloon port was then inserted into this space to maintain insufflation pressures of 8 to 10 mm Hg. Two additional 5 mm ports were then placed at the level of the umbilicus of the posterior axillary line and another just above the inguinal ligament lateral to the umbilicus. Under direct visualization, the potential space between the external and internal oblique muscle was cleared from costal margin down to the inguinal ligament. The external oblique aponeurosis was released starting at the costal margin to the level of the inguinal ligament using coagulation scissors (Fig. 3).

One potential limitation of this approach is the absence of skin flaps, which might reduce the fascial advancement one could obtain. To better characterize these issues, a porcine model was created in which the advancement gained from the minimally invasive component separation was compared with an open component separation [34]. This study revealed that the minimally invasive component separation provided 86% of the myofascial advancement obtained with an open release. The authors' initial human series of seven patients undergoing resection of infected prosthetic mesh and single-stage abdominal wall reconstruction was reported recently [35]. The mean abdominal wall defect in this series of patients was 338 cm^2, after

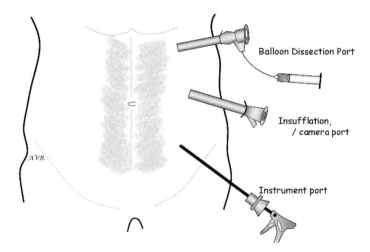

Fig. 1. Placement of trocars for laparoscopic component separation.

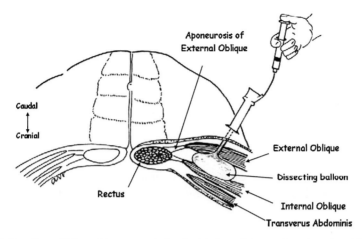

Fig. 2. Insertion of bilateral laparoscopic inguinal balloon between the external and internal oblique muscles. (*From* Rosen MJ, Williams CP, Jin J, et al. Laparoscopic versus open-component separation: a comparative analysis in a porcine model. Am J Surg 2007;194:385–9; with permission.)

the completion of component separation primary fascial closure was achieved in all patients. No mortality was noted in the postoperative period, but two cases of superficial surgical site infection and hematoma were reported. There was no hernia recurrence in a follow up period of 4.5 months. This preliminary study demonstrated the feasibility of this novel technique with minimal wound complications in these very complex

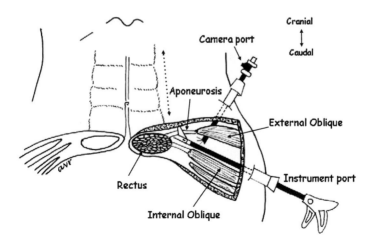

Fig. 3. Release of external oblique aponeurosis from linea semilunaris. (*From* Rosen MJ, Williams CP, Jin J, et al. Laparoscopic versus open-component separation: a comparative analysis in a porcine model. Am J Surg 2007;194:385–9; with permission.)

patients. Long-term results are necessary to validate the efficacy of this minimally invasive approach.

Another study also investigated an alternative laparoscopically assisted component separation technique for ventral hernia repair. Milburn's and colleagues [36] took a modified approach of incising only the transversus abdominus fascia and posterior rectus sheath in the open abdomen of cadavers and repeated the procedure laparoscopically. They noted equal amount of release when compared with the traditional Ramirez component separation technique. Although the results were encouraging, this technique did not require the creation of the potential space between internal oblique and transversus abdominus muscle, and without allowing the medial movement of the external and internal oblique muscles, it was not a true component separation.

Special considerations for ventral hernia repair

Obesity

Obesity has long been considered a risk factor for hernia formation and hernia recurrence, as it predisposes the patient for postoperative wound complications [37]. The extensive tissue dissection required for most open ventral hernia repairs can lead to tissue ischemia and necrosis, resulting in increased incidence of wound infection. Hernia recurrence rates can be as high as 50% [38] in the obese populations when compared with the less than 20% recurrence rate in the nonobese population. In the past, laparoscopic ventral hernia repair has been relatively contraindicated in patients who were obese because of the perceived technical challenges and surgeon inexperience. With the improvement in technology and surgeon expertise, however, laparoscopic repair in this special group of patients is now feasible, and may even be superior to the open approach in terms of postoperative complications. This advantage already has been shown in laparoscopic cholecystectomy [39] and appendectomy [40] in patients who are obese.

Birgisson and colleagues [41] first reported their experience with laparoscopic ventral hernia repair in 46 obese (body mass index [BMI] >30 kg/m^2) or morbidly obese (BMI >40 kg/m^2) patients. Although the operative time for the obese and morbidly obese groups was significantly longer compared with the nonobese group (146 versus 99 minutes, $P<.05$), the defect size and length of stay for these groups were not statistically different. No patients in the morbidly obese group required conversion to open procedure. The postoperative complication rate was 17% in the obese group and 22% in the nonobese group, and consisted of mostly seroma and superficial wound infections. Two cases of enterotomy occurred in two patients. One patient had laparoscopic repair and placement of antibacterial-soaked mesh without any postoperative adverse events. The other patient had gross spillage of enteric content and underwent laparoscopic small bowel repair with postponement of the hernia repair. At a mean follow-up of 8.5 months, one patient in the obese and morbidly obese group had a hernia recurrence. This was the first study that demonstrated the feasibility of laparoscopic hernia repair in obese patients with fewer wound complications and reduced overall perioperative morbidity. Another study by Novitsky and colleagues [42] reported the results of a larger group of patients (n = 163), in which 109 (67%) patients had BMIs greater than 35 kg/m^2. In this study, the mean operative time was 178 minutes, and five patients (3%) required conversion to an open repair secondary to dense adhesions (n = 2), small bowel enterotomy (n = 1), inability to reduce an incarcerated omentum/bowel (n = 1), and a fistula in a previously placed mesh (n = 1). No perioperative mortality was noted in this study. Twenty patients (12.3%) experienced postoperative complications that included persistent abdominal discomfort, urinary tract infections, pulmonary complications, and mesh infections. Two patients required removal of the prosthetic meshes because of wound infections. Although most patients experienced early postoperative wound seromas, they were managed conservatively and resolved without any interventions. The hernia recurrence rate was 5.5% (n = 9) after a mean follow-up of 25 months. This study suggested that prior failed ventral hernia repairs appear to be a predictive factor for future hernia repair failure in both nonobese and obese populations. Novitsky noted a hernia recurrence rate of 1.4% in his obese patients undergoing their first hernia repair, much lower than the 5.5% reported in the overall population. Therefore, the author advocates the use of laparoscopic approach in obese patients undergoing their initial hernia repair to avoid future failures of multiple open procedures. This has the great potential of reducing future patient morbidities associated with multiple failed repairs.

Novitsky's study was followed by another large study by Ramshaw's group [43]. In this study, 901 patients were stratified into two groups of BMI greater (n = 134) or less (n = 767) than 40 kg/m^2. The morbidly obese group had longer operative time (154 versus 119 minutes, $P<.01$) and hospital stay (3.6 versus 2.4 days, $P = .03$). The peri-operative complication rates in the two groups were comparable (19.7% versus 15.3%, $P = .46$). For a mean follow-up of 19 months, the hernia recurrence rate was 8.3% in the morbidly obese group and 2.9% in the nonmorbidly obese group ($P = .003$). These two larger studies verified the early results reported by Birgisson and colleagues, that laparoscopic repairs did not result in more adverse events in patients who are obese compared with nonobese patients. Overall several studies have reported perioperative morbidities in the range of 3% to 31% and hernia recurrence rate of 0% to 7.8% in the obese population [41–44]. When comparing these results with nonobese patients who underwent laparoscopic hernia repairs, they are within the acceptable range and sometimes even more improved. However, no study specifically has evaluated a laparoscopic versus an open approach to ventral hernia repair in morbidly obese patients.

Elderly

As the life expectancy of the general population continues to increase, the management of ventral hernias in the elderly population deserves special attention. Ventral hernias that were treated conservatively in the past may now require surgical operations because of the increasing risk of bowel incarceration or strangulation as patients continue to live longer. The additional comorbidities, in particular, pulmonary and cardiovascular, are mainly responsible for the morbidities and mortalities associated with older patients postoperatively. Although the laparoscopic ventral hernia repair has been shown to decrease the inflammatory response to surgery, many surgeons remain reluctant to perform laparoscopic ventral hernia repairs in patients who are elderly. This is partly because of the concern of tolerating the hemodynamic and ventilatory changes associated with laparoscopy, and the longer operative times and frequent steep Trendelenburg position used during laparoscopic surgery [45,46].

Although little information is available for the use of laparoscopy in ventral hernia repairs in the elderly, it has been studied extensively in laparoscopic colorectal surgery. In general, laparoscopic colorectal surgery in the elderly takes longer to perform but results in less intraoperative blood loss and has less postoperative infectious complications and shorter hospital stay [47,48]. Perhaps even more important is the ability of the elderly patients to return to independent living significantly faster than those patients undergoing open colon procedures [48].

To date, there have been only two studies evaluating the outcome of elderly patients undergoing laparoscopic ventral hernia repair. The first one by Tessier and colleagues [49] evaluated 97 patients undergoing laparoscopic ventral hernia repair with 76% of patients being older than 60 years. Although the older patients group (greater than or equal to 60 years) had more comorbidities, this group demonstrated comparable postoperative length of hospital stay and complication rates when compared with the younger group (younger than 60 yrs). Lee's group [50] conducted a retrospective study comparing the clinical outcome of 117 patients undergoing laparoscopic ventral hernia repairs with mesh in two age groups (younger than 55 years versus greater than or equal to 55 yrs). The postoperative complications were higher in the elderly group (12.9% versus 4.8%), and the recurrence rate was also higher in the older group (3.7% versus 1.6%). These differences, however, were not statistically significant. Despite these apparent differences between the two groups, the overall outcomes in the elderly patients are encouraging. Future prospective studies are necessary to validate the results shown by these two retrospective studies.

Complications of ventral hernia repair

Enterotomy

Bowel injuries can occur during open and laparoscopic ventral hernia repairs. Perhaps one of the most important management strategies in dealing with these situations is to avoid them. In the laparoscopic approach, one should have a low threshold for conversion to an open procedure. In certain cases where a small area of bowel adhesions is too difficult to lyse laparoscopically, the surgeon can make a small open incision, exteriorize the bowel, complete the adhesiolysis, return the bowel to the abdomen, and reinsufflate and complete the procedure laparoscopically. If one recognizes an enterotomy during a laparoscopic procedure, there are several options for its management. It is difficult to provide a clear algorithm in these situations, because it must rely on the skill level of the surgeon, whether there was gross spillage, and the segment of bowel injured. Options include: opening the abdomen, repairing the injury, and performing a primary hernia repair; using a biologic mesh as a reinforcement, or in special circumstances, place a synthetic mesh. Another option is to repair the injury laparoscopically; complete the adhesiolysis, admit the patient to the hospital and return to the operating room in 2 to 6 days for mesh placement. Although the impact of an enterotomy is significant, the outcome of a missed enterotomy is one of the most devastating complications of hernia surgery. In one study, a recognized enterotomy was associated with a mortality rate of 1.7%; however, this rate increased to 7.7% when missed [51]. This is a significant increase, given that the mortality rate of uncomplicated ventral hernia is only 0.05%. One of the most important aspects of ventral hernia repair is that the patients understand these implications preoperatively and have a clear understanding of the need to convert to an open procedure and the possibility that they still may have their hernia at the conclusion of the procedure.

Seroma

Postoperative seroma formation is one of the most common complications after open and laparoscopic ventral hernia repair. In the laparoscopic repair, because the mesh is placed intraperitoneally, the hernia sac is not resected; therefore, essentially all patients develop a postoperative seroma. Typically, these fluid collections resolve within 6 to 8 weeks, although some remain and can become problematic. The cause of seroma formation is likely multifactorial, involving specific patient characteristics, surgical techniques, and the physical and biochemical make-up of the mesh used. Symptomatic seromas that do not resolve can be aspirated using sterile techniques. These collections can become infected and result in eventual mesh infection and removal. Preoperative discussion with patients explaining the likelihood of postoperative seromas may reduce the concerns the patients might have in noticing the persistent early postoperative bulge and not associating that with a recurrence.

Summary

Ventral hernia repair remains one of the most common general surgery procedures performed in the United States. The controversy that surrounds most of the approaches to this challenging surgical problem is a result of the lack of well-designed prospective comparative trials. As this article points out, there is a significant area for contributions of best practice approaches to the disease of ventral herniation. In design of these important trials, specific answers to the difficult question of whether laparoscopic or open approaches provide superior patient outcomes, or which is the most appropriate approach for obese, elderly, or multiply recurrent hernias must be answered. In addition, the role of rectus muscle medialization in re-creation of a functional dynamic abdominal wall with the use of minimally invasive component separation and its role in routine and complex ventral hernia repair must be addressed. As the field of abdominal wall reconstruction after ventral herniation continues to grow, significant improvements in patient quality of life and reduction in recurrence rates should be expected.

References

[1] Santora TA, Rosylin JJ. Incisional hernia. Surg Clin North Am 1993;73:557–70.
[2] Pollock AV, Evans M. Early prediction of late incisional hernia. Br J Surg 1989;76:953–4.
[3] Anthony T, Bergen PC, Kim LT, et al. Factors affecting recurrences following incisional herniorrhaphy. World J Surg 2000;24:95–100 [discussion: 101].
[4] Yahchouchy-Chouillard E, Aura T, Picone O, et al. Incisional hernias. I. Related risk factors. Dig Surg 2003;20:3–9.
[5] Si Z, Bhardwaj R, Rosch R, et al. Impaired balance of type I and type III procollage mRNA in cultured fibroblasts of patients with incisional hernia. Surgery 2002;131:324–31.
[6] Zheng H, Si Z, Kasperk R, et al. Recurrent inguinal hernia: disease of the collagen matrix? World J Surg 2002;26(4):401–8.
[7] Rosch R, Junge K, Knops M, et al. Analysis of collagen-interacting proteins in patients with incisional hernias. Langenbecks Arch Surg 2003;387:427–32.
[8] Stumpf M, Cao W, Klinge U, et al. Collagen distribution and expression of matrix metalloproteinases 1 and 13 in patients with anastomotic leakage after large-bowel surgery. Langenbecks Arch Surg 2002;386(7):502–6.
[9] Cannon DJ, Read RC. Metastatic emphysema: a mechanism for acquiring inguinal herniation. Ann Surg 1981;194:270–8.
[10] Cobb WS, Kercher KW, Heniford BT. Laparoscopic repair of incisional hernias. Surg Clin North Am 2005;85(1):91–103.
[11] Burger JW, Luijendijk RW, Hop WC, et al. Long-term follow-up of a randomized controlled trial of suture versus mesh repair of incisional hernia. Ann Surg 2004;240:578–83.
[12] Usher FC, Ochsner J, Tuttle LL Jr. Use of marlex mesh in the repair of incisional hernias. Am Surg 1958;24(12):967–74.
[13] Klinge U, Conze J, Krones C, et al. Incisional hernia: open techniques. World J Surg 2005; 29:1066–72.

[14] Awad ZT, Puri V, LeBlanc K, et al. Mechanism of ventral hernia recurrence after mesh repair and a new proposed classification. J Am Coll Surg 2005;201:132–40.

[15] LeBlanc KA, Booth WV. Laparoscopic repair of incisional abdominal hernia using expanded polytetrafluoroethylene: preliminary findings. Surg Laparosc Endosc 1993;3: 39–41.

[16] Carbonell AM. A gold standard for measuring defects during ventral hernia repair. Presented at: Hernia Repair 2007. Hollywood (FL), March 7–11, 2007.

[17] Heniford BT, Park A, Ramshaw BJ, et al. Laparoscopic repair of ventral hernias: nine years' experience with 850 consecutive hernias. Ann Surg 2003;238:391–400.

[18] Nimeri AA, Brunt LM. Laparoscopic ventral hernia repair: 5 mm port and alternative mesh insertion method. J Am Coll Surg 2006;202:708–10.

[19] Carlson MA, Peterson A. Technique for the insertion of large mesh during minimally invasive incisional herniorrhaphy. Surg Endosc 2007;21:1243–4.

[20] LeBlanc KA. The critical technical aspects of laparoscopic repair of ventral and incisional hernias. Am Surg 2001;67:809–12.

[21] LeBlanc KA, Booth WV, Whitaker JM, et al. Laparoscopic incisional and ventral herniorrhaphy: our initial 100 patients. Hernia 2001;5:41–5.

[22] Leber GE, Garb JI, Alexander AI, et al. Long-term complications associated with prosthetic repair of incisional hernias. Arch Surg 1998;133:378–82.

[23] Park A, Birch DW, Lovrics P. Laparoscopic and open incisional hernia repair: a comparative study. Surgery 1998;124:816–22.

[24] Wright BE, Niskanene BD, Peterson DJ, et al. Laparoscopic ventral hernia repair: are there comparative advantages over traditional methods of repair? Am Surg 2002;68:291–6.

[25] Ramshaw BJ, Esartia P, Schwab J, et al. Comparison of laparoscopic and open ventral herniorrhaphy. Am Surg 1999;65:823–31.

[26] van't Riet M, Vrijland WW, Lange JF, et al. Mesh repair of incisional hernia: comparison of laparoscopic and open repair. Eur J Surg 2002;168:684–9.

[27] McGreevy JM, Goodney PP, Birkmeyer CM, et al. A prospective study comparing the complication rates between laparoscopic and open ventral hernia repairs. Surg Endosc 2003;17: 1778–80.

[28] Lomanto D, Iyer SG, Shabbir A, et al. Laparoscopic versus open ventral hernia mesh repair: a prospective study. Surg Endosc 2006;20:1030–5.

[29] Birgener J, Buck L, Richards M, et al. Long-term outcomes in laparoscopic vs open ventral hernia repair. Arch Surg 2007;142:562–7.

[30] Olmi S, Scaini A, Cesana GC, et al. Laparoscopic versus open incisional hernia repair: an open randomized controlled study. Surg Endosc 2007;21:555–9.

[31] Jin J, Rosen MJ, Blatnik J, et al. Use of acellular dermal matrix for complicated ventral hernia repair: does technique affect outcomes? J Am Coll Surg 2007;205:654–60.

[32] Alder AC, Alder SC, Livingston EH, et al. Current opinions about laparoscopic incisional hernia repair: a survey of practicing surgeons. Am J Surg 2007;194:659–62.

[33] Ramirez OM, Ruas E, Dellan AL. Components separation method for closure of abdominal wall defects: an anatomic and clinical study. Plast Reconstr Surg 1990;86:519–26.

[34] Rosen MJ, Williams C, Jin J, et al. Laparoscopic versus open-component separation: a comparative analysis in a porcine model. Am J Surg 2007;194:385–9.

[35] Rosen MJ, Jin J, McGee MF, et al. Laparoscopic component separation in the single-stage treatment of infected abdominal wall prosthetic removal. Hernia 2007;11:435–40.

[36] Milburn ML, Shah PK, Friedman EB, et al. Laparoscopically assisted component separation technique for ventral incisional hernia repair. Hernia 2007;11(2):157–61.

[37] Sugerman HJ, Kellum JM, Reines HD, et al. Greater risk of incisional hernia with morbidly obese than steroid-dependent patients and low recurrence with prefascial polypropylene mesh. Am J Surg 1996;171:80–4.

[38] Hesselink VJ, Luijendiik RW, de Wilt JH, et al. An evaluation of risk factors in incisional hernia recurrence. Surg Gynecol Obstet 1993;176:228–34.

[39] Miles RH, Carballo RE, Prinz RA, et al. Laparoscopy: the preferred method of cholecystectomy in the morbidly obese. Surgery 1992;112:818–22.

[40] Memon MA. Laparoscopic appendectomy: current status. Ann R Coll Surg Engl 1997;79: 393–402.

[41] Birgisson G, Park AE, Mastrangelo MJ, et al. Obesity and laparoscopic repair of ventral hernias. Surg Endosc 2001;15:1419–22.

[42] Novitsky YW, Cobb WS, Kercher KW, et al. Laparoscopic ventral hernia repair in obese patients, a new standard of care. Arch Surg 2006;141:57–61.

[43] Tsereteli Z, Pryor BA, Heniford BT, et al. Laparoscopic ventral hernia repair (LVHR) in morbidly obese patients. Hernia 2007;12:233–8.

[44] Raftopoulos I, Courcoulas AP. Outcome of laparoscopic ventral hernia repair in morbidly obese patients with a body mass index exceeding 35 kg/m2. Surg Endosc 2007;21:2293–7.

[45] Gebhardt H, Bautz H, Ross M, et al. Pathophysiological and clinical aspects o the CO2 pneumoperitoneum. Surg Endosc 1997;11:864–7.

[46] Bannenberg JJ, Rademaker BM, Grundeman PF, et al. Hemodynamic during laparoscopy in the supine or prone positio. Surg Endosc 1995;9:125–7.

[47] Frasson M, Braga M, Vignali A, et al. Benefits of laparoscopic colorectal resections are more pronounced in elderly patients. Dis Colon Rectum 2008;51:296–300.

[48] Vignali M, Di Palo S, Tamburini A, et al. Laparoscopic vs open colectomies in octogenarians: a case-matched control study. Dis Colon Rectum 2005;48:2070–5.

[49] Tessier DJ, Swain JM, Harold KL. Safety of laparoscopic ventral hernia repair in older patients. Hernia 2006;10:53–7.

[50] Lee YK, Iqbal A, Vitamvas M, et al. Is it safe to perform laparoscopic ventral hernia repair with mesh in elderly patients? Hernia 2007;10:53–7.

[51] LeBlanc KA, Elieson MJ, Corder JM III. Enterotomy and mortality rates of laparoscopic incisional and ventral hernia repair: a review of the literature. JSLS 2007;11:408–14.

ELSEVIER
SAUNDERS

SURGICAL
CLINICS OF
NORTH AMERICA

Surg Clin N Am 88 (2008) 1101–1119

Recent Advances and Controversies in Pediatric Laparoscopic Surgery

Emily T. Durkin, MD[a], Aimen F. Shaaban, MD[b],*

[a]*Department of Surgery, University of Wisconsin School of Medicine and Public Health, 600 Highland Ave, Madison, WI 53792, USA*
[b]*Department of Surgery, University of Iowa Carver College of Medicine, 1500 JCP, 200 Hawkins Drive, Iowa City, IA 52242, USA*

The field of minimally invasive surgery (MIS) is the fastest growing area of surgical innovation. Each year as new techniques and tools are developed, more patients benefit from surgical procedures previously associated with a significantly more invasive approach. Pediatric patients represent a naturally appealing population of patients who are likely to benefit greatly from MIS for a variety of reasons specific to this population. Shorter hospital stays, less painful incisions, a faster return to normal activity, and a shorter recovery period are just a few of the advantages that MIS offers to the pediatric age group. Current barriers to advancement of this field include limited case volume for complex procedures, inappropriate "adult-sized" instrumentation, and lack of outcome documentation.

Most pediatric surgical training programs, however, now include a curriculum in MIS. This critical element should have the greatest impact on advancement of this field. Additionally, many pediatric surgeons in the academic and private sectors are finding creative ways to approach pediatric surgical problems from a minimally invasive perspective. As these techniques become more widespread, the need for smaller and more specialized equipment is recognized. Laparoscopic instruments designed specifically for smaller bodies have made MIS techniques possible in even the tiniest of infants. Lastly, as a result of a broader experience and strong leadership from the national pediatric surgical organizations, prospective multicenter trials are emerging to guide further application of MIS in the treatment of childhood surgical disease. This article summarizes the recent advances and controversies within the field of pediatric MIS. Issues unique to the

* Corresponding author.
E-mail address: shaaban@surgery.wisc.edu (A.F. Shaaban).

0039-6109/08/$ - see front matter © 2008 Elsevier Inc. All rights reserved.
doi:10.1016/j.suc.2008.05.014

pediatric population and to the disease entities frequently encountered in the surgical treatment of children in particular are addressed.

Pediatric thoracic surgery

The surgical treatment of all the organs within the chest, with the exception of the heart, remains within the scope of practice of most pediatric surgeons. Traditionally, video-assisted thoracoscopic surgery (VATS) was developed to provide biopsy specimens of thoracic structures in immuno-compromised patients when a definitive diagnosis otherwise could not be obtained [1]. Although this continues to be used widely in the pediatric population, an increasing number of pediatric surgical conditions also are being addressed using a thoracoscopic approach.

Pectus repair

The emergence of minimally invasive pectus repair (MIPR) represents an ideal case study in the development, evaluation, and widespread acceptance of a new technique in MIS that addresses a common pediatric surgical condition. Originally reported by Nuss and colleagues [2] with nearly a decade of outcome data at the time of its initial presentation, MIPR established a new paradigm in the treatment of pectus excavatum. The subsequent decade since that report has yielded several reports comparing the MIPR to a modified Ravitch repair [3,4]. With increasing experience, similar outcomes have been demonstrated in the two approaches in regard to perioperative morbidity, hospital length of stay, and cosmetic result. In contrast to modified Ravitch repair, MIPR does not seem associated with a decrease in static or exercise cardiopulmonary capacity [5,6]. It is theorized that this observation results from less chest wall scar formation with MIPR.

The current MIPR technique remains similar to that originally described by Nuss. Only minor modifications in the way in which the crossbar is passed or stabilized have been proposed. Although the risk for significant mediastinal injury with bar passage is extremely low, the addition of unilateral or bilateral thoracoscopy may help to minimize these significant events. Bar rotation remains the Achilles heel of MIPR. A clinically insignificant degree of bar rotation can be expected in up one third of patients whereas significant bar rotation requiring reoperation should be limited to less than 3% of patients [3,7]. The incidence of this complication is highest in the first 3 months after MIPR. Despite being a correctable problem in most situations, reoperations for bar rotation are a significant source of emotional and physical hardship for patients and their families. The use of side stabilizers, dual crossbars, and rib-encircling fixation sutures may reduce the likelihood of this complication. The implementation of all of these added maneuvers may be appropriate in older teenagers or adults in whom the chest wall has more rigidity or in the situation of significant asymmetry.

Empyema

Probably the most common application for thoracoscopy in the pediatric population is the treatment of complicated empyema by thoracoscopic drainage and pleural decortication. Despite being a relatively common pediatric condition, however, the management and indications for surgical intervention remain somewhat controversial [8]. Currently, a multitude of treatment algorithms exist for the treatment of pediatric empyema. The major drawback for thoracoscopic drainage when compared with tube thoracostomy is the stringent need for general anesthesia. It may be argued, however, that heavy sedation or general anesthesia is routinely needed for tube thoracostomy placement in children and carries similar risks albeit with inferior outcomes. In a recent review by Engum, the results of multiple pediatric empyema trials comparing VATS decortication with traditional closed chest drainage and antibiotic therapy were summarized [9]. Thoracopscopic intervention is associated with significantly shorter hospital stays and shorter antibiotic duration and results in fewer invasive procedures overall. It is the authors' preference to intervene thoracoscopically for pediatric empyema at the earliest possible juncture. This emergency room to operating room approach relies on an institutional practice consensus and the authors believe sets the stage for the best possible outcomes [8].

Bronchopulmonary-foregut malformations

The largest experience with congenital lung anomalies (bronchopulmonary sequestration, cystic adenomatoid malformation, and lobar emphysema) and foregut malformations (bronchogenic cysts and esophageal duplications) continues to exist within pediatric surgical practice. Although some areas of controversy remain, operative resection routinely is performed shortly after diagnosis in most cases to reduce chronic infectious complications and to prevent malignant transformation [10]. Many case series document the relatively straightforward resection of extralobar thoracic lesions [11–13]. Despite the publication of several small case series, however, the long-term outcomes of thoracoscopic lobectomy in the pediatric population are not well documented [14–17]. Albanese and Rothenberg recently reported their combined experience with thoracoscopic lobectomy over 10 years [18]. Only four perioperative complications and no long-term morbidity were observed in a series of 144 patients who had extended follow-up. These results highlight the safety of thoracoscopic lobectomy but underscore the need for prospective controlled trials to document improved outcomes and to characterize the learning curve for these highly technical procedures.

Congenital diaphragmatic hernia

Few problems in pediatric surgery are as clinically challenging as the treatment of congenital diaphragmatic hernia (CDH). MIS was first believed more safely applied to those hernias presenting in a delayed fashion later in childhood [19–21]. In the past few years, there has been increasing interest in attempting minimally invasive repair in the early neonatal period for children born with CDH. Selection criteria for thoracoscopic CDH repair in newborns are poorly developed; however, several parameters recently were suggested by Yang and colleagues [22]. Infants selected for thoracoscopic repair were required to have a preoperative peak inspiratory pressure less than 24 mm Hg and demonstration of the nasogastric tube tip within the abdomen. The rationale for the former requirement was to include only patients who had some pulmonary reserve that would tolerate an applied pneumothorax during the procedure. The latter requirement predicted an intact esophageal hiatus enhancing the feasibility of completing the repair thoracoscopically without the use of a patch. Using this approach, the investigators were able to complete the thoracoscopic repair in all of the patients (n = 7) without significant complication. Not all patients who have CDH are good candidates for thoracoscopic repair and prospective controlled trials are needed to help define selection criteria and document outcomes.

Another question is whether or not a thoracoscopic or laparoscopic approach is best suited for the correction of CDH. Although no direct comparisons have been performed, the advantages of thoracoscopic approach are emphasized in several studies [22–25]. The ability to use lower insufflation pressures, the presence of more working space for hernia repair after intestinal reduction, and a gentle no-touch technique for reducing the intestinal contents are cited as reasons most pediatric surgeons favor a thoracoscopic approach [26].

Esophageal atresia and tracheoesophageal fistula

Another complicated surgical problem unique to the pediatric population is the repair of esophageal atresia and distal tracheoesophageal fistulas. Until recently, only a few reports, all from single institutions, had been published detailing individual surgeons' experiences with thoracoscopic repair of this anomaly [27–29]. The first multicenter, multisurgeon review of all pediatric patients undergoing thoracoscopic repair of a tracheoesophageal fistula was detailed in a recent series by Holcomb and colleagues [30] and included 104 neonates. Their results demonstrated that thoracoscopic repair of esophageal atresia and tracheoesophageal fistulas can be accomplished safely in neonates with results and complication rates comparable to those done via thoracotomy. The proposed benefits of thoracoscopy were a reduction in the long-term musculoskeletal sequellae seen after thoracotomy and an enhanced visualization of the anatomy through the thoracoscope. The investigators and others caution that the procedure itself has a steep learning curve, however, and should be performed only by experienced pediatric endoscopic surgeons [30,31].

Thymectomy

Thoracoscopy continues to be used to address disorders of the pediatric mediastinum with good results. Thoracoscopic resection of the thymus has been reported in children suffering from juvenile myasthenia gravis (MG) [32–34]. Recently Wagner and colleagues [35] published long-term results for relatively small cohorts of children who underwent an open or thoracoscopic thymectomy for MG. Mean operating times were surprisingly nearly identical in both groups. The thoracoscopic group had outcomes equal to the open group in regards to induction of remission and the added benefits of less blood loss, shorter hospital stay, and improved cosmesis. Concerns regarding the potential inability to maximally resect the thymus via thoracoscopy leading to lower rates of disease remission or a higher incidence of recurrence have not materialized in this and other long-term studies. As such, thoracoscopic thymectomy for MG has been adopted as the preferred approach by most pediatric surgeons.

Pathology of the great vessels

Thoracoscopy also lends itself nicely to pediatric pathology involving the great vessels within the chest. The minimally invasive approach can simplify the intraoperative procedure and the time for children undergoing aortopexy, vascular ring division, or patent ductus arteriosus (PDA) ligation. Complete resolution of chronic airway symptoms is reported after thoracoscopic aortopexy in neonates, older children, and adolescents [36,37]. Good outcomes also have been observed with thoracoscopic division of vascular rings in children [38,39]. Despite these encouraging results, prospective controlled trials are not yet reported with either of these approaches.

Conversely, thoracoscopic PDA ligation has been well studied. Vanamo and colleagues [40] published a recent comparison of 50 cases of VATS PDA ligation documented in a prospective fashion and compared these results to a historical cohort ligated via thoracotomy. The outcomes were mixed as the VATS group experienced a higher rate of recurrent laryngeal nerve injury (12%) but required shorter operative times, fewer days of pleural drainage, and shorter neonatal ICU and overall hospital stays. Although these results seem promising, this report and others excluded patients who had large ductal diameters and very low-birth-weight premature infants who had hemodynamic instability [41,42]. Additionally, the application of this approach in older children must take into consideration the excellent results seen with coil occlusion [43,44]. Therefore, VATS PDA ligation seems best suited for hemodynamically stable infants and older children who may be at high risk for complications after coil occlusion.

Congenital cardiac malformations

The field of robotic surgery continues to progress exponentially, and robotic instruments increasingly are considered for implementation in pediatric surgery because of their ability to articulate increasing surgeon dexterity while working in small spaces. Particularly exciting are the opportunities for implementation of robotics to aid in the correction of congenital cardiac anomalies [45]. Until now, the complexity of these operations and the large scale of all commercially available robotic equipment have limited its usefulness in congenital cardiac surgery, which typically is performed in the neonate. Additionally, the necessity of cardiopulmonary bypass to adequately visualize intracardiac pathology limits the applicability of robotics in many cardiac procedures. Recently, an exciting report described the thoracoscopic-assisted repair of an atrial septal defect in a 14-year-old patient using hypothermic fibrillation and robotic instruments [46]. Subsequent case series are likely to follow and hopefully will provide more guidance for the use of VATS or robotics in pediatric cardiac disease.

Pediatric abdominopelvic laparoscopy

Gastroesophageal reflux disease

Over the past few years, laparoscopic fundoplication has become the treatment of choice for pediatric gastroesophageal reflux. Similar to outcomes in adult patients, laparoscopic fundoplication in children imparts a faster return to normal feeding and activity, less postoperative pain, and a shorter hospital stay [47]. Long-term prospective controlled trials in comparison to open Nissen fundoplication have revealed nearly identical outcomes in regard to symptom control and recurrent reflux; however, higher rates of wrap herniation occasionally occur in laparoscopic fundoplication [48–50].

One of the current challenges of laparoscopic fundoplication comes in the treatment of recurrent reflux disease after operation, particularly in the setting of neurologic impairment [51]. These cases not only are technically difficult but also can be a source of increased morbidity for this already vulnerable pediatric population. Therefore, there has been interest in even less invasive ways of controlling reflux that do not require reoperation, such as the use of radiofrequency ablation at the lower esophageal sphincter or endoscopic fundoplication [52,53].

Pediatric obesity surgery

As the number of obese children continues to increase, there has been interest among several bariatric surgeons in developing bariatric surgical treatment options for obese children and adolescents [54,55]. The development of laparoscopic adjustable gastric banding imparts a potential advantage for pediatric patients specifically because it seems to avoid many of the chronic nutritional derangements of traditional gastric bypass. Although this technique has not yet received Food and Drug Administration approval for use in children, several studies recently were published that evaluate the safety and efficacy of this procedure in obese children [56–59]. One prospective study of a cohort of 73 obese adolescents, ranging in age from 13 to 17 years old, found that gastric banding not only resulted in excellent weight loss at 1 and 2 years but also reduced comorbid conditions present in these children by nearly 70% [60]. With a growing problem of pediatric obesity, it is imperative that standardized protocols for bariatric surgery in children be established and included in the curriculum for pediatric surgical training.

Pyloric stenosis

Laparoscopic pyloromyotomy is a well-established and successful approach to the treatment of hypertrophic pyloric stenosis. Kim and colleagues [61] reported their results comparing laparoscopic pyloromyotomy to the traditional Ramstedt open pyloromyotomy and periumbilical open pyloromyotomy. The laparoscopic group had shorter operating times without higher complications or cost. A meta-analysis by Hall and colleagues [62], however, found that overall the complication rate for laparoscopic pyloromyotomy was higher (including mucosal perforation and incomplete pyloromyotomy) with similar operative times, although the laparoscopic group still had a shorter recovery.

Splenectomy

Laparoscopic splenectomy is a well-established procedure in children for a variety of nontraumatic pathologies. This approach allows for the removal of a large spleen without the added morbidity and postoperative pain associated with a larger incision. A large single institution series evaluating outcomes in children undergoing laparoscopic splenectomy recently was reported [63]. In a cohort of 223 children undergoing laparoscopic splenectomy for a variety of pathologies, the investigators reported a low morbidity rate (11%) and an impressive early discharge rate, with 70% of children going home on the first postoperative day. Laparoscopic partial splenectomy also is described and can be of particular benefit in young children who have hereditary spherocytosis, children who have hypersplenism, and children who have symptomatic splenic cysts [64]. Unroofing of isolated splenic cysts has been accomplished laparoscopically but shown to result in an unacceptably high rate of recurrence in one analysis [65,66].

Biliary disease

Laparoscopic cholecystectomy remains the standard of care in children who have cholecystitis, symptomatic cholelithiasis, and biliary dyskinesia with benefits and outcomes similar to those seen in adults [67–69]. Over the past few years, there have been intriguing advancements in developing laparoscopic approaches to the treatment of congenital and acquired biliary diseases previously considered too complex for laparoscopy. Laparoscopic cystgastrostomy and Roux-en-Y cystjejunostomy are described in the treatment of pediatric pancreatic pseudocysts [70,71]. Several case series exist for the laparoscopic treatment of biliary atresia and choledochal cysts with acceptable outcomes [72]. Pediatric biliary disease also is treated with robotic techniques that may help to simplify complex biliary reconstruction procedures that are challenging for even experienced laparoscopic surgeons [73–75].

Small intestinal pathology

MIS has been used to treat a variety of pediatric small intestinal pathology successfully, including Crohn's disease, Meckel's diverticulum, malrotation, and intussusception [76,77]. Some controversy exists in the use of laparoscopy to reduce intussusception when air enema has failed [78,79]. Two separate studies recently were published evaluating the safety and efficacy of laparoscopic reduction of intussusception [80,81]. Both groups reported success with laparoscopic reduction in 72% to 85% of cases in which enema reduction was unsuccessful. Laparoscopic-assisted bowel resection was performed via the umbilical port site in cases in which a pathologic lead point was encountered [82]. Operative time and complication rates were similar in the open and laparoscopic groups, with the additional benefit of a quicker return of bowel function and a shorter length of stay in the laparoscopic group.

Appendicitis

Appendectomy is the most common pediatric surgical procedure for pathology and frequently is performed in children and adolescents by pediatric and adult general surgeons. For this reason, laparoscopic appendectomy was one of the earliest MIS procedures performed in children [83]. In recent years, many innovative techniques have been described for the laparoscopic treatment of appendicitis in children. These approaches include intra- and extracorporeal resection, transection of the appendiceal stump with stapling or ligature devices, and an overall trend toward reduction in the number of port sites placed [84–86]. Many studies have compared the results of open versus laparoscopic appendectomy in children with conflicting results [87–90]. Several recent studies, however, including a large meta-analysis, have demonstrated laparoscopic appendectomy in the pediatric population associated with fewer complications, such as wound infection and ileus, when compared with open appendectomy [90–92].

Even more controversy exists for laparoscopic appendectomy in cases of perforated appendicitis in children. Some reports have suggested that the laparoscopic approach contributes to a higher rate of abscess formation in children who have perforated appendicitis [87,93]. Nadler and colleagues [94], however, recently reported no difference in infectious complications and a lower overall rate of perioperative complications in their patient cohort with perforated appendicitis treated laparoscopically. Overall, studies comparing laparoscopic versus open appendectomy in children who have complicated appendicitis or perforation are lacking.

Large intestine pathology

Laparoscopic segmental resection and complete laparoscopic proctocolectomy are well described in the treatment of pediatric inflammatory bowel disease [76,95,96]. Technical details and clinical outcomes essentially are the same as those reported for these procedures performed in adults. Meier and colleagues [97] recently published their experience with a completely minimally invasive approach in a cohort of pediatric patients. Their operative times were not significantly longer than an open approach; however, the investigators did report an increased number of postoperative obstructive complications at the ileostomy site, which they attributed to the use of a laparoscopic port site for the stoma.

The treatment of pediatric colonic aganglionosis or Hirschsprung's disease also has been revolutionized by MIS. What once was considered a three-stage operation consisting of a diverting colostomy, resection of the aganglionic bowel segment, and subsequent restoration of bowel continuity, now is largely replaced with a single-stage operation at most centers [98]. A laparoscopic Duhamel procedure was first described by Smith and colleagues [99]. Subsequently several techniques of laparoscopic-assisted Soave-type endorectal pull-through were described [100]. Eventually, De la Torre-Mondragón and colleagues [101] reported the technique of a completely transanal endorectal pull-through. This technique requires no specialized laparoscopic equipment and takes advantage of the relative proximity and compliance of the pelvic anatomy found in infants. This approach has become popular among pediatric surgeons worldwide and also is used in older children who have late diagnosis of Hirschsprung's disease and in long-segment disease in combination with laparoscopic assistance [98,102]. Subsequent multicenter trials comparing this technique to an open endorectal pull-through revealed superior results in regard to shorter hospital length of stay, earlier return to full feedings, reduced pain, fewer postoperative small bowel obstructions, and lower overall costs [103,104]. No differences were observed in operative time, blood loss, or recurrent enterocolitis. Some residual concerns regarding the impact of operative retraction on anal sphincter physiology have little support in the available literature and likely relate to subtle variations in the operative technique.

Anorectal malformations

Similar to the pull-through procedure for Hirschsprung's disease, the treatment of the anorectal malformations has followed a trend of primary neonatal repair. Traditionally, patients required a decompressive colostomy shortly after birth followed by a distal study to define the anatomy and identify fistulous connections. The pull-through then followed and lastly intestinal continuity restored. Many centers now prefer a single-stage operation for repair of imperforate anus without a diverting colostomy. Laparoscopic repair of imperforate anus was first described by Georgeson and colleagues [105] in 2000. The proposed advantages include less pain, easier identification, and control of the fistula and a more accurate localization of the anus within the center of the sphincter complex. Because of its seemingly technical complexity and a lack of long-term outcome data, this procedure has been slow to gain acceptance amongst pediatric surgeons. As experience is accumulating, however, several comparative studies now exist and the laparoscopic approach is gaining momentum.

In a recent study by Ichijo and colleagues [106], the outcomes of 15 laparoscopic Georgeson-type repair of high or intermediate anorectal malformations were compared with nine posterior sagittal anorectoplasty (PSARP)-type repairs. Diverting colostomy was performed in all patients and pull-through performed several months later. In follow-up, the central location of the anus within the sphincter complex was assessed by anal endosonography and MRI. Continence was assessed by questionnaire. The investigators found the anus centrally located with similar frequency using either procedure. Continence scores were better for the laparoscopic group and reached statistical significance after 3 years. The PSARP group, however, included two men with a bladder neck fistula, which may have biased the continence comparison to favor the laparoscopic group. These results are encouraging, however, and warrant further investigation.

The application of the laparoscopic approach seems most appropriate in men who have high or intermediate types of anorectal malformation. The advantage is in identification and control of rectourethral and rectovesical fistulae. In this regard, Vick and colleagues [107] published a series of six male neonates born at term who underwent a laparoscopic single-stage procedure for high imperforate anus malformations. The investigators reported excellent visualization and control of fistulous connections in all cases and superb overall results in their small series. Long-term follow-up in this group of patients will be essential to evaluate continence.

Urologic and gonadal abnormalities

Pediatric urologists and surgeons have embraced MIS techniques for the diagnosis and treatment of certain benign and even certain malignant gonadal abnormalities. Radmayr and colleagues [108] reported the long-term results of a cohort of 84 children who underwent a primary or two-stage laparoscopic procedure for a total of 108 undescended testes. Their mean follow-up time for all patients was 6.2 years and none of the testes managed with a primary laparoscopic procedure became atrophic, and only two managed by a two-stage laparoscopic procedure atrophied during the follow-up period. Laparoscopic treatment of pediatric varicocele has also been performed with good results, but postoperative hydrocele formation is common, and approximately 10% to 15% of patients ultimately require additional surgical intervention [109,110].

In female pediatric patients, laparoscopy can be diagnostic and therapeutic in chronic abdominal pain caused by gonadal pathology. MIS is helpful especially in the diagnosis of suspected ovarian torsion because of the difficulties and delays associated with noninvasive imaging in the pediatric population [111]. Detorsion and oophoropexy results in salvage of the ovary in most cases [112]. Concomitant ovarian cystectomy should be performed as indicated. Surgeons should proceed with caution, however, when partially decompressing ovarian cysts to facilitate a laparoscopic resection, especially in premenarchal patients. The authors prefer to perform the cystectomy in any but the simplest cases through a small Pfannenstiel's or lower midline incision. In addition to serum markers (such as bHCG, AFP, and CA125) and the gross appearance of the cyst, additional parameters, such as the presence of pain or ascites, can be used to assess the likelihood of malignancy [113]. The relative rarity of malignant germ cell or epithelial tumors supports attempts at ovarian salvage when malignancy is not suspected. In the rare situation in which malignancy is histologically discovered after the operation, reoperation can be performed for salpingoophorectomy and staging if needed. This easily can be done laparoscopically even if an open cystectomy was performed.

Minimally invasive repair of ureteropelvic junction obstruction in infants and children has been reported by many groups as safe and efficacious. Until recently, no study had directly compared the transperitoneal laparoscopic approach to the retroperitoneoscopic approach. Canon and colleagues [114] compared these two surgical procedures in a series of 49 consecutive patients, crossing over from the retroperitoneoscopic approach to the transperitoneal laparoscopic approach after the first 20 patients. Both procedures were identical with regards to length of stay and postoperative analgesia requirement. There was a significantly longer operative length with the retroperitoneoscopic procedure, which the investigators attributed to a learning curve effect. They concluded that both procedures are safe and efficacious and should be performed in accordance with surgeon preference and individual experience level.

Inguinal hernia repair

The use of laparoscopic hernia repair in the pediatric population has been championed to increase identification of contralateral hernias, decrease trauma to the gonadal vessels and vas deferens, and reduce the amount of postoperative analgesia needed [115,116]. A slightly increased recurrence rate and postoperative hydrocele formation for laparoscopic inguinal herniorrhaphy, however, is reported [115]. With greater reported experience, the laparoscopic approach to repair of inguinal hernias in children is gaining acceptance among pediatric surgeons [117]. Several techniques are described in the pediatric surgical literature. One recent report describes one center's experience with 300 hernia repairs using a subcutaneous endoscopically assisted ligation of the internal ring via a single-port technique [118]. The investigators reported a recurrence rate of 4.3%, which improved with more experience.

Laparoscopy for pediatric malignancy

Because MIS is well documented as safe and efficacious in the pediatric population for surgical procedures in the thorax and abdomen, there may be a significant role for MIS in the diagnosis and treatment of pediatric malignancy. The use of MIS to establish a definitive diagnosis in children who have suspected malignancy first was described by Holcomb and colleagues [119] in 1995. Several questions, however, regarding the safety and appropriateness of MIS in the setting of pediatric malignancies remain. To date, only small case series have been published evaluating the feasibility of MIS for resection of pediatric solid organ tumors, specifically neuroblastoma, and these techniques have been slow to gain acceptance among pediatric surgeons [120–122]. Metzelder and colleagues [123] published an intriguing study this year of a cohort of 307 children who had diagnosed malignancy at their institution that underwent minimally invasive treatment for their cancer. This report represents a valuable first step in evaluating the potential for MIS therapy in childhood cancer. Furthermore, the study further reinforced the feasibility and safety of MIS for diagnosis and staging of malignancy and evaluation of recurrent disease. In addition to reducing postoperative pain, the use of MIS may facilitate an earlier initiation of chemotherapy.

Laparoscopy for pediatric trauma

Given the advances in MIS that have been made in recent years for the treatment of surgical disorders in children, it is logical that this technology also be applied in the setting of injured children. Traditionally, the application of MIS in the presence of intra-abdominal traumatic injury has been limited by surgeon preference and familiarity and its ability to thoroughly evaluate injury; however, several studies recently have been published evaluating the applicability of MIS for trauma in children [124,125]. One potentially useful application of laparoscopy in the treatment of blunt trauma is in those cases in which free fluid is present but no solid organ injury can be identified. A report published by Feliz and colleagues [126] evaluated exactly this situation in a series of 32 children. Not surprisingly, because these children had significantly lower injury severity scores and higher Glasgow Coma Scale scores, they experienced significantly fewer ICU admission days and shorter overall lengths of hospital stay. Laparoscopic intervention, however, was diagnostic and therapeutic in nearly 20% of these children and almost 60% of those who underwent laparoscopy avoided the additional morbidity of a laparotomy. Lastly, as technical expertise is developing, reports evaluating laparoscopy in the treatment of penetrating trauma in children are emerging [127].

Summary

The next decade in pediatric health care likely will be characterized in part by an exponential growth of MIS. Innovative techniques are being used for increasingly complex and challenging operations in the pediatric population. As a general approach, MIS is being embraced by all generations of pediatric surgeons around the world. In many instances, it already has become the standard of care. Exciting innovations in the field of pediatric MIS continue to be reported in the pediatric literature each year and presented at conferences, which are increasingly dedicated to advancing the field of pediatric endosurgery. Another impetus for growth is that most pediatric surgical practices now have publicly viewable Web sites designed specifically for parents, thereby increasing the visibility of pediatric MIS. Families are better informed with regard to various surgical options for their children and increasingly demand cutting-edge therapy. Large and well-conducted prospective trials comparing laparoscopic with traditional open procedures in children are desperately needed to guide appropriate counseling in the face of these expectations. Challenges that remain include difficulties with institutional review board approval for studies involving pediatric patients, single-institution studies, and low treatment group numbers that make randomization difficult. These problems are aggravated by market-driven limitations in instrumentation, which diminish the practicality of pediatric MIS in many centers. As popular demand for less invasive procedures in children increases, however, and minimally invasive instrumentation is reduced in scale, the design and execution of these essential trials will become more feasible. Ultimately, the benefits of MIS for the treatment of a myriad of pediatric surgical conditions cannot be overstated and no doubt will be the driving force behind its growth in the next decade.

References

[1] Rodgers BM, Talbert JL. Thoracoscopy for diagnosis of intrathoracic lesions in children. J Pediatr Surg 1976;11(5):703–8.
[2] Nuss D, Kelly RE Jr, Croitoru DP, et al. A 10-year review of a minimally invasive technique for the correction of pectus excavatum. J Pediatr Surg 1998;33(4):545–52.
[3] Kelly RE Jr, Shamberger RC, Mellins RB, et al. Prospective multicenter study of surgical correction of pectus excavatum: design, perioperative complications, pain, and baseline pulmonary function facilitated by internet-based data collection. J Am Coll Surg 2007; 205(2):205–16.

 [4] Hosie S, Sitkiewicz T, Petersen C, et al. Minimally invasive repair of pectus excavatum—the Nuss procedure. A European multicentre experience. Eur J Pediatr Surg 2002;12(4):235–8.
 [5] Borowitz D, Cerny F, Zallen G, et al. Pulmonary function and exercise response in patients with pectus excavatum after Nuss repair. J Pediatr Surg 2003;38(4):544–7.
 [6] Bawazir OA, Montgomery M, Harder J, et al. Midterm evaluation of cardiopulmonary effects of closed repair for pectus excavatum. J Pediatr Surg 2005;40(5):863–7.
 [7] Park HJ, Chung WJ, Lee IS, et al. Mechanism of bar displacement and corresponding bar fixation techniques in minimally invasive repair of pectus excavatum. J Pediatr Surg 2008; 43(1):74–8.
 [8] Cremonesini D, Thomson AH. How should we manage empyema: antibiotics alone, fibrinolytics, or primary video-assisted thoracoscopic surgery (VATS)? Semin Respir Crit Care Med 2007;28(3):322–32.
 [9] Engum SA. Minimal access thoracic surgery in the pediatric population. Semin Pediatr Surg 2007;16(1):14–26.
[10] Laberge JM, Puligandla P, Flageole H. Asymptomatic congenital lung malformations. Semin Pediatr Surg 2005;14(1):16–33.
[11] Suda T, Hasegawa S, Negi K, et al. Video-assisted thoracoscopic surgery for extralobar pulmonary sequestration. J Thorac Cardiovasc Surg 2006;132(3):707–8.
[12] Jesch NK, Leonhardt J, Sumpelmann R, et al. Thoracoscopic resection of intra- and extralobar pulmonary sequestration in the first 3 months of life. J Pediatr Surg 2005;40(9): 1404–6.
[13] de Lagausie P, Bonnard A, Berrebi D, et al. Video-assisted thoracoscopic surgery for pulmonary sequestration in children. Ann Thorac Surg 2005;80(4):1266–9.
[14] Rothenberg SS. Experience with thoracoscopic lobectomy in infants and children. J Pediatr Surg 2003;38(1):102–4.
[15] Albanese CT, Sydorak RM, Tsao K, et al. Thoracoscopic lobectomy for prenatally diagnosed lung lesions. J Pediatr Surg 2003;38(4):553–5.
[16] Koontz CS, Oliva V, Gow KW, et al. Video-assisted thoracoscopic surgical excision of cystic lung disease in children. J Pediatr Surg 2005;40(5):835–7.
[17] Emil S, Su W. Thoracoscopic upper lobectomies for symptomatic congenital lung cysts. J Laparoendosc Adv Surg Tech A 2008;18(1):174–8.
[18] Albanese CT, Rothenberg SS. Experience with 144 consecutive pediatric thoracoscopic lobectomies. J Laparoendosc Adv Surg Tech A 2007;17(3):339–41.
[19] Becmeur F, Jamali RR, Moog R, et al. Thoracoscopic treatment for delayed presentation of congenital diaphragmatic hernia in the infant. A report of three cases. Surg Endosc 2001; 15(10):1163–6.
[20] van der Zee DC, Bax NM. Laparoscopic repair of congenital diaphragmatic hernia in a 6-month-old child. Surg Endosc 1995;9(9):1001–3.
[21] Arca MJ, Barnhart DC, Lelli JL Jr, et al. Early experience with minimally invasive repair of congenital diaphragmatic hernias: results and lessons learned. J Pediatr Surg 2003;38(11): 1563–8.
[22] Yang EY, Allmendinger N, Johnson SM, et al. Neonatal thoracoscopic repair of congenital diaphragmatic hernia: selection criteria for successful outcome. J Pediatr Surg 2005;40(9): 1369–75.
[23] Becmeur F, Reinberg O, Dimitriu C, et al. Thoracoscopic repair of congenital diaphragmatic hernia in children. Semin Pediatr Surg 2007;16(4):238–44.
[24] Kohno M, Ikawa H, Okamoto S, et al. Laparoscopic repair of late-presenting Bochdalek hernia in 2 infants. Surg Laparosc Endosc Percutan Tech 2007;17(4):317–21.
[25] Nguyen TL, Le AD. Thoracoscopic repair for congenital diaphragmatic hernia: lessons from 45 cases. J Pediatr Surg 2006;41(10):1713–5.
[26] Schaarschmidt K, Strauss J, Kolberg-Schwerdt A, et al. Thoracoscopic repair of congenital diaphragmatic hernia by inflation-assisted bowel reduction, in a resuscitated neonate: a better access? Pediatr Surg Int 2005;21(10):806–8.

[27] Lobe TE, Rothenberg SS, Waldschidt J, et al. Thoracoscopic repair of esophageal atresia in an infant: a surgical first. Ped Endosurg Innov Techniques 1999;3:141–8.
[28] Rothenberg SS. Thoracoscopic repair of tracheoesophageal fistula in newborns. J Pediatr Surg 2002;37(6):869–72.
[29] Bax KM, van Der Zee DC. Feasibility of thoracoscopic repair of esophageal atresia with distal fistula. J Pediatr Surg 2002;37(2):192–6.
[30] Holcomb GW III, Rothenberg SS, Bax KM, et al. Thoracoscopic repair of esophageal atresia and tracheoesophageal fistula: a multi-institutional analysis. Ann Surg 2005; 242(3):422–8 [discussion: 428–30].
[31] Nguyen T, Zainabadi K, Bui T, et al. Thoracoscopic repair of esophageal atresia and tracheoesophageal fistula: lessons learned. J Laparoendosc Adv Surg Tech A 2006;16(2): 174–8.
[32] Lobe TE. Pediatric thoracoscopy. Semin Thorac Cardiovasc Surg 1993;5(4):298–302.
[33] Kolski H, Vajsar J, Kim PC. Thoracoscopic thymectomy in juvenile myasthenia gravis. J Pediatr Surg 2000;35(5):768–70.
[34] Skelly CL, Jackson CC, Wu Y, et al. Thoracoscopic thymectomy in children with myasthenia gravis. Am Surg 2003;69(12):1087–9.
[35] Wagner AJ, Cortes RA, Strober J, et al. Long-term follow-up after thymectomy for myasthenia gravis: thoracoscopic vs open. J Pediatr Surg 2006;41(1):50–4 [discussion: 50–4].
[36] van der Zee DC, Bax NM. Thoracoscopic tracheoaortopexia for the treatment of life-threatening events in tracheomalacia. Surg Endosc 2007;21(11):2024–5.
[37] Durkin ET, Krawiec ME, Shaaban AF. Thoracoscopic aortopexy for primary tracheomalacia in a 12-year-old. J Pediatr Surg 2007;42(7):E15–7.
[38] Al-Bassam A, Saquib Mallick M, Al-Qahtani A, et al. Thoracoscopic division of vascular rings in infants and children. J Pediatr Surg 2007;42(8):1357–61.
[39] Koontz CS, Bhatia A, Forbess J, et al. Video-assisted thoracoscopic division of vascular rings in pediatric patients. Am Surg 2005;71(4):289–91.
[40] Vanamo K, Berg E, Kokki H, et al. Video-assisted thoracoscopic versus open surgery for persistent ductus arteriosus. J Pediatr Surg 2006;41(7):1226–9.
[41] Villa E, Vanden Eynden F, Le Bret E, et al. Paediatric video-assisted thoracoscopic clipping of patent ductus arteriosus: experience in more than 700 cases. Eur J Cardiothorac Surg 2004;25(3):387–93.
[42] Nezafati MH, Soltani G, Vedadian A. Video-assisted ductal closure with new modifications: minimally invasive, maximally effective, 1,300 cases. Ann Thorac Surg 2007;84(4):1343–8.
[43] Jacobs JP, Giroud JM, Quintessenza JA, et al. The modern approach to patent ductus arteriosus treatment: complementary roles of video-assisted thoracoscopic surgery and interventional cardiology coil occlusion. Ann Thorac Surg 2003;76(5):1421–7 [discussion: 1427–8].
[44] Dutta S, Mihailovic A, Benson L, et al. Thoracoscopic ligation versus coil occlusion for patent ductus arteriosus: a matched cohort study of outcomes and cost. Surg Endosc 2007;22(7):1643–8.
[45] Cannon JW, Howe RD, Dupont PE, et al. Application of robotics in congenital cardiac surgery. Semin Thorac Cardiovasc Surg Pediatr Card Surg Annu 2003;6:72–83.
[46] Baird CW, Stamou SC, Skipper E, et al. Total endoscopic repair of a pediatric atrial septal defect using the da Vinci robot and hypothermic fibrillation. Interact Cardiovasc Thorac Surg 2007;6(6):828–9.
[47] Rothenberg SS. Laparoscopic Nissen procedure in children. Semin Laparosc Surg 2002; 9(3):146–52.
[48] Rothenberg SS. The first decade's experience with laparoscopic Nissen fundoplication in infants and children. J Pediatr Surg 2005;40(1):142–6 [discussion: 147].
[49] Graziano K, Teitelbaum DH, McLean K, et al. Recurrence after laparoscopic and open Nissen fundoplication: a comparison of the mechanisms of failure. Surg Endosc 2003; 17(5):704–7.

[50] Celik A, Loux TJ, Harmon CM, et al. Revision Nissen fundoplication can be completed laparoscopically with a low rate of complications: a single-institution experience with 72 children. J Pediatr Surg 2006;41(12):2081–5.

[51] Capito C, Leclair MD, Piloquet H, et al. Long-term outcome of laparoscopic Nissen-Rossetti fundoplication for neurologically impaired and normal children. Surg Endosc 2007;22(4):875–80.

[52] Islam S, Geiger JD, Coran AG, et al. Use of radiofrequency ablation of the lower esophageal sphincter to treat recurrent gastroesophageal reflux disease. J Pediatr Surg 2004;39(3): 282–6 [discussion: 282–6].

[53] Thomson M, Antao B, Hall S, et al. Medium-term outcome of endoluminal gastroplication with the EndoCinch device in children. J Pediatr Gastroenterol Nutr 2008;46(2):172–7.

[54] Inge TH, Zeller MH, Lawson ML, et al. A critical appraisal of evidence supporting a bariatric surgical approach to weight management for adolescents. J Pediatr 2005;147(1):10–9.

[55] Inge TH, Lawson L. Treatment considerations for severe adolescent obesity. Surg Obes Relat Dis 2005;1(2):133–9.

[56] Holterman AX, Browne A, Dillard BE III, et al. Short-term outcome in the first 10 morbidly obese adolescent patients in the FDA-approved trial for laparoscopic adjustable gastric banding. J Pediatr Gastroenterol Nutr 2007;45(4):465–73.

[57] Dillard BE III, Gorodner V, Galvani C, et al. Initial experience with the adjustable gastric band in morbidly obese US adolescents and recommendations for further investigation. J Pediatr Gastroenterol Nutr 2007;45(2):240–6.

[58] Nadler EP, Youn HA, Ginsburg HB, et al. Short-term results in 53 US obese pediatric patients treated with laparoscopic adjustable gastric banding. J Pediatr Surg 2007;42(1): 137–41 [discussion: 141–2].

[59] Al-Qahtani AR. Laparoscopic adjustable gastric banding in adolescent: safety and efficacy. J Pediatr Surg 2007;42(5):894–7.

[60] Nadler EP, Youn HA, Ren CJ, et al. An update on 73 US obese pediatric patients treated with laparoscopic adjustable gastric banding: comorbidity resolution and compliance data. J Pediatr Surg 2008;43(1):141–6.

[61] Kim SS, Lau ST, Lee SL, et al. Pyloromyotomy: a comparison of laparoscopic, circumumbilical, and right upper quadrant operative techniques. J Am Coll Surg 2005;201(1):66–70.

[62] Hall NJ, Van Der Zee J, Tan HL, et al. Meta-analysis of laparoscopic versus open pyloromyotomy. Ann Surg 2004;240(5):774–8.

[63] Rescorla FJ, West KW, Engum SA, et al. Laparoscopic splenic procedures in children: experience in 231 children. Ann Surg 2007;246(4):683–7 [discussion: 687–8].

[64] Hery G, Becmeur F, Mefat L, et al. Laparoscopic partial splenectomy: indications and results of a multicenter retrospective study. Surg Endosc 2008;22(1):45–9.

[65] Brown MF, Ross AJ III, Bishop HC, et al. Partial splenectomy: the preferred alternative for the treatment of splenic cysts. J Pediatr Surg 1989;24(7):694–6.

[66] Schier F, Waag KL, Ure B. Laparoscopic unroofing of splenic cysts results in a high rate of recurrences. J Pediatr Surg 2007;42(11):1860–3.

[67] Siddiqui S, Newbrough S, Alterman D, et al. Efficacy of laparoscopic cholecystectomy in the pediatric population. J Pediatr Surg 2008;43(1):109–13 [discussion: 113].

[68] Siddiqui T, MacDonald A, Chong PS, et al. Early versus delayed laparoscopic cholecystectomy for acute cholecystitis: a meta-analysis of randomized clinical trials. Am J Surg 2008; 195(1):40–7.

[69] St Peter SD, Keckler SJ, Nair A, et al. Laparoscopic cholecystectomy in the pediatric population. J Laparoendosc Adv Surg Tech A 2008;18(1):127–30.

[70] Seitz G, Warmann SW, Kirschner HJ, et al. Laparoscopic cystojejunostomy as a treatment option for pancreatic pseudocysts in children–a case report. J Pediatr Surg 2006;41(12): e33–5.

[71] Saad DF, Gow KW, Cabbabe S, et al. Laparoscopic cystogastrostomy for the treatment of pancreatic pseudocysts in children. J Pediatr Surg 2005;40(11):e13–7.

[72] Aspelund G, Ling SC, Ng V, et al. A role for laparoscopic approach in the treatment of biliary atresia and choledochal cysts. J Pediatr Surg 2007;42(5):869–72.
[73] Meehan JJ. Robotic repair of congenital duodenal atresia: a case report. J Pediatr Surg 2007;42(7):E31–3.
[74] Dutta S, Woo R, Albanese CT. Minimal access portoenterostomy: advantages and disadvantages of standard laparoscopic and robotic techniques. J Laparoendosc Adv Surg Tech A 2007;17(2):258–64.
[75] Woo R, Le D, Albanese CT, et al. Robot-assisted laparoscopic resection of a type I choledochal cyst in a child. J Laparoendosc Adv Surg Tech A 2006;16(2):179–83.
[76] Rothenberg SS. Laparoscopic segmental intestinal resection. Semin Pediatr Surg 2002; 11(4):211–6.
[77] Mattei P. Minimally invasive surgery in the diagnosis and treatment of abdominal pain in children. Curr Opin Pediatr 2007;19(3):338–43.
[78] Kia KF, Mony VK, Drongowski RA, et al. Laparoscopic vs open surgical approach for intussusception requiring operative intervention. J Pediatr Surg 2005;40(1):281–4.
[79] van der Laan M, Bax NM, van der Zee DC, et al. The role of laparoscopy in the management of childhood intussusception. Surg Endosc 2001;15(4):373–6.
[80] Bailey KA, Wales PW, Gerstle JT. Laparoscopic versus open reduction of intussusception in children: a single-institution comparative experience. J Pediatr Surg 2007;42(5):845–8.
[81] Burjonrappa SC. Laparoscopic reduction of intussusception: an evolving therapeutic option. JSLS 2007;11(2):235–7.
[82] Prasad TR, Chui CH, Jacobsen AS. Laparoscopic-assisted resection of Meckel's diverticulum in children. JSLS 2006;10(3):310–6.
[83] Gilchrist BF, Lobe TE, Schropp KP, et al. Is there a role for laparoscopic appendectomy in pediatric surgery? J Pediatr Surg 1992;27(2):209–12 [discussion: 212–4].
[84] Ates O, Hakguder G, Olguner M, et al. Single-port laparoscopic appendectomy conducted intracorporeally with the aid of a transabdominal sling suture. J Pediatr Surg 2007;42(6): 1071–4.
[85] Visnjic S. Transumbilical laparoscopically assisted appendectomy in children: high-tech low-budget surgery. Surg Endosc 2007;22(7):1667–71.
[86] Wehrman WE, Tangren CM, Inge TH. Cost analysis of ligature versus stapling techniques of laparoscopic appendectomy in children. J Laparoendosc Adv Surg Tech A 2007;17(3): 371–4.
[87] Oka T, Kurkchubasche AG, Bussey JG, et al. Open and laparoscopic appendectomy are equally safe and acceptable in children. Surg Endosc 2004;18(2):242–5.
[88] Vernon AH, Georgeson KE, Harmon CM. Pediatric laparoscopic appendectomy for acute appendicitis. Surg Endosc 2004;18(1):75–9.
[89] Khan MN, Fayyad T, Cecil TD, et al. Laparoscopic versus open appendectomy: the risk of postoperative infectious complications. JSLS 2007;11(3):363–7.
[90] Aziz O, Athanasiou T, Tekkis PP, et al. Laparoscopic versus open appendectomy in children: a meta-analysis. Ann Surg 2006;243(1):17–27.
[91] Schmelzer TM, Rana AR, Walters KC, et al. Improved outcomes for laparoscopic appendectomy compared with open appendectomy in the pediatric population. J Laparoendosc Adv Surg Tech A 2007;17(5):693–7.
[92] Tsao KJ, St Peter SD, Valusek PA, et al. Adhesive small bowel obstruction after appendectomy in children: comparison between the laparoscopic and open approach. J Pediatr Surg 2007;42(6):939–42 [discussion: 942].
[93] McKinlay R, Neeleman M, Klein R, et al. Intraabdominal abscess following open and laparoscopic appendectomy in the pediatric population. Surg Endosc 2003;17(5):730–3.
[94] Nadler EP, Reblock KK, Qureshi FG, et al. Laparoscopic appendectomy in children with perforated appendicitis. J Laparoendosc Adv Surg Tech A 2006;16(2):159–63.
[95] Dutta S, Rothenberg SS, Chang J, et al. Total intracorporeal laparoscopic resection of Crohn's disease. J Pediatr Surg 2003;38(5):717–9.

[96] Simon T, Orangio G, Ambroze W, et al. Laparoscopic-assisted bowel resection in pediatric/ adolescent inflammatory bowel disease: laparoscopic bowel resection in children. Dis Colon Rectum 2003;46(10):1325–31.

[97] Meier AH, Roth L, Cilley RE, et al. Completely minimally invasive approach to restorative total proctocolectomy with j-pouch construction in children. Surg Laparosc Endosc Percutan Tech 2007;17(5):418–21.

[98] Georgeson KE, Robertson DJ. Laparoscopic-assisted approaches for the definitive surgery for Hirschsprung's disease. Semin Pediatr Surg 2004;13(4):256–62.

[99] Smith BM, Steiner RB, Lobe TE. Laparoscopic Duhamel pullthrough procedure for Hirschsprung's disease in childhood. J Laparoendosc Surg 1994;4(4):273–6.

[100] Georgeson KE, Fuenfer MM, Hardin WD. Primary laparoscopic pull-through for Hirschsprung's disease in infants and children. J Pediatr Surg 1995;30(7):1017–21 [discussion: 1021–2].

[101] De la Torre-Mondragon L, Ortega-Salgado JA. Transanal endorectal pull-through for Hirschsprung's disease. J Pediatr Surg 1998;33(8):1283–6.

[102] Elhalaby EA, Hashish A, Elbarbary MM, et al. Transanal one-stage endorectal pull-through for Hirschsprung's disease: a multicenter study. J Pediatr Surg 2004;39(3):345–51 [discussion: 345–51].

[103] Langer JC, Durrant AC, de la Torre L, et al. One-stage transanal Soave pullthrough for Hirschsprung disease: a multicenter experience with 141 children. Ann Surg 2003;238(4):569–83 [discussion: 583–5].

[104] El-Sawaf MI, Drongowski RA, Chamberlain JN, et al. Are the long-term results of the transanal pull-through equal to those of the transabdominal pull-through? A comparison of the 2 approaches for Hirschsprung disease. J Pediatr Surg 2007;42(1):41–7 [discussion: 47].

[105] Georgeson KE, Inge TH, Albanese CT. Laparoscopically assisted anorectal pull-through for high imperforate anus–a new technique. J Pediatr Surg 2000;35(6):927–30 [discussion: 930–1].

[106] Ichijo C, Kaneyama K, Hayashi Y, et al. Midterm postoperative clinicoradiologic analysis of surgery for high/intermediate-type imperforate anus: prospective comparative study between laparoscopy-assisted and posterior sagittal anorectoplasty. J Pediatr Surg 2008;43(1):158–62 [discussion: 162–3].

[107] Vick LR, Gosche JR, Boulanger SC, et al. Primary laparoscopic repair of high imperforate anus in neonatal males. J Pediatr Surg 2007;42(11):1877–81.

[108] Radmayr C, Oswald J, Schwentner C, et al. Long-term outcome of laparoscopically managed nonpalpable testes. J Urol 2003;170(6 Pt 1):2409–11.

[109] Koyle MA, Oottamasathien S, Barqawi A, et al. Laparoscopic Palomo varicocele ligation in children and adolescents: results of 103 cases. J Urol 2004;172(4 Pt 2):1749–52 [discussion: 1752].

[110] Pini Prato A, MacKinlay GA. Is the laparoscopic Palomo procedure for pediatric varicocele safe and effective? Nine years of unicentric experience. Surg Endosc 2006;20(4):660–4.

[111] Hurh PJ, Meyer JS, Shaaban A. Ultrasound of a torsed ovary: characteristic gray-scale appearance despite normal arterial and venous flow on Doppler. Pediatr Radiol 2002;32(8):586–8.

[112] Cass DL. Ovarian torsion. Semin Pediatr Surg 2005;14(2):86–92.

[113] Morowitz M, Huff D, von Allmen D. Epithelial ovarian tumors in children: a retrospective analysis. J Pediatr Surg 2003;38(3):331–5 [discussion: 331–5].

[114] Canon SJ, Jayanthi VR, Lowe GJ. Which is better—retroperitoneoscopic or laparoscopic dismembered pyeloplasty in children? J Urol 2007;178(4 Pt 2):1791–5 [discussion: 1795].

[115] Gorsler CM, Schier F. Laparoscopic herniorrhaphy in children. Surg Endosc 2003;17(4):571–3.

[116] Schier F. Laparoscopic surgery of inguinal hernias in children—initial experience. J Pediatr Surg 2000;35(9):1331–5.

[117] Antonoff MB, Kreykes NS, Saltzman DA, et al. American Academy of Pediatrics Section on Surgery hernia survey revisited. J Pediatr Surg 2005;40(6):1009–14.

[118] Ozgediz D, Roayaie K, Lee H, et al. Subcutaneous endoscopically assisted ligation (SEAL) of the internal ring for repair of inguinal hernias in children: report of a new technique and early results. Surg Endosc 2007;21(8):1327–31.

[119] Holcomb GW III, Tomita SS, Haase GM, et al. Minimally invasive surgery in children with cancer. Cancer 1995;76(1):121–8.

[120] Spurbeck WW, Davidoff AM, Lobe TE, et al. Minimally invasive surgery in pediatric cancer patients. Ann Surg Oncol 2004;11(3):340–3.

[121] Iwanaka T, Arai M, Kawashima H, et al. Endosurgical procedures for pediatric solid tumors. Pediatr Surg Int 2004;20(1):39–42.

[122] Sailhamer E, Jackson CC, Vogel AM, et al. Minimally invasive surgery for pediatric solid neoplasms. Am Surg 2003;69(7):566–8.

[123] Metzelder ML, Kuebler JF, Shimotakahara A, et al. Role of diagnostic and ablative minimally invasive surgery for pediatric malignancies. Cancer 2007;109(11):2343–8.

[124] Streck CJ, Lobe TE, Pietsch JB, et al. Laparoscopic repair of traumatic bowel injury in children. J Pediatr Surg 2006;41(11):1864–9.

[125] Reynolds EM, Curnow AJ. Laparoscopic distal pancreatectomy for traumatic pancreatic transection. J Pediatr Surg 2003;38(10):E7–9.

[126] Feliz A, Shultz B, McKenna C, et al. Diagnostic and therapeutic laparoscopy in pediatric abdominal trauma. J Pediatr Surg 2006;41(1):72–7.

[127] Garg N, St Peter SD, Tsao K, et al. Minimally invasive management of thoracoabdominal penetrating trauma in a child. J Trauma 2006;61(1):211–2.

SURGICAL
CLINICS OF
NORTH AMERICA

Surg Clin N Am 88 (2008) 1121–1130

Robotic Surgery

Dmitry Oleynikov, MD

Minimally Invasive and Computer Assisted Surgery,
983280 Nebraska Medical Center, Omaha, NE 68198-3280, USA

The minimally invasive surgical revolution of the early nineties ushered in an era in which a surgeon did not have to have his or her hands directly on the human body. Once long instruments were placed between the surgeon and the patient, robotic integration became inevitable. If one can reach for a small incision with a long instrument, why cannot one do that with a robotic arm? Commercial robotic systems followed shortly thereafter. The concept behind robotics was to improve the surgeon's sense of touch characteristics and to allow more fluid, minimally invasive surgical procedures to be performed; however, with any new technologies, increased costs and difficulty of use arise. The next generation of robots are being built smaller, smarter, and less expensively.

This article discusses the developments that led up to robotic surgical systems as well as what is on the horizon for new robotic technology. Topics include how robotics is enabling new types of procedures, including natural orifice translumenal endoscopic surgery (NOTES) in which one cannot reach by hand under any circumstances, and how these developments will drive the next generation of robots.

Commercial systems

The daVinci Surgical System (dVSS) was developed by Intuitive Surgical (Sunny Valley, California). It became the first surgical robotics system cleared in 2000 by the US Food and Drug Administration (FDA) for use in general laparoscopic surgery. After several years the FDA also approved the dVSS for thorascopic, urologic, and gynecologic surgeries, as well as an adjunct to some cardiac procedures. Currently, over 800 dVSS are installed in hospitals worldwide.

E-mail address: doleynik@unmc.edu

0039-6109/08/$ - see front matter. Published by Elsevier Inc.
doi:10.1016/j.suc.2008.05.012 *surgical.theclinics.com*

The system has three-dimensional visualization of the operating field, a 7-degree range of motion, tremor elimination, and comfortable seated operating posture [1]. These advantages allow surgeons handlike dexterity and enhanced precision through minimally invasive techniques. The shortcomings of surgical robotics are the lack of haptic feedback while operating, the inability to switch instruments as well as operating field during the procedure, the large size of the robot with bulky arms, and the high cost of the technology [2]. Nevertheless, the dVSS has proved useful for a wide variety of applications in cardiothoracic, urologic, and general surgery [3–5].

Urologists have been especially pleased with the added dexterity provided by the dVSS in removal of the prostate. The operative field is typically in the deep pelvis, and the need for wristlike dexterity is hard to duplicate with conventional laparoscopic techniques. Suturing is especially challenging in the narrow male pelvis, and the dVSS excels in the area. Multiple studies have shown that, with enough experience, robotic prostatectomy is safe and effective for men who have prostate cancer [6].

Other robotic systems on the market today include RoboDoc, an orthopedic surgery system developed at the University of California Davis and commercialized by Integrated Surgical Systems (Sacramento, California). The implementation of this device gave orthopedic surgeons improved accuracy of drilling the femur shaft from 75% to 96% while preparing the bones for prosthetic implants. A similar system known as the Acrobat has been designed by Limited (London, England) for complicated total knee arthroplasty. The significant difference made by these devices led to the acceptance and realization that information technology could be applied to other fields in surgery.

There is a long delay between the idea and commercialization of products, and robotic surgery is only in its infancy. Several fascinating new developments may change how we use the robotics in the near future. These new technologies are still in an experimental stage but offer a glimpse of what the next generation of robots will offer. Miniaturization of robotic technology appears to be the theme of the new generation of devices. Robots that are smaller than current systems have a natural advantage because they are easier to deploy and can be used in more settings. The University of Washington group has developed a smaller prototype machine that has the capability of being mounted on the patient and controlled remotely (Fig. 1). This robot, named RAVEN, has been prototyped and tested in the field. Due to its smaller size and updated enhancements it can be deployed in remote areas and teleoperated [7]. Other robotic technology allows the surgeon to make rounds while sitting in a remote location. This device developed by Dr. Yulun Wang is called the RP-7 (In Touch Health, Santa Barbara, California) and is a mobile robotic platform that enables the physician to be remotely present by controlling robot movements via the Internet. Patients surveyed felt that the encounter was a positive one and were able to completely believe that they were communicating with their

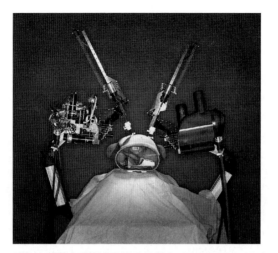

Fig. 1. University of Washington RAVEN.

physician in person even if the physician was far removed from the patient's bedside [8].

Robotics provides a unique possibility of separating the surgeon from the patient. This separation can be measured in feet or in thousands of miles. Telesurgery along with telementoring has been now been tested in several environments and has been shown to be feasible and beneficial. The removal of a gallbladder across the Atlantic Ocean and the mentoring of surgeons in Canada [9] are examples of how technology is rapidly approaching the day when any surgeon can be connected to a number of colleagues who may be able to consult and in some cases assist during complex surgical procedures.

As minimally invasive surgical techniques continually develop toward reducing the invasiveness of surgical procedures, robotics technology becomes more crucial. Natural orifice translumenal endoscopic surgery (NOTES) is a new approach to abdominal surgery that promises to further reduce invasiveness by accessing the peritoneal cavity from a natural orifice. Theoretically, the elimination of external incisions avoids wound infections, further reduces pain, and improves cosmetics and recovery times [10]. NOTES is currently being demonstrated in human studies. The first transvaginal assisted cholecystectomy in the United States was performed in March 2007 [11]. Subsequently, the first transgastric cholecystectomy, also in the United States, was performed in June 2007 using the EndoSurgical Operating System (USGI Medical, San Capistrano, California) [12]. Significant limitations have been identified with the use of conventional endoscopic tools. For example, it is difficult to perform NOTES procedures using a limited two-dimensional image of the surgical environment when the exact orientation of the flexible endoscope is not intuitively obvious. Furthermore, the lack of triangulation between the image and the tools limits depth perception and reduces surgical dexterity [13]. New tools are needed to perform such procedures because simply slipping a hand inside is not possible. Robotics offers the best solutions under these circumstances.

Flexible endoscopy platform

A flexible endoscopy platform for natural orifice surgery with robotic actuation and visualization enhancement is the next area of development. Work has been performed toward the development of an endoluminal robotic system for providing visualization and dexterous instrumentation for the performance of endoluminal surgeries [14]. A first-generation device for teleoperated endoluminal surgery, the ViaCath System, has been developed by EndoVia Medical (Norwood, Massachusetts). The device consists of a console and two flexible instruments located alongside a standard endoscope. Each instrument, together with the positioning arm, provides 7 degrees of freedom. Several end effectors have been developed specifically for this device, including a needle holder, grasper, scissors, and electrocautery knife. A second-generation robotics system shown in Fig. 2 is currently being developed at Purdue University.

A four-channel platform scope (TransPort, USGI Medical, San Capistrano, California) based on the ShapeLock locking overtube has been developed [15]. This device incorporates independent steering of the distal tip such that, once the endoscope is positioned, the base of the endoscope can be frozen while still allowing four-way movement of the tip. Furthermore, the sizing of the working channels allows for the insertion of 5 mm graspers, similar to those used with existing laparoscopic tools, for a more aggressive retraction of organs. The EndoSurgical Operating System, including the TransPort Multi-lumen Operating Platform, is currently

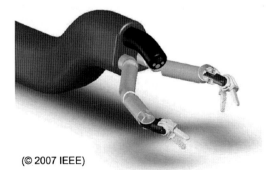

(© 2007 IEEE)

Fig. 2. Robotic endoluminal surgical system being developed at Purdue University. (*From* Abbott DJ, Becke C, Rothstein RI, et al. Design of an endolumenal NOTES robotic system. In: Proceedings of the IEEE/RSJ International Conference on Intelligent Robots and Systems. San Diego, CA: October 29-November 2, 2007. p. 412; with permission. Copyright © 2007 IEEE.)

available commercially. Instruments based on the robotic flexible endoscopy platform demonstrate the potential for improving surgical dexterity for natural orifice procedures; however, these devices remain constrained by the size of the natural orifice and do not provide a sufficient platform for visualization and application of off-axis forces.

Miniature robot platform

Miniaturization of robotic tools and the ability to place robots entirely inside the peritoneal cavity offers significant benefits in natural orifice procedures. Once inserted, the robots can be used inside the peritoneum without the typical constraints of an externally actuated flexible endoscopic device. The robots can be positioned to provide visualization and tissue manipulation within each quadrant of the peritoneal cavity. Multiple miniature robots can be placed inside the peritoneal cavity, with the number of devices not limited by the small diameter of the natural orifice. Such robots equipped with stereoscopic imaging could provide much needed depth perception for the surgeon and could allow triangulation between the image plane and the motion of the tools.

Mobile miniature robots provide a remotely controlled platform for vision and surgical task assistance. The basic design of a mobile robot consists of two independently driven wheels with a helical profile allowing for forward, reverse, and turning motions. A tail is used to prevent counterrotation. The capabilities of robots with a mobile platform have been demonstrated in multiple porcine model procedures as shown in Fig. 3. A mobile robot with an adjustable-focus camera has provided the sole visual feedback for a laparoscopic gallbladder removal without damage to peritoneal structures [16]. The ability of a robot with a mobile platform to provide task assistance has also been demonstrated through the successful biopsy of three samples of hepatic tissue [17]. The onboard camera provided visualization for locating an adequate biopsy site, and the mobile platform enabled the robot to traverse the peritoneal cavity to the chosen site. The feasibility of using in vivo mobile robots for NOTES procedures has been successfully demonstrated in a porcine model [18]. A mobile robot was introduced through the esophageal opening and was inserted into the stomach through a sterile overtube using a standard upper endoscope. It was able to explore the gastric cavity before advancement into the peritoneal cavity through a transgastric incision. Once fully inserted, an endoscope was advanced to view the mobile robot as it maneuvered within the peritoneal cavity. The robot was then retracted into the gastric cavity, and the transgastric incision was closed. The ability to navigate the peritoneal cavity while not restrained from the outside was very advantageous and led to the next set of experiments in which multiple robots could be used.

The insertion of multiple tools is limited by the size of the natural orifice, and the tools must be entirely flexible for insertion through the complex

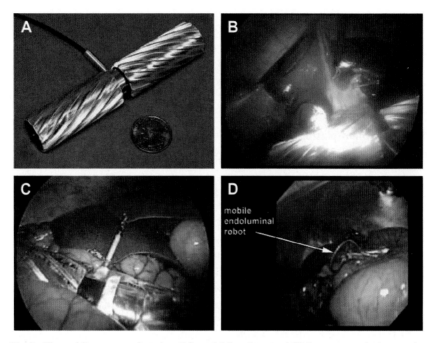

Fig. 3. The mobile camera robot viewed from (*A*) benchtop and (*B*) laparoscope during porcine cholecystectomy. A mobile robot demonstrates (*C*) liver biopsy and (*D*) translumenal peritoneal exploration.

geometry of the natural lumen. In a nonsurvivable in vivo procedure in a porcine model, the feasibility of using multiple miniature robots for improving spatial orientation and providing task assistance was demonstrated [19]. This cooperative procedure used three miniature in vivo robots, shown in Fig. 4, including a peritoneum-mounted imaging robot, a lighting robot, and a retraction robot in cooperation with a standard upper endoscope to demonstrate various capabilities for NOTES procedures.

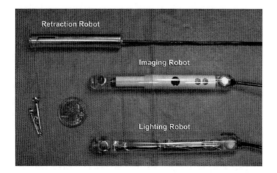

Fig. 4. Retraction, imaging, and lighting robots used in cooperative NOTES procedure.

The peritoneum-mounted imaging robot provides a stable, reposition-able, adjustable focus imaging platform for minimally invasive surgery. The basic design of the robot consists of an inner housing containing the lens and focusing mechanism, two LEDs for lighting, and a permanent mag-net direct current motor for rotating the inner housing within the clear outer housing. Each end of the imaging robot is fitted with a magnetic cap. The robot is held to the upper abdominal wall using the interaction of magnets housed in the robot and those contained in an external magnetic handle. The handle can be moved along the exterior surface of the abdomen for gross positioning and panning of the robot. The video feedback from the imaging robot is displayed on a standard monitor in the operating room.

The external housing for the lighting consists of a clear outer tube that contains six white LEDs and is fitted on each end with a magnetic cap. Sim-ilar to the imaging robot, the lighting robot is held to the interior abdominal wall using the interaction of the magnetic end caps with magnets housed in an external handle. The retraction robot is designed to enable tissue retrac-tion for natural orifice procedures. The basic design of the retraction robot consists of an external housing with two embedded magnets for fixation and a tethered grasping device. A permanent magnet direct current motor coupled with a drum is contained within the external housing. As the motor rotates, the tether is wound and unwound about the drum to raise and lower the grasping device. Endoscopic or laparoscopic tools are currently used to actuate the grasper device. In the near future, this task will be accomplished using a cooperative robot.

A nonsurvivable NOTES procedure in a porcine model was performed us-ing the imaging robot, lighting robot, and a retraction robot in cooperation with a standard upper endoscope. The endoscope was used via a gastrotomy into the peritoneal cavity. Once inserted, each robot was independently se-cured to and positioned along the upper abdominal wall using the external magnetic handles. The video feedback from the imaging robot guided the exploration of the peritoneal cavity and provided visualization for endoscopic manipulation of the bowel and gallbladder. The retraction robot provided access for the endoscope to the surgical target.

This procedure demonstrated the feasibility of providing a stable, reposi-tionable platform for NOTES procedures through using multiple miniature in vivo robots with appropriate capabilities. The stable image and additional lighting were key to the surgeon's ability to visualize and manipulate within the peritoneal cavity for this NOTES procedure. A multi-armed dexterous miniature in vivo robot with stereovision capabilities has been developed to provide the surgeon with a stable, repositionable platform for visualiza-tion and tissue manipulation for performing NOTES procedures in the peritoneal cavity [20]. The basic design of the robot, shown in Fig. 5, consists of two "arms," with each connected to a central "body" by a rota-tional "shoulder" joint. Each arm consists of an upper arm and a lower arm fitted with either a forceps or cautery end effector.

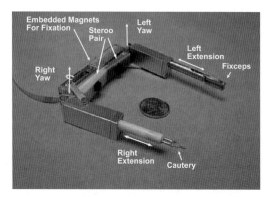

Fig. 5. University of Nebraska mini robot.

The body of the robot is held to the upper abdominal wall using magnets housed in the body of the robot and an external magnetic handle which can be moved along the outer surface of the abdomen throughout a procedure to reposition the robot internally. This handle enables the surgeon to position the robot to obtain alternative views and workspaces within each quadrant of the peritoneal cavity without requiring an additional incision or a retroflexed configuration. The NOTES robot successfully demonstrated

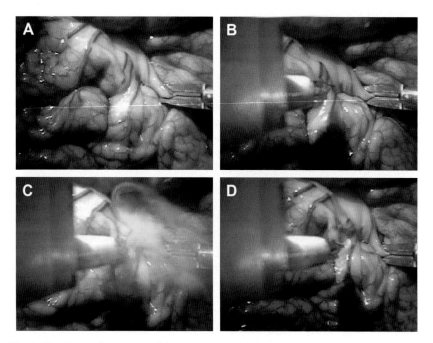

Fig. 6. View from robot camera of tissue grasping (*A*), cautery arm positioning (*B*), and cautery (*C, D*).

various capabilities in a nonsurvivable procedure in a porcine model. Through a standard endoscopically created gastrotomy, the robot was inserted into the peritoneal cavity and magnetically attached to the anterior abdominal wall. Using the video feedback from the on-board cameras, the surgeon explored the peritoneal cavity, identified the target for tissue manipulation, and positioned the robot to provide a suitable workspace for visualization and tissue manipulation. A small bowel dissection was then performed, as shown in Fig. 6. The forceps arm was extended toward the small bowel and was used to grasp the tissue. The arm was then retracted to provide access to the tissue for the cautery arm. The shoulder of the cautery arm was then rotated and the lower arm was extended to cauterize the small bowel. The visualization and dexterity are very similar to that in routine laparoscopy but without abdominal wall incisions.

Summary

The dVSS remains the only commercially available therapeutic robotic system currently available. It has allowed surgeons to perform procedures that previously were thought to be either too complicated or too risky to be performed in a laparoscopic fashion. New technology has since improved, allowing one to reach areas that could not be reached before and to perform operations without scars, such as natural orifice surgery. With the development of new types of devices that are smaller, cheaper, and based on more modular components, each device will be tailored to a given operation. New technologies are sure to follow along, and this field will not look the same in 10 to 15 years. It can be expected that we will continue to move toward more automation, more computer interface, and more mechanical assist and further away from the open surgical techniques that were pioneered in the years before.

References

[1] Intuitive Surgical. 2004. Available at: www.intuitivesurgical.com. Accessed March 19, 2008.
[2] Hanly EJ, Zand J, Bachman SL, et al. Value of the SAGES learning center in introducing new technology. Surg Endosc 2005;19(4):477–83 [Epub 2005 Feb 10].
[3] Ahlering T, Skarecky D, Lee D, et al. Successful transfer of open surgical skills to a laparoscopic environment using a robotic interface: initial experience with laparoscopic radical prostatectomy. J Urol 2003;170:1738–41.
[4] Perez A, Zinner M, Ashley S, et al. What is the value of telerobotic technology in gastrointestinal surgery? Surg Endosc 2003;17:811–3.
[5] Tatooles AJ, Pappas PS, Gordon PJ, et al. Minimally invasive mitral valve repair using the da Vinci Robotic System. Ann Thorac Surg 2004;77:1978–84.
[6] Pasticier G, Rietbergen JB, Guillonneau B, et al. Robotically assisted laparoscopic radical prostatectomy: feasibility study in men. Eur Urol 2001;40(1):70–4.
[7] Lum MJH, Rosen J, King H, et al. Telesurgery via unmanned aerial vehicle (UAV) with a field deployable surgical robot. In: Proceedings of Medicine Meets Virtual Reality (MMVR 15), Long Beach, California, February 6–9, 2007. p. 313–5.

[8] Ellison LM, Nguyen M, Fabrizio MD, et al. Postoperative robotic telerounding: a multicenter randomized assessment of patient outcomes and satisfaction. Arch Surg 2007;142(12): 1177–81 [discussion: 1181].

[9] Sebajang H, Trudeau P, Dougall A, et al. The role of telementoring and telerobotic assistance in the provision of laparoscopic colorectal surgery in rural areas. Surg Endosc 2006; 20(9):1389–93 [Epub 2006, Jul 3].

[10] ASGE, SAGES. ASGE/SAGES working group on natural orifice translumenal endoscopic surgery white paper, October 2005. Gastrointest Endosc 2006;63:199–203.

[11] Department of Surgery. Incisionless surgery with natural orifice techniques [online] 2007. Available at: http://www.columbiasurgery.org/news/2007_notes.html. Accessed March 19, 2008.

[12] USGI Medical. USGI announces first NOTES transgastric cholecystectomy procedures [online] 2007. Available at: http://www.usgimedical.com/pr_transgastric_cholecystectomy. html. Accessed March 19, 2008.

[13] Ko CW, Kalloo AN. Peroral transgastric abdominal surgery. Chin J Dig Dis 2006;7:67–70.

[14] Abbott DJ, Becke C, Rothstein RI, et al. Design of an endolumenal NOTES robotic system. In: Proceedings of the IEEE/RSJ International Conference on Intelligent Robots and Systems. San Diego, CA: October 29-November 2, 2007. p. 410–6.

[15] Swanstrom LL, Whiteford M, Khajanchee. Developing essential tools to enable transgastric surgery. Surg Endosc 2008;22:600–4.

[16] Rentschler ME, Dumpert J, Platt SR, et al. Mobile in vivo camera robots provide sole visual feedback for abdominal exploration and cholecystectomy. Surg Endosc 2006;20(1):135–8.

[17] Rentschler M, Dumpert J, Platt S, et al. An in vivo mobile robot for surgical vision and task assistance. ASME J Med Devices 2007;1(1):23–9.

[18] Rentschler ME, Dumpert J, Platt SR, et al. Natural orifice surgery with an endoluminal mobile robot. Surg Endosc 2007;21(7):1212–5.

[19] Lehman AC, Berg KA, Dumpert J, et al. Surgery with cooperative robots. Comput Aided Surg 2008;13:95–105.

[20] Lehman AC, Dumpert J, Wood NA, et al. Natural orifice translumenal endoscopic surgery with a miniature in vivo surgical robot. Presented at the 2008 Annual Meeting of the Society of American Gastrointestinal and Endoscopic Surgeons; Philadelphia, PA: April 9–12, 2008.

ELSEVIER
SAUNDERS

Surg Clin N Am 88 (2008) 1131–1148

SURGICAL
CLINICS OF
NORTH AMERICA

Natural Orifice Translumenal Endoscopic Surgery

Simon Bergman, MD[a,b], W. Scott Melvin, MD[b,c],*

[a]Department of Surgery, The Ohio State University School of Medicine
and Public Health, 410 West 10th Avenue, Columbus, OH 43210, USA
[b]Center for Minimally Invasive Surgery, The Ohio State University School of Medicine
and Public Health, N729 Doan Hall, 410 West 10th Avenue, Columbus, OH 43210, USA
[c]Division of General Surgery, The Ohio State University School of Medicine and Public
Health, N729 Doan Hall, 410 West 10th Avenue, Columbus, OH 43210, USA

Since Kalloo's [1] initial description of transgastric peritoneoscopy in 2004, natural orifice translumenal endoscopic surgery (NOTES) has captured the imagination of surgeons and gastroenterologists worldwide and has progressed exponentially in a short period of time. A multitude of additional reports have surfaced detailing increasingly complex surgical procedures in animal models through a variety of approaches, including the esophagus, stomach, colon, vagina, and bladder [2]. As the NOTES experience grew, it became increasingly evident that endoscopic translumenal surgery was feasible, and, today, human procedures ignited by Rao's transgastric appendectomy [3] are being reported from throughout the international community. In North America, human work was initiated at the Ohio State University evaluating the ability of transgastric peritoneoscopy to appropriately stage pancreatic malignancies.

Although it has yet to be examined in comparative studies, patient benefit is implied from the laparoscopic surgery body of knowledge. If smaller incisions lead to less pain, faster recovery, and decreased rates of hernias, adhesive disease, and wound infections as well as better cosmesis, it seems reasonable that a complete lack of incisions would be even superior [4,5]. When surveyed, most patients would prefer a transgastric over a laparoscopic cholecystectomy, citing improved pain and cosmesis as major deciding factors, but only if the safety profile was comparable to the that of the laparoscopic approach [6,7]. Sixty-eight percent of women would undergo

---

* Corresponding author. The Ohio State University School of Medicine and Public Health, N729 Doan Hall, 410 West 10th Avenue, Columbus, OH 43210-1228.
  E-mail address: scott.melvin@osumc.edu (W.S. Melvin).

0039-6109/08/$ - see front matter © 2008 Elsevier Inc. All rights reserved.
doi:10.1016/j.suc.2008.05.011
surgical.theclinics.com

a transvaginal procedure over a laparoscopic procedure to avoid postoperative pain and hernias [8]. Fueled by patient interest if not patient demand, by industry, and by the fear of being left behind, the interest in NOTES in the medical and surgical communities is undeniable. Nevertheless, despite this enthusiasm, there are insufficient data to determine safety and benefit.

In an effort to facilitate the safe introduction of translumenal surgical techniques in a controlled and ethical manner, the Society of American Gastrointestinal and Endoscopic Surgeons and the American Society of Gastrointestinal Endoscopy have joined forces to form the Natural Orifice Surgery Consortium for Assessment and Research (NOSCAR) and published a white paper establishing the potential barriers to the clinical practice of NOTES (Box 1) [9,10]. This article provides an overview of the currently available animal data on NOTES on the topics of translumenal access and closure, iatrogenic intraperitoneal complications, especially infection and overinsufflation, spatial orientation, and the development of enabling technologies. Human trials to date are also reviewed and discussed.

Terminology

The new lexicon of terms surrounding NOTES needs to be carefully described and scrutinized as the field continues to expand. A variety of new surgical techniques and approaches are being evaluated, and until standard terminology is developed, this will result in a confusing use of terms and abbreviations. Currently, NOTES should be strictly understood to represent

---

Box 1. Potential barriers to clinical practice [9,10]

- Access to peritoneal cavity
- Gastric (intestinal) closure
- Prevention of infection
- Development of suturing device
- Development of anastomotic (nonsuturing) device
- Spatial orientation
- Development of a multitasking platform to accomplish procedures
- Control of intraperitoneal hemorrhage
- Management of iatrogenic intraperitoneal complications
- Physiologic untoward events
- Compression syndromes
- Training other providers

Data from Rattner D, Kallo A. ASGE/SAGES working group on natural orifice translumenal endoscopic surgery. Surg Endosc 2006;20:329–33; and Kallo A, Rattner D. ASGE/SAGES working group on natural orifice translumenal endoscopic surgery. Gastrointest Endosc 2006;63(2):199–203.

diagnostic or therapeutic interventions performed via existing orifices of the human body (mouth, anus, urethra, vagina). Transabdominal approaches such as single port systems are really only a modification of laparoscopy and not a subset of NOTES. In addition, multiple hybrid procedures including combined endolumenal and transabdominal approaches will continue to confuse the terminology. Endolumenal technology, even in the context of a full-thickness opening of the hollow viscus, may be described in a variety of ways that may or may not be appropriately called NOTES. At present, it will be left to the discerning reader and author to understand and describe surgical approaches by using the correct terminology.

Access

Peritoneoscopy has been performed via transgastric, transcolonic, transvesical, and transvaginal approaches with variable human and animal experience. Recently, transesophageal mediastinoscopy and thoracoscopy have been described. The choice of approach should be guided by surgeon familiarity with the access organ, location of the target organ, the diameter and length of necessary instruments, the ease of closure and infectious considerations, as well as the potential of injury to surrounding organs (Table 1). The latter risk can be minimized using several techniques, including extreme positioning, preliminary insufflation using a Veress needle [11], and image-guided techniques such as endoscopic ultrasound [12–14] or image registered technology [15].

Transgastric approaches

The peroral transgastric approach has been used to perform liver biopsies [1], cholecystectomies and cholecystogastric anastamoses [16], distal pancreatectomies [17], splenectomies [18], gastrojejunostomies [19], ventral hernia repairs [20], enteric anastamoses [21], and oophorectomies and tubal ligations [22,23] in animal models. The acidic environment of the stomach and consequent diminished bacterial load and excellent blood supply make it an organ forgiving to injury. Furthermore, its location offers excellent access and visualization of lower abdominal and pelvic structures. With

Table 1
Comparison of translumenal approaches

Parameter	Esophageal	Gastric	Colic	Vesical	Vaginal
Bacterial load	+	+	+++	−	+
Size	++	++	+++	+	+++
Injury potential	+++	+	++	+++	++
Access to upper abdomen	−	+	+++	+++	+++
Access to lower abdomen	−	+++	+	+	+
Animal data	+	+++	++	+	++
Human data	−	++	+	+	+++

Abbreviations: +, relative benefits; −, relative risks

meticulous technique, other than minor injury to the liver and abdominal wall, the risk of injury to surrounding organs is minimal. The major disadvantage of this approach is access to the upper abdomen, because the necessary retroflexion provides a counterintuitive view and makes endoscopic manipulations more difficult and sometimes impossible. This disadvantage can be overcome in part by innovative devices that allow greater stability, such as the ShapeLock device [24], or improved articulation or range of motion, such as the R-scope [25]. Furthermore, the size of instruments and overtubes is limited by the diameter of the cricopharyngeus.

The authors' preferred transgastric peritoneal access technique is through the anterior gastric wall, identified by external palpation. A needle-knife is used to create a gastrotomy, and a radially dilating balloon exchanged over a guidewire is used to dilate the tract. The balloon and endoscope are finally pushed out of the gastric lumen as a unit. Alternatively, a sphicterotome over a guidewire may be used to incise the gastric wall over several centimeters [1]. The former technique may be superior in that the dilation may be less traumatic then a sphicterotome incision, and because the muscle fibers spring back together following endoscope withdrawal, closure may be simplified [26]. Other peritoneal access techniques include PEG-like percutaneous puncture and guidewire insertion into the stomach before gastrotomy creation [27]. The self-approximating translumenal access and submucosal endoscopy with mucosal flap techniques involve blunt creation of a 6- to 12-cm submucosal tunnel followed by muscular fiber incision and endoscope exit. In an animal model, Sumiyama and colleagues [25,28,29] reported a small bowel injury and two deaths, including air embolism, using this technique.

Genitourinary approaches

Low peritoneal access via the genitourinary tract affords surgeons a straight shot to most abdominal structures. The vaginal and bladder closures are easy to perform and manage owing to low bacterial counts and low risks of infectious complications such as leaks or fistulas. Transvaginal access can be gained using a needle-knife incision on the anterior vaginal wall and a dilating balloon [30] or a standard rigid trocar or overtube inserted through the posterior vaginal wall [31,32]. Although this access is relatively safe, a rectal injury was reported by Scott and colleagues [32] while performing a cholecystectomy. Transvesical access is gained under cystoscopic guidance. An opening in the bladder is created on the ventral bladder wall with a urethral catheter, which is then exchanged over a guidewire for a 5-mm overtube. Through this approach, Lima and colleagues [33] performed peritoneoscopy and liver biopsy. In contrast to the vagina, which can accommodate large overtubes and multiple instruments, the size of the urethra is a severe limitation making this approach more suitable for dual access NOTES techniques. Via a urethral overtube, rigid instrumentation such as ultrasonic shears or clip appliers were used to perform hybrid transgastric/transvesical nephrectomies and cholecystectomies [34,35].

Transcolonic approaches

Because of its high bacterial load, the colon is not an ideal conduit for translumenal procedures; however, it may be selected in cases when therapy is directed toward the colon or when the colon must be entered for other reasons. Additionally, via the transrectal approach the upper rectum can be repaired using standard techniques. To maintain a tight seal around their endoscope, Pai and colleagues [36] while performing transcolic cholecystectomy created a subcentimetric colostomy 15 to 20 cm from the anal verge and then, over a catheter, pushed the larger endoscope through. This technique was also used to perform a hepatic wedge resection [37]. In a dual approach transcolic/transvaginal distal pancreatectomy, T-tags were placed in lieu of a purse-string suture with equal success [38]. Others have placed a 12-mm trocar through the rectum to perform a dual approach transgastric/transrectal small bowel resection [39]. Wilhelm and colleagues [40] have devised an innovative sigmoid access to limit bacterial contamination. Fluid is first instilled into the pelvis via a Veress needle, pushing the small bowel out of the pelvis as it floats on top of this artificial ascites. An appropriate entry point is identified using transrectal ultrasound, and a purse-string suture is placed in the colon wall via a modified transanal endoscopic microsurgery approach. A guide tube is then inserted peranal through the colon wall, creating a sterile endoscope conduit.

Transesophageal approaches

Perhaps because of the poor blood supply to the esophagus, the lack of serosa, difficult closure techniques, and the disastrous consequences of an esophageal leak and resultant mediastinitis, not until recently has the esophagus been investigated as a potential NOTES access point. Nevertheless, the limited experience is encouraging. Following access to the mediastinum using a submucosal tunneling technique, mediastinoscopy and thoracoscopy were performed as were mediastinal lymph node and lung biopsies [41–43]. In the survival study by Gee and colleagues [41], all animals survived, and the only complications were pneumothorax and lung bruising. Under esophageal ultrasound guidance, Fritscher and colleagues [14] created an esophagostomy using a needle-knife and exited directly into the mediastinum. They were able to perform lymph node biopsies, pericardial fenestration, and myocardial saline injections without any complications.

Closure

Given the excellent safety profile of current laparoscopic techniques, translumenal closure techniques must approach 100% reliability before embarking on human trials studying translumenal peritoneoscopy. In humans, any degree of morbidity, let alone mortality, from this aspect of the procedure should be considered completely unacceptable. Significant animal work has been performed in this field, mostly with respect to gastrotomies, which remain the most challenging to close in a reliable way.

It has been suggested that gastrotomies may not require closure. This lack of the need for closure may be true in certain species such as canines and swine that may be more resistant to infectious insults than humans. The authors' laboratory has shown 100% survival in dogs with endoscopic gastrotomies left to heal without treatment [44]. Similar results were found in a swine colon perforation model. All control animals recovered fully, and, at the time of necropsy, perforations were found to have healed spontaneously [45]. In humans, conservative nonoperative management of perforated gastroduodenal ulcers is considered by some to be part of the treatment algorithm [46]. Several comparative studies, including one randomized controlled study, report success rates of 50% to 90% with equivalent morbidity and mortality to surgical management [47–50]. Factors that predict the failure of this approach are generally absent in the healthy, non-diseased stomach subjected to endoscopic enterotomies, that is, age greater than 70 years, a history longer than 9 to 24 hours before treatment, the use of immunosuppression or non-steroidal anti-inflammatory drugs, concomitant illness, the presence of shock, or a large pneumo- or hydroperitoneum [48–53]. These risk factors represent a significant issue for investigators in this field who must address the need for appropriate animal models and control groups as well as more sensitive outcome measures to rigorously establish the superiority of one closure technique over another.

Gastrotomy closure techniques

Current gastrotomy closure techniques involve plug and patch or reapproximation techniques and require either "through-the-scope" or "out-of-scope" devices. The authors' group has recently published results demonstrating the success of the former approach with endoscopic placement of a bioabsorbable mesh plug in 12 canines having undergone transgastric peritoneoscopy. All of the canines survived without leakage for 2 weeks [44]. Similarly, in a rat gastric perforation model, a porcine-derived small intestine submucosal patch was used successfully for closure in all animals. Histologic examination revealed the patch to be an effective scaffolding agent as evidenced by early regeneration of normal gastric mucosa at its edges [54]. A nitinol self-expandable double umbrella-shaped device with an inner nonpermeable polyethylene terephthalate patch was deployed in gastrotomies following endoscopic transgastric peritoneoscopy. Five of six animals thrived for several weeks and one died of sepsis [55].

Through-the-scope reapproximation techniques are usually simple and do not require bulky or expensive devices. In their seminal study, Kalloo and colleagues [1] performed gastrotomy closure with endoscopic clips and all animals recovered uneventfully. Excellent results have also been reported after reapproximation of the gastric edges using several endoscopic loop applications [56]. Others have described pulling omentum into the gastrotomy and clipping it in place to provide a conceptually similar repair to the Graham patch [57]. The argument against such repairs is that, despite their success, endoscopic clips and loops provide only superficial mucosal reapproximation of the gastric wall, violating the surgical dogma that seromuscular apposition is necessary for proper healing. Swain and colleagues [58] have developed a promising full-thickness T-tag tissue apposition system that can be passed down the working channel of a gastroscope. This system was used to close a Heineke-Mikulicz pyloroplasty in a porcine model, with six of seven animals surviving without complications. Furthermore, it was successfully used in humans for endoscopic repair of a perforated duodenal ulcer and a gastroenteroanastamotic leak [59].

Flexible linear staplers introduced alongside the scope have been used in a pig model to provide full-thickness stapled gastrotomy closure with good success; however, the investigators commented on some difficulty with instrument handling and positioning due to its size and lack of articulation [60]. This device has also been used in the clinical setting for endoscopic full-thickness gastric wall resections for early gastric adenocarcinoma with excellent clinical outcomes [61]. The NDO Plicator, initially designed for endoscopic gastroesophageal junction plication in the treatment of gastroesophageal reflux, is also effective [62]. Other prototypes in different stages of development such as the Eagle Claw [63], the g-Prox (USGI, San Clemente, California), and the SewRite (LSI Solutions, Victor, New York) also offer endoscopic seromuscular suturing capabilities and are currently being studied [64,65].

Genitourinary tract closure techniques

Little morbidity stems from an unrepaired injury to the vaginal wall, and it can be closed easily with simple sutures only. This ease of closure has been demonstrated in the animal laboratory [30–32] and in the clinical arena in the context of transvaginal surgery [66]. Similarly, following transvesical peritoneoscopy, holes in the bladder were left open with transurethral urinary drainage for 4 days. In three of four pigs, excellent healing was seen at 15 days, whereas the catheter was accidentally exteriorized in one animal [33]. Other transvesical studies did not detail the closure technique.

Colotomy closure techniques

Pai and colleagues successfully closed four of five colotomies using a combination of endoscopic clips and loops. These animals survived 2 weeks until necropsy, at which time the incisions were found to be well healed. One animal could not be closed and was euthanized 48 hours later with septic complications [36]. The clip closure configuration may have an impact on success as documented by Raju and colleagues [67] in a nonsurvival pig study designed to look exclusively at closure techniques. Transverse clip closure of a colotomy leaked in three of three pigs, whereas longitudinal clip closure resulted in a leak-proof seal in six of seven. Other groups have had success in all animals closed using T-tags and endoloops following transcolic peritoneoscopy [38]. In four pigs, the colonic incision was created by using a prototype incision and closure device from LSI Solutions. Under endoscopic visualization, the device is passed alongside the endoscope to the desired area of colotomy. When fired, a full-thickness purse-string suture is deployed, and a 20-mm incision is made automatically. The purse-string suture is then secured with a titanium knot [68]. An alternative for serosa-to-serosa approximation is the over-the-scope Eagle Claw endoscopic suturing device. This closure technique was used in ten pigs. It was successful in seven animals and unsuccessful in two. Despite surviving following the procedure, one animal showed repair dehiscence at necropsy [69].

Esophagotomy closure techniques

When a submucosal tunnel technique is used, the proximal mucosal incision has either been closed with regular endoscopic mucosal clips or left to seal on its own, and the distal muscular incision, covered by a so-called "mucosal flap," has usually been left untouched [41,43]. At 2 weeks using this closure technique Sumiyama and colleagues [42] demonstrated healed mucosal entry sites without ulceration. The distal myotomy defect had remained open but was effectively sealed with the overlying mucosal flap.

Unique NOTES-related complications

As peritoneal access changes and instruments and platforms are modified, and as procedures are refined or reinvented, one will see a shift in the profile of certain complications much like when comparing open and laparoscopic surgery. For example, hernias and wound infections may give way to "compression syndromes" and intra-abdominal infections. Surgeons embarking on NOTES must understand and recognize these changes in iatrogenic complications to avoid them or manage them appropriately.

Insufflation

The classic systemic hemodynamic effects of increased intra-abdominal pressure have been well described in multiple animal and human studies. These effects are tachycardia, an increase in arterial blood pressure, peripheral vasoconstriction, decreased stroke volume and cardiac output, and decreased renal blood flow, particularly with intra-abdominal pressure above 15 mm Hg [70–73]. As demonstrated in an animal model, similar physiologic derangements occurring with pneumoperitoneum are seen in the context of a simple gastroscopy as large amounts of air are insufflated into the stomach and small bowel [74]. Although insufflation pressures can be regulated during laparoscopic surgery, this is not true with standard endoscopic insufflators.

During transgastric peritoneoscopy with standard on-demand endoscopic insufflation, intra-abdominal pressure, although maintaining an acceptable mean of 12 mm Hg throughout the procedure, peaked above 15 mm Hg and 20 mm Hg 21% to 31% and 17% of the time, respectively. These periods of high pressure when recognized by the endoscopist (less than 50% of the time) were associated with temporary loss of visualization as air was suctioned out to attempt correction. There was an inverse relationship between the cardiac index, which decreased during the procedure, and intra-abdominal pressure. On the other hand, in control animals undergoing standard laparoscopic autoregulated insufflation, pressures only rose above 15 mm Hg 2% of the time, and the cardiac index was kept stable [75,76]. Similarly, Meirless and colleagues [77] showed wide variations in pressures between 4 and 32 mm Hg for on-demand insufflation compared with 8 to 15 mm Hg with autoregulated insufflation. With prolonged NOTES procedures and in patients with comorbidities or less physiologic reserve, there is certainly a potential, albeit transient, risk of renal injury, hypoventilation, and cardiovascular collapse. Furthermore, intra-abdominal pressure variability and attempts at manual correction by the surgeon could lead to iatrogenic injury.

Several techniques have been developed to address these issues. The first is to place a percutaneous conduit, either in the form of an angiocatheter or a Veress needle, to monitor intra-abdominal pressure and act as a vent. Alternatively, autoregulated insufflators can be connected to these conduits to provide better control of intra-abdominal pressure. Autoregulated insufflation may be used by connecting a laparoscopic insufflator to the working ports of the endoscope, although insufflation may be limited when obstructing those channels with instruments. A solution is to connect an autoregulated source to tubing that is fixed alongside the endoscope and ends at or near its tip [76,78].

Infection

Potential sources of infection are numerous when considering translumenal endoscopic surgery. During access, the peritoneal cavity may become contaminated from contact with a non-sterile endoscope alone or from its passage through a contaminated orifice. Furthermore, the seal between the wall of the access organ and the scope may be inadequate and allow leakage, which could also occur postoperatively following improper closure. As is true with any approach, spillage from the target organ can occur, or the peritoneal cavity may experience secondary contamination from bacteremia [79]. When including all survival animal NOTES studies, the overall infection rate is 10% to 20% [2,79]. The contribution of each of these components to the overall risk of infection is unknown, and few data exist concerning optimal methods of prevention.

Many groups have successfully prevented postoperative infectious complications following transgastric peritoneoscopy by using antibiotic solution gastric lavage, prophylactic parenteral antibiotics, and high-level endoscope disinfection [19,22,23]. In the first two survival animals of their series without antibiotic gastric lavage, Kalloo and colleagues [1] reported intra-abdominal microabcesses at necropsy in both pigs. When antibiotic lavage was used, the following three animals had no signs of infection. Despite similar prophylactic regimens, there are several reports of intra-abdominal infection. In a study by Pauli and colleagues [28], two of five transgastric NOTES animals had abscesses in their abdominal cavities at necropsy. Likewise, Merrifield and colleagues [80] reported two of five deaths from purulent peritonitis in animals having undergone transgastric hysterectomy. In contrast, others have shown that forgoing antibiotic lavage does not always have infectious consequences [21]. In fact, the authors' experience with transgastric human NOTES trial suggests that this prevention method may not be necessary at all [81,82].

Another factor that requires consideration is the impact of proton pump inhibitors on gastric flora. In a controlled rat model, animals were pretreated with proton pump inhibitors and their gastric contents aspirated and reinjected into their own peritoneal cavities. Two weeks later, bacterial cultures were positive in 20% of rats in the control group compared with 60% in the group treated with proton pump inhibitors [83]. Following transgastric peritoneoscopy, increased intraperitoneal bacterial growths in patients on proton pump inhibitors have also been demonstrated in the authors' human data, although there was no cross-contamination between the gastric lumen and peritoneal cavity [81]. The clinical significance and true risk of proton pump inhibitor therapy in NOTES remains to be determined.

Prophylaxis in transcolonic peritoneoscopy usually consists of cefazolin and betadine enemas, which have been shown to eliminate over 80% of colonic bacteria [84]. In ex vivo gastric colonic tissue, combining that type of preparation with parenteral cefazolin before the procedure decreased bacteria loads from 1.2×10^6 CFUs/cm^2 to 0 CFUs/cm^2 [85]. Using this strategy as well as high-level disinfection of the endoscopes, Pai and colleagues [36] reported euthanasia in only one animal because of septic deterioration. Although the remaining four survived to necropsy, all had serosal and subserosal microabcesses. Another study by the same group yielded similar results. Microabcesses were identified in six of six pigs 14 days after the transcolonic procedure [68]. On the other hand, following Wilhelm and colleagues' [40] innovative sterile sigmoid approach, five survival animals did not show any sign of infection.

The clinical significance of the microabcesses found at necropsy in animals that otherwise are healthy and thriving remains unclear. This self-limiting pathology can probably be found in a significant number of animals and humans during normal surgical recovery. The data are conflicting, and this avenue requires further investigation at the basic science level and in the context of clinical comparative studies before any recommendations can be made.

Spatial orientation

Additional challenges exist because of the unusual orientation and the atypical site of access to visualization systems that are currently being employed for NOTES. Traditional surgery, followed closely by laparoscopic surgery, uses a relatively stable and manageable imaging platform that can be easily controlled because it is relatively short, and most are designed to be rigid and require little manipulation. This arrangement is significantly perturbed when long flexible scopes without the ability to effectively maintain an upright image and rotation are used. The disorientation caused by this phenomenon needs to be overcome. Although a variety of algorithms have been attempted to deal with this problem, currently, none are seen as optimal. A solution to the unusual image rotation may be an automatic "righting" system that is created by the installation of an artificial horizon that can always be selected as the upright situation in the electronic image. Experience gained with these scopes and the learning that occurs when the scope is outside the intestinal lumen allow one to accommodate for these disorienting changes. Because of the disorientation and lack of outside anatomic landmarks, a steep learning curve exists. This problem is being addressed by many investigators and corporate entities who are all working on enabling technology. The broad concepts that are being addressed fall into several categories—delivery platforms, technology, instrumentation, and imaging and navigation systems.

Delivery platforms, technology, and navigation systems

Flexible endoscopes have been designed and modified to operate effectively in a relatively stable close-quarter environment and to illuminate a hollow viscus. When the scope enters a relatively open and dynamic environment such as the abdominal cavity, the effectiveness of the device is diminished. When multiple operators are required to use the device and complex instruments are place via the device, the situation is further complicated. The direct coupling of the imaging system to the effector instruments is confounding as well. One group has developed and tested a "direct drive" endoscope device which completely replaces the traditional dual-wheel scope and allows a distance between the imaging operator and the instrument operators [86]. A unique approach has also been described and developed by Oleynikov and his group [87]. They have prototyped and developed telerobotic devices that can be deployed and even assembled within the body cavities. Currently, small tethers connect the devices to

1142   BERGMAN & MELVIN

the external power source, controlling imaging and visualization devices. "Robots" are mobile or can be fixed to the abdominal wall with magnets or transabdominal needles, or left to be mobile and self-prevailed in the abdominal cavity. In the future, safe completion of NOTES procedures will most likely not rely on the current reconfigured flexible endoscope. Laparoscopic surgery has matured through the development of multiple instruments that allow complex tasks to be completed, including energy devices for hemostasis, staplers, and suturing devices. These types of devices will be enabling technology to allow complex tasks to be completed to access long flexible devices. Some of these instruments are traditional devices such as bipolar electrocautery, some are modified laparoscopic instruments such as the flexible endostich (Covidien, New Haven, Connecticut), and others are entirely new and unique to the field of NOTES and therapeutic endoscopy (ie, g-Prox).

Automatic devices could potentially be beneficial as well and potentially include magnetic anastomotic devices and battery-powered light sources. Although surgical robots in the current form will not be beneficial, the surgeon/patient interface may be similar to allow control of the device via long flexible or articulated instruments that can be remotely controlled to provide intracavitary therapeutic procedures. These devices could be placed via natural orifices, percutaneously, or even intravascularly.

A variety of different solutions for navigation during NOTES have been suggested. None of these possibilities are clinically in use. One allows virtual registration of the tip of the instrument so that in a separate video display the tip can be displayed in relationship to other previously registered fiduciaries. Other schemes have attempted to combine the actual image with preoperative imaging modalities, essentially combining the real-time actual image with MRI or CT.

Human work

NOTES techniques have been evaluated for the most part in large human models as previously described. The early launch into human experience has captivated investigators and clinicians. Currently, human experience is limited to case reports and small case series, although data are currently accumulating. Limited data are available to determine any clinical benefit or even delineate the danger of these novel approaches. Since the initial report by Rao and coworkers, this group has completed an additional 14 NOTES cases, mostly diagnostic procedures and appendectomies. The ongoing experience is rapidly growing. In April of 2008, Zorron [88] presented the active Brazilian database of 160 human cases, with more cases currently accruing. These cases are mostly transgastric and transvaginal procedures for appendicitis, gynecologic indications, and cholecystectomy. The US experience remains relatively small and was launched in October 2006 by the authors' group at Ohio State to evaluate the role of transgastric peritoneoscopy for the staging of pancreatic malignancies [89]. This experience now includes 20 patients with malignancies and an additional 25 patients with previous surgery who underwent diagnostic peritoneoscopy for the safe placement of laparoscopic trocars [90]. Therapeutic experience with NOTES in the United States was presented initially by Bessler and his group [91] in the fall of 2007, describing a transvaginal cholecystectomy with laparoscopic guidance. This experience increased when Horgan's group at the University of California at San Diego cooperated with an international group and reported several transvaginal cholecystectomies and expanded their approach to include transvaginal appendectomy for acute appendicitis (S. Horgan, personal communication, April 2008). Swanstrom and his group [92] have completed four hybrid transgastric cholecystectomies without complications.

Despite the rapid accrual of human cases, currently, no conclusion can be made about the efficacy, safety, or potential benefits of NOTES based on the objective evidence in humans. Careful controlled studies to obtain more data are needed to delineate these factors.

Training

Considerable debate is ongoing as to whether NOTES is a surgical or medical specialty. Leading investigators currently fall under both categories, with most successful groups being composed of several members with a diverse background and training. It is clear that current training programs have significant limitations. Primary gastroenterology training requires the background of internal medicine; therefore, it fails to include the basic principles of surgical care including advanced anatomy, tissue handling and dissecting techniques, the care of complications, and the physiologic response to surgical injury. In primary surgical training, many situations fail to provide the adequate technical training in flexible endoscopy, with many surgical programs failing to even achieve minimum numbers for diagnostic endoscopy to allow for credentialing at most hospitals.

This dilemma can be solved by a variety of techniques and training. Ponsky [93] has proposed a new paradigm in training, developing a new "gastrointestinal interventionalist." Others have suggested that the future of NOTES training lies in the concept of cross-training, or hybrid training, culminating in the formation of "interventional digestivists" [94]. It is imperative that individuals who embark in the field of NOTES have the ability to understand surgery as well as perform the technical aspects of therapeutic endoscopy. Improved training of surgeons by the addition of flexible endoscopic training to surgical training can likely resolve this issue. The authors' center has addressed this need by working closely with surgeons who have advanced fellowship training in therapeutic endoscopy, and a fellowship has been developed for advanced training in therapeutic endoscopy, training the educators for future surgical trainees.

Summary

In the late 1980s, the concept of minimally invasive surgery rapidly changed the field of abdominal surgery, and the growth was dramatic and, at times, unsafe. The expansion was fueled by the profound benefit provided to the patient by a well-trained minimally invasive surgeon. The field of minimally invasive surgery has matured but continues to evolve with the addition of technology and innovation. NOTES is a new modification of minimally invasive therapeutic interventions that may evolve into a category of procedures and technology that will improve patient care. With adequate assessment, background research, protocol development, as well as data collection, NOTES may demonstrate improvement in patient care; however, the current level of investigation in technology development is insufficient to support the concept of advanced therapy performed by translumenal techniques. With investigation and technology development, the field of minimally invasive surgery will continue to evolve.

References

[1] Kalloo AN, Singh VK, Jagannath SB, et al. Flexible transgastric peritoneoscopy: a novel approach to diagnostic and therapeutic interventions in the peritoneal cavity. Gastrointest Endosc 2004;60(1):114–7.

[2] Della Flora E, Wilson TG, Martin IJ, et al. A review of natural orifice translumenal endoscopic surgery (NOTES) for intra-abdominal surgery: experimental models, techniques, and applicability to the clinical setting. Ann Surg 2008;247(4):583–602.

[3] Rao GV. Transgastric appendectomy results and follow up (SAGES transgastric surgery panel). Presented at the SAGES Meeting; Dallas, TX: 2006.

[4] Duepree H-J, Senagore AJ, Delaney CP, et al. Does means of access affect the incidence of small bowel obstruction and ventral hernia after bowel resection? Laparoscopy versus laparotomy. J Am Coll Surg 2003;197:177–81.

[5] Lourenco T, Murray A, Grant A, et al. Laparoscopic surgery for colorectal cancer: safe and effective? A systematic review. Surg Endosc 2007, in press.

[6] Shyam Varadarajulu S, Tamhane A, Drelichman ER, et al. Patient perception of natural orifice transluminal endoscopic surgery as a technique for cholecystectomy. Gastrointest Endosc, in press.

[7] Volckmann ET, Hungness ES, Soper NJ, et al. Patient perceptions of natural orifice transluminal surgery (NOTES). Surg Endosc 2007;21(1):S349.

[8] Peterson CY, Andrews B, Ramamoorthy S, et al. Women's perception of transvaginal NOTES surgery. Surg Endosc 2008;22(1):S238.

[9] Rattner D, Kallo A. ASGE/SAGES working group on natural orifice translumenal endoscopic surgery. Surg Endosc 2006;20:329–33.

[10] Kallo A, Rattner D. ASGE/SAGES working group on natural orifice translumenal endoscopic surgery. Gastrointest Endosc 2006;63(2):199–203.

[11] Ko CW, Shin EJ, Buscaglia JM, et al. Preliminary pneumoperitoneum facilitates transgastric access into the peritoneal cavity for natural orifice transluminal endoscopic surgery: a pilot study in a live porcine model. Endoscopy 2007;39:849–53.

[12] Wagh MS, Merrifield BF, Thompson CC. Endoscopic transgastric abdominal exploration and organ resection: initial experience in a porcine model. Clin Gastroenterol Hepatol 2005;3:892–6.

[13] Panzer S, Harris M, Berg W, et al. Endoscopic ultrasound in the placement of a percutaneous endoscopic gastrostomy tube in the non-transilluminated abdominal wall. Gastrointest Endosc 1995;42:88–90.

[14] Fritscher-Ravens A, Patel K, Ghanbari A, et al. Natural orifice transluminal endoscopic surgery (NOTES) in the mediastinum: long-term survival animal experiments in transesophageal access, including minor surgical procedures. Endoscopy 2007;39:870–5.

[15] Vosburgh KG, San Jose Estepar R. Natural orifice transluminal endoscopic surgery (NOTES): an opportunity for augmented reality guidance. Studies in Health Technology and Informatics 2007;125:485–90.

[16] Park PO, Bergstrom M, Ikeda K, et al. Experimental studies of transgastric gallbladder surgery: cholecystectomy and cholecystogastric anastamosis. Gastrointest Endosc 2005;61(4): 601–6.

[17] Matthes K, Yusuf TE, Willingham FF, et al. Feasibility of endoscopic transgastric distal pancreatectomy in a porcine animal model. Gastrointest Endosc 2007;66(4):762–6.

[18] Kantsevoy SV, Hu B, Jagannath SB, et al. Transgastric endoscopic splenectomy: is it possible? Surg Endosc 2006;20(3):522–5.

[19] Kantsevoy SV, Jagannath SB, Niiyama H, et al. Endoscopic gastrojejunostomy with survival in a porcine model. Gastrointest Endosc 2005;62(2):287–92.

[20] Hu B, Kalloo AN, Chung SS, et al. Peroral transgastric endoscopic primary repair of a ventral hernia in a porcine model. Endoscopy 2007;39:390–3.

[21] Bergstrom M, Ikeda K, Swain P, et al. Transgastric anastamosis by using flexible endoscopy in a porcine model. Gastrointest Endosc 2006;63(2):307–12.

[22] Wagh MS, Merrifield BF, Thompson CC. Survival studies after endoscopic transgastric oophorectomy and tubectomy in a porcine model. Gastrointest Endosc 2006;63(3):473–8.

[23] Jagannath SB, Kantsevoy SV, Vaughn CA, et al. Peroral transgastric endoscopic ligation of fallopian tubes with long-term survival in a porcine model. Gastrointest Endosc 2005;61(3): 449–53.

[24] Swain P. The ShapeLock system adapted to intragastric and transgastric surgery. Endoscopy 2007;39:466–70.

[25] Sumiyama K, Gostout CJ, Rajan E, et al. Transgastric cholecystectomy: transgastric accessibility to the gallbladder improved with the SEMF method and a novel multibending therapeutic endoscope. Gastrointest Endosc 2007;65:1028–34.

[26] Sumiyama K, Gostout CJ. Techniques for transgastric access to the peritoneal cavity. Gastrointest Endosc Clin N Am 2008;18:235–44.

[27] Kantsevoy SV, Jagannath SB, Niiyama H, et al. A novel safe approach to the peritoneal cavity for peroral transgastric endoscopic procedures. Gastrointest Endosc 2007;65(3): 497–500.

[28] Pauli EM, Moyer MT, Haluck RS, et al. Self-approximating transluminal access technique for natural orifice transluminal endoscopic surgery: a porcine survival study. Gastrointest Endosc 2008;67(4):690–7.

[29] Sumiyama K, Gostout CJ, Rajan E, et al. Submucosal endoscopy with mucosal flap safety valve. Gastrointest Endosc 2007;65(4):688–94.

[30] Tsakayannis D, Ilias S. Transvaginal NOTES cholecystectomy in the porcine model. Gastrointest Endosc 2007;65(5):AB291.

[31] Matthes K, Menke D, Koehler P, et al. Feasibility of endoscopic transgastric (ETGN) and transvaginal (ETVN) nephrectomy. Gastrointest Endosc 2007;65(5):AB290.

[32] Scott DJ, Tang SJ, Fernandex ER, et al. Completely transvaginal NOTES cholecystectomy using magnetically anchored intruments. Surg Endosc 2007;21:2308–16.

[33] Lima E, Rolanda C, Pego JM, et al. Transvesical endoscopic peritoneoscopy: a novel 5 mm port for intra-abdominal scarless surgery. J Urol 2006;176:802–5.

[34] Rolanda C, Lima E, Pego JM, et al. Third generation cholecystectomy by natural orifices: transgastric and transvesical combined approach (video). Gastrointest Endosc 2007;65: 111–7.

[35] Lima E, Rolanda C, Pego JM, et al. Third-generation nephrectomy by natural orifice trans-
     luminal endoscopic surgery. J Urol 2007;178:2648–54.
[36] Pai RD, Fong DG, Bundga ME, et al. Transcolonic endoscopic cholecystectomy: a NOTES
     survival study in a porcine model. Gastrointest Endosc 2006;64:428–34.
[37] Fong DG, Pai RD, Fishman DS. Transcolonic hepatic wedge resection in a porcine model.
     Gastrointest Endosc 2006;63(5):AB102.
[38] Ryou M, Fong DG, Pai ED, et al. Dual-port distal pancreatectomy using a prototype endo-
     scope and endoscopic stapler: a natural orifice transluminal endoscopic surgery (NOTES)
     survival study in porcine model. Endoscopy 2007;39(10):881–7.
[39] Mintz Y, Horgan S, Cullen J, et al. Dual-lumen natural orifice translumenal endoscopic
     surgery (NOTES): a new method for performing a safe anastomosis. Surg Endosc 2008;
     22(2):348–51.
[40] Wilhelm D, Meining A, von Delius S, et al. An innovative, safe and sterile sigmoid access
     (ISSA) for NOTES. Endoscopy 2007;39:401–6.
[41] Gee DG, Willingham FF, Singh AK. Natural orifice transesophageal mediastinoscopy and
     thoracoscopy: a survival series in swine. Surg Endosc 2008;22(1):S156.
[42] Sumiyama K, Gostout CJ, Rajan E, et al. Transesophageal mediastinoscopy by submucosal
     endoscopy with mucosal flap safety valve technique. Gastrointest Endosc 2007;65(4):679–83.
[43] Willingham FF, Gee DG, Lauwers GY, et al. Natural orifice transesophageal mediastino-
     scopy and thoracoscopy. Surg Endosc 2007;20(1):S349.
[44] Bergman S, Fix DJ, Volt K, et al. Gastrotomies do not require repair following endoscopic
     transgastric peritoneoscopy: a controlled study. Surg Endosc 2008;20(1):S242.
[45] Raju GS, Ijaz A, Xiao SY, et al. Controlled trial of immediate endoluminal closure of colon
     perforations in a porcine model by use of a novel clip device. Gastrointest Endosc 2006;64:
     989–97.
[46] Putcha RV, Burdick S. Management of iatrogenic perforation. Gastroenterol Clin North
     Am 2003;32:1289–309.
[47] Kristensen ES. Conservative management of 155 cases of perforated peptic ulcer. Acta Chir
     Scand 1980;146:189–93.
[48] Songne B, Jean F, Foulatier O, et al. Nonoperative treatment for perforated peptic ulcer:
     results of a prospective study. Ann Chir 2004;129:578–82.
[49] Dascalescu C, Andriescu L, Bulat C, et al. Taylor's method: a therapeutic alternative for
     perforated gastroduodenal ulcer. Hepatogastroenterology 2006;53:543–6.
[50] Crofts TJ, Park KGM, Steele RJC, et al. A randomised trial of nonoperative treatment for
     perforated peptic ulcer. N Engl J Med 1989;320:970–3.
[51] Anonymous. Conservative management of perforated peptic ulcer. Lancet 1989;2(8677):
     1429–30.
[52] Buchler P, Oulhaci W, Morel P, et al. Results of conservative treatment for perforated gas-
     troduodenal ulcers in patients not eligible for surgical repair. Swiss Med Wkly 2007;137:
     337–40.
[53] Irvin T. Mortality and perforated peptic ulcer: case for risk stratification in elderly patients.
     Br J Surg 1989;76:215–8.
[54] de la Fuente SG, Gottfried MR, Lawson DC, et al. Evaluation of porcine-derived small in-
     testine submucosa as a biodegradable graft for gastrointestinal healing. J Gastrointest Surg
     2003;7:96–101.
[55] Perretta S, Sereno S, Forgione A, et al. A new method to close the gastrotomy by using a car-
     diac septal occluder: long-term survival study in a porcine model. Gastrointest Endosc 2007;
     66:809–13.
[56] Katsarelias D. Endoloop application as an alternative method for gastrotomy closure in
     experimental transgastric surgery. Surg Endosc 2007;21:1862–5.
[57] Feretis C, Kalantzopoulos D, Koulouris P, et al. Endoscopic transgastric procedures in
     anesthetized pigs: technical challenges, complications, and survival. Endoscopy 2007;39:
     394–400.

[58] Park PO, Bergstrom M, Ikeda K, et al. Endoscopic pyloroplasty with full-thickness transgastric and transduodenal myotomy with sutured closure. Gastrointest Endosc 2007;66:116–20.

[59] Bergstrom M, Swain P, Park PO. Early clinical experience with a new flexible endoscopic suturing method for natural orifice transluminal endoscopic surgery and intraluminal endosurgery. Gastrointest Endosc 2008;67:528–33.

[60] Magno P, Giday SA, Dray X, et al. A new stapler-based full-thickness transgastric access closure: results from an animal pilot trial. Endoscopy 2007;39:876–80.

[61] Kähler GF, Collet PH, Grobholz R, et al. Endoscopic full-thickness gastric resection using a flexible stapler device. Surg Technol Int 2007;16:61–5.

[62] McGee MF, Marks JM, Onders RP, et al. Complete endoscopic closure of gastrotomy after natural orifice translumenal endoscopic surgery using the NDO Plicator. Surg Endosc 2008; 22:214–20.

[63] Hu B, Chung SC, Sun LC, et al. Endoscopic suturing without extracorporeal knots: a laboratory study. Gastrointest Endosc 2005;62(2):230–3.

[64] Sclabas GM, Swain P, Swanstrom LL. Endoluminal methods for gastrotomy closure in natural orifice transenteric surgery (NOTES). Surg Innov 2006;13:23–30.

[65] Ryou M, Pai RD, Sauer JS, et al. Evaluating an optimal gastric closure method for transgastric surgery. Surg Endosc 2007;21:677–80.

[66] Shen CC, Hsu TY, Huang FJ, et al. Comparison of one- and two-layer vaginal cuff closure and open vaginal cuff during laparoscopic-assisted vaginal hysterectomy. J Am Assoc Gynecol Laparosc 2002;9(4):474–80.

[67] Raju GS, Ahmed I, Shibukawa G, et al. Endoluminal clip closure of a circular full-thickness colon resection in a porcine model. Gastrointest Endosc 2007;65(3):503–9.

[68] Fong DG, Pai RD, Thompson CC. Transcolonic endoscopic abdominal exploration: a NOTES survival study in a porcine model. Gastrointest Endosc 2007;65:312–8.

[69] Pham BV, Raju GS, Ahmed I, et al. Immediate endoscopic closure of colon perforation by using a prototype endoscopic suturing device: feasibility and outcome in a porcine model. Gastrointest Endosc 2006;64:113–9.

[70] Joris JL, Noirot DP, Legrand MJ, et al. Hemodynamic changes during laparoscopic cholecystectomy. Anesth Analg 1993;76(5):1067–71.

[71] McLaughlin JG, Scheeres DE, Dean RJ, et al. The adverse hemodynamic effects of laparoscopic cholecystectomy. Surg Endosc 1995;9(2):121–4.

[72] Bergman S, Nutting A, Feldman LS, et al. Elucidating the relationship between cardiac preload and renal perfusion under pneumoperitoneum. Surg Endosc 2006;20(5):794–800.

[73] Chiu AW, Chang LS, Birkett DH, et al. A porcine model for renal hemodynamic study during laparoscopy. J Surg Res 1996;60(1):61–8.

[74] von Delius S, Karagianni A, Henke J, et al. Changes in intra-abdominal pressure, hemodynamics, and peak inspiratory pressure during gastroscopy in a porcine model. Endoscopy 2007;39:962–8.

[75] von Delius S, Huber W, Feussner H, et al. Effect of pneumoperitoneum on hemodynamics and inspiratory pressures during natural orifice transluminal endoscopic surgery (NOTES): an experimental, controlled study in an acute porcine model. Endoscopy 2007;39:854–9.

[76] Bergström M, Swain P, Park P-O. Measurements of intraperitoneal pressure and the development of a feedback control valve for regulating pressure during flexible transgastric surgery (NOTES). Gastrointest Endosc 2007;66(1):174–8.

[77] Meirles O, Kantsevoy SV, Kalloo AN, et al. Comparison of intra-abdominal pressures using the gastroscope and laparoscope for transgastric surgery. Surg Endosc 2007;21:998–1001.

[78] McGee MF, Rosen MJ, Marks J. A reliable method for monitoring intra-abdominal pressure during natural orifice translumenal endoscopic surgery. Surg Endosc 2007;21:672–6.

[79] Kantsevoy SV. Infection prevention in NOTES. Gastrointest Endosc Clin N Am 2008;18: 291–6.

[80] Merrifield B, Wagh M, Thompson C. Peroral transgastric organ resection in the abdomen: a feasibility study in pigs. Gastrointest Endosc 2006;63:693–7.

[81] Narula VK, Hazey JW, Renton DB, et al. Transgastric instrumentation and bacterial contamination of the peritoneal cavity. Surg Endosc 2008;22:605–11.

[82] Narula VK, Happel LC, Volt K, et al. Transgastric endoscopic peritoneoscopy does not require decontamination of the stomach in humans. Surg Endosc 2008;22(1):S157.

[83] Ramamoorthy SL, Lee JK, Mintz Y, et al. The impact of proton pump inhibitors on intraperitoneal sepsis. Surg Endosc 2008;22(1):S159.

[84] Bachman SL, Sporn E, Furrer JL. Colonic sterilization for NOTES procedures: a comparison of two decontamination protocols. Surg Endosc 2008;22(1):S157.

[85] Ryou M, Hazan R, Rahme L, et al. The effectiveness of current sterility techniques in natural orifice transluminal endoscopic surgery (NOTES). Gastrointest Endosc 2007;65(5):AB290.

[86] Thompson CC, Ryou M, Rothstein RI, et al. Stomach—direct drive endoscopic system for endoluminal and NOTES applications. The DAVE project. Available at: http://daveproject. org/viewfilms.cfm?film_id=612. Accessed April 21. 2008.

[87] Rentschler ME, Dumpert J, Platt SR, et al. Surg Endosc 2007;21(7):1212–5.

[88] Zorron R. Human work to date, an international perspective [oral presentation]. In: Update on NOTES. The SAGES Annual Meeting, April 10, 2008.

[89] Hazey JW, Narula VK, Renton DB, et al. Natural orifice transgastric endoscopic peritoneoscopy in humans: initial clinical trial. Surg Endosc 2008;22:16–22.

[90] Happel LC, Needleman BJ, Mikami DJ, et al. Transgastric peritoneoscopy for evaluation of the abdominal wall to direct laparoscopic trocar placement. Surg Endosc 2008;20(1):S240.

[91] Bessler M, Steven PD, Milone L, et al. Transvaginal laparoscopic assisted endoscopic cholecystectomy: a hybrid approach to natural orifice surgery. Gastrointest Endosc 2007;66(6): 1243–5.

[92] Swanstrom LL, Soper NJ, Hungness ES. Early experience with transgastric NOTES cholecystectomy in humans. Surg Endosc 2008;22(1):S034.

[93] Ponsky JL. Gastroenterologists as surgeons: what they need to know. Gastrointest Endosc 2005;61(3):454.

[94] Hawes RII. Advanced endoscopy and endosurgical procedures: do we need a new subspecialty? Gastrointest Endosc Clin N Am 2007;17:635–9.

ELSEVIER
SAUNDERS

Surg Clin N Am 88 (2008) 1149–1157

SURGICAL
CLINICS OF
NORTH AMERICA

Index

Note: Page numbers of article titles are in **boldface** type.

A

Abdominal laparoscopy surgery, pediatric, 1106–1112. See also *Minimally invasive surgery (MIS), in children, abdominal laparoscopic surgery.*

ACS. See *American College of Surgeons (ACS).*

Adenocarcinoma, of esophagus
Barrett's esophagus and, 954
incidence of, 979

Adrenal gland tumors, laparoscopic surgery of, 1035–1038

Adrenalectomy, laparoscopic. See *Laparoscopic adrenalectomy.*

Age, as factor in PEH, 959

Aldosteronoma(s), laparoscopic adrenalectomy for, 1036

AMA. See *American Medical Association (AMA).*

American College of Radiology, on laparoscopic cholecystectomy, 930

American College of Surgeons (ACS)
accreditation of Educational Institutes by, 930
Committee on Emerging Surgical Technology and Education of, on laparoscopic cholecystectomy, 928–930
Division of Education of, on laparoscopic cholecystectomy, 928–930
on evaluation of obese patient for bariatric surgery, 993

American Medical Association (AMA), Current Procedural Terminology of, 935–936

American Society for Bariatric Surgery, 992–993

American Society for Metabolic and Bariatric Surgery (ASMBS), 992–993

American Society of Gastrointestinal Endoscopy, 1132

Anastomosis(es), cervical, thoracoscopic-laparoscopic esophagectomy with, for malignant and premalignant diseases of esophagus, 984–986

Anorectal malformations, in children, laparoscopic surgery for, 1109–1110

Antireflux surgery (ARS), **943–958**
for Barrett's esophagus, 955
for GERD, **943–958**
goal of, 947–948
laparoscopic Nissen fundoplication, 948–949
outcomes of, 950–951
patient selection for, 944, 946–947
postoperative care, 950
principles of, 947–950
technique of, 947–950
Toupet fundoplication, 949

Appendicitis, in children, laparoscopic surgery for, 1108–1109

ARS. See *Antireflux surgery (ARS).*

ASMBS. See *American Society for Metabolic and Bariatric Surgery (ASMBS).*

Atresia(s), esophageal, in children, MIS of, 1104

B

Barcelona trial, on minimally invasive colon cancer surgery, 1048–1050

Bariatric surgery, 991–1007. See also specific techniques, e.g., *Roux-en-Y gastric bypass (RYGB).*
candidates for, 992

doi:10.1016/S0039-6109(08)00130-8   *surgical.theclinics.com*

Moving?

Make sure your subscription moves with you!

To notify us of your new address, find your **Clinics Account Number** (located on your mailing label above your name), and contact customer service at:

E-mail: elspcs@elsevier.com

800-654-2452 (subscribers in the U.S. & Canada)
1-407-563-6020 (subscribers outside of the U.S. & Canada)

Fax number: 407-363-9661

Elsevier Periodicals Customer Service
6277 Sea Harbor Drive
Orlando, FL 32887-4800

*To ensure uninterrupted delivery of your subscription, please notify us at least 4 weeks in advance of move.

United States Postal Service

Statement of Ownership, Management, and Circulation
(All Periodicals Publications Except Requestor Publications)

1. Publication Title	2. Publication Number								3. Filing Date
Surgical Clinics of North America	5	2	9	-	8	0	0	0	9/15/08

4. Issue Frequency	5. Number of Issues Published Annually	6. Annual Subscription Price
Feb, Apr, Jun, Aug, Oct, Dec	6	$238.00

7. Complete Mailing Address of Known Office of Publication (Not printer) (Street, city, county, state, and ZIP+4)

Elsevier Inc.
360 Park Avenue South
New York, NY 10010-1710

Contact Person
Stephen Bushing

Telephone (Include area code)
215-239-3688

8. Complete Mailing Address of Headquarters or General Business Office of Publisher (Not printer)

Elsevier Inc., 360 Park Avenue South, New York, NY 10010-1710

9. Full Names and Complete Mailing Addresses of Publisher, Editor, and Managing Editor (Do not leave blank)
Publisher (Name and complete mailing address)

John Schrefer, Elsevier, Inc., 1600 John F. Kennedy Blvd. Suite 1800, Philadelphia, PA 19103-2899
Editor (Name and complete mailing address)

Catherine Bewick, Elsevier, Inc., 1600 John F. Kennedy Blvd. Suite 1800, Philadelphia, PA 19103-2899
Managing Editor (Name and complete mailing address)

Catherine Bewick, Elsevier, Inc., 1600 John F. Kennedy Blvd. Suite 1800, Philadelphia, PA 19103-2899

10. Owner (Do not leave blank. If the publication is owned by a corporation, give the name and address of the corporation immediately followed by the names and addresses of all stockholders owning or holding 1 percent or more of the total amount of stock. If not owned by a corporation, give the names and addresses of the individual owners. If owned by a partnership or other unincorporated firm, give its name and address as well as those of each individual owner. If the publication is published by a nonprofit organization, give its name and address.)

Full Name	Complete Mailing Address
Wholly owned subsidiary of	4520 East-West Highway
Reed/Elsevier, US holdings	Bethesda, MD 20814

11. Known Bondholders, Mortgagees, and Other Security Holders Owning or Holding 1 Percent or More of Total Amount of Bonds, Mortgages, or Other Securities. If none, check box. ☐ None

Full Name	Complete Mailing Address
N/A	

12. Tax Status (For completion by nonprofit organizations authorized to mail at nonprofit rates) (Check one)
The purpose, function, and nonprofit status of this organization and the exempt status for federal income tax purposes:
☐ Has Not Changed During Preceding 12 Months
☐ Has Changed During Preceding 12 Months (Publisher must submit explanation of change with this statement)

PS Form 3526, September 2006 (Page 1 of 3 (Instructions Page 3)) PSN 7530-01-000-9931 **PRIVACY NOTICE:** See our Privacy policy in www.usps.com

13. Publication Title	14. Issue Date for Circulation Data Below	
Surgical Clinics of North America	August 2008	

15. Extent and Nature of Circulation		Average No. Copies Each Issue During Preceding 12 Months	No. Copies of Single Issue Published Nearest to Filing Date
a. Total Number of Copies (Net press run)		5300	5300
b. Paid Circulation (By Mail and Outside the Mail)	(1) Mailed Outside-County Paid Subscriptions Stated on PS Form 3541. (Include paid distribution above nominal rate, advertiser's proof copies, and exchange copies)	2209	2059
	(2) Mailed In-County Paid Subscriptions Stated on PS Form 3541 (Include paid distribution above nominal rate, advertiser's proof copies, and exchange copies)		
	(3) Paid Distribution Outside the Mails Including Sales Through Dealers and Carriers, Street Vendors, Counter Sales, and Other Paid Distribution Outside USPS®	1881	1793
	(4) Paid Distribution by Other Classes Mailed Through the USPS (e.g. First-Class Mail®)		
c. Total Paid Distribution (Sum of 15b (1), (2), (3), and (4))	▲	4090	3852
d. Free or Nominal Rate Distribution (By Mail and Outside the Mail)	(1) Free or Nominal Rate Outside-County Copies Included on PS Form 3541	103	99
	(2) Free or Nominal Rate In-County Copies Included on PS Form 3541		
	(3) Free or Nominal Rate Copies Mailed at Other Classes Mailed Through the USPS (e.g. First-Class Mail)		
	(4) Free or Nominal Rate Distribution Outside the Mail (Carriers or other means)		
e. Total Free or Nominal Rate Distribution (Sum of 15d (1), (2), (3) and (4))	▲	103	99
f. Total Distribution (Sum of 15c and 15e)	▲	4193	3951
g. Copies not Distributed (See instructions to publishers #4 (page #3))	▲	1107	1349
h. Total (Sum of 15f and g)	▲	5300	5300
i. Percent Paid (15c divided by 15f times 100)		97.54%	97.49%

16. Publication of Statement of Ownership

☐ If the publication is a general publication, publication of this statement is required. Will be printed ☐ Publication not required
in the **October 2008** issue of this publication.

17. Signature and Title of Editor, Publisher, Business Manager, or Owner

Jean Jauvibe (signature)

Jean Jauviber, Executive Director of Subscription Services

Date
September 15, 2008

I certify that all information furnished on this form is true and complete. I understand that anyone who furnishes false or misleading information on this form or who omits material or information requested on the form may be subject to criminal sanctions (including fines and imprisonment) and/or civil sanctions (including civil penalties).

PS Form 3526, September 2006 (Page 2 of 3)